Health Empowerment of Women

HEALTH EMPOWERMENT OF WOMEN

A DESIRABLE STRATEGY IN 21ST CENTURY HOSPITALS –

VOLUME - I
GENERAL HEALTH

Editors

DR. AMARJEET SINGH
DR. VANITA SURI
DR. SUKHPAL KAUR

KALPAZ

ISBN: 978-93-5324-050-9 (Vol. I)
978-93-5324-024-0 (Set)

First Published, 2020

Published by

Kalpaz Publications
C-30, Satyawati Nagar,
Delhi – 110052
Ph.: 011-47034999, 9811692060
www.kalpazpublications.com
E-mail: kalpaz@hotmail.com

Printed at: G. Print Process, Delhi

Contents

Foreword

The life expectancy of women is more than that of men. Though, both are at equal risk of developing various communicable as well as non communicable diseases, women experience earlier, and more severe diseases with poorer outcomes than men. Some of the health issues that affect both men and women can affect women differently. Various reasons attributed to this include biological, social and behavioural conditions. Women are more likely to die following a heart attack and show more signs of depression and anxiety than men. The effects of sexually transmitted diseases can be more serious in women. Osteoarthritis affects more in women than men. They are more likely to have urinary tract problems. There is a higher burden of disability due to NCDs. Women experience many unique health issues related to reproduction and sexuality which are responsible for one third of all health problems experienced by them during their reproductive years. These include pregnancy, menopause, and conditions of the female organs. Breast cancer and cervical cancer are the most common cancers and are substantial contributors to compromised quality of life in women.

Women provide healthcare worldwide, both in the formal healthcare setting as well as in the informal sector and at home. Yet their own needs for health care are poorly addressed, especially among rural and poor communities. They have traditionally been disadvantaged in terms of economic and social status, particularly in the developing countries. This in turn reduces their access to the necessities of life including health care.

The current book on **"Health Empowerment of Women"** has been very well compiled by the editors. The uniqueness of the book is that it is an entirely indigenous product, i.e., based on the work of the students and faculty of PGIMER, Chandigarh. Another strong point of the book is that it highlights quite effectively the role nurses can play in improving the quality of services in Indian hospitals as well as in community settings. Due importance is given to patients as well as family caregivers' satisfaction through their empowerment in self-care, which ought to be the ultimate test of efforts in the provision of medical care .

The concept of self-care was evolved to empower patients to enable them to take care of their routine lives so that they are not dependent on doctor/ nurses. Implementation of this concept requires that the health care professionals impart skills of self-care to the women. Nurses and midwives have an important role in this endeavor. Dissemination of health related information to the family and community has been projected as one of the primary functions of the nurses / midwives in promoting the health of antenatal women and helping them to attain their optimum state of well-being.

In the era of evidence based medicine this book showcases the evidences regarding effects of a variety of interventions related to various day to day issues of women health including menstruation; polycystic ovary syndrome; infertility management; minor disorders in pregnancy; ante and post-natal care; behavior therapy for urine leakage; pelvic organ prolapse; menopause related problems; prevention and management of low back pain; non-surgical interventions and exercises for knee osteoarthritis etc. Dealing with congenital malformations and genetic disorders as well as prevention and management of complications related to various treatment modalities amongst the women suffering from cancer of breast and cervix have also been very aptly written.

I am pleased to write foreword for the great initiative being taken by the authors and the editors to write and compile various easy to understand self care interventions regarding the day to day and very sensitive health issues of women health. I congratulate the authors for undertaking this commendable work. I earnestly hope that this book will empower women in all walks of their life to have a healthy and productive life.

Dr. Sandhya Ghai

Principal, NINE, PGIMER,
Chandigarh

Preface

In the field of women's health maternal mortality ratio / rate (MMR) is usually is the most discussed / used indicator .Most of the decisions and the attention of the health care planners continue to be focused on the end point i.e. maternal mortality. Other aspects of women's reproductive health have not received the desired attention. In particular, the consumer perspective has been altogether ignored. The client i.e. the woman, needs intimate, empathetic as well as sympathetic and sensitive care. Sadly, these aspects are grossly missing in the existing system / setup of hospital based care which is a product of modernization. With substantial improvement in the life expectancy all over the world, mortality data should no more be the major criteria for evaluating health services. Health care provision should focus on improving the quality of lives of the patients and the morbidities faced by them. From women's point of view, reproductive health problems are the major morbidities which remain un-noticed given the associated "culture of silence". In developing countries situation is further aggravated by the constraints from living conditions- particularly for women. Use of health service by them is naturally less than desirable and is usually delayed. The "culture of tolerance", dictates women to keep on suffering these maladies in silence. So much so that they are rather forced to internalize a "concept of normality" through which they start accepting such problems as a part of 'being a woman'! These issues assume enormous dimension in countries like India where majority of women do not get an opportunity for appropriate and adequate treatment of their reproductive health problems.

Against this background, Dr Santosh Sharma's PhD thesis work on Impact of behavior therapy on urinary incontinence was a godsend opportunity that came my way. In fact, there was a blessing in disguise when her earlier PhD thesis protocol on uterine prolapse / hysterectomy prevalence was rejected by the Dean's doctoral committee as it was considered unworthy of a PhD level work! So, we sent a revised protocol involving an RCT on impact of behavior therapy on urinary incontinence (UI). And the rest is history! Since, the seeds/

idea of this book originated through Dr Santosh Sharma's work, it would be worthwhile to summarize her study conclusions:

- Prevalence of UI was 11.6% in the study area.
- 3/4th women had UI for more than 1 year. Bulk of them felt embarrassed due to UI.
- Main activities affected by UI were traveling for more than 30 minutes.
- Consultation rate was 20%.
- Main reasons for non-consultation were- 'considered it normal', 'did not take it seriously' and 'shyness'.

Impact of behavior therapy: -

- 62% cases felt much better after intervention.
- In the RCT urge incontinence cases decreased from 16 to 2, stress UI from 29 to 9 and mixed UI from 33 to 17. Mild UI cases increased to 19 from 13, moderate case reduced from 24 to 6 and severe cases reduced to 3 from 41.
- Immediately after intervention, 30 (73%) cases became continent.
- At the end of follow-up 41 (52.5%) cases were continent.
- Those who had more than 75% compliance with behavior therapy had more than 75% reduction in the leakage episodes in more than 90% cases. Among those whose compliance was less than 50% half had no relief.

  Overall, it was concluded that behavior therapy was successful in managing UI.

It was clear that such a therapy would prove to be an empowerment mechanism for hapless incontinent women who are rather forced to tolerate this easily treatable yet significantly image – damaging malady, may be because of the fear of surgery, shame or shortage of money'. It is a low-tech therapy. But why has pelvic floor exercises received so little attention so far? One plausible explanation is that it does not fit the medical model of high tech intervention. Adopting exercises and bladder training for UI does not require the professional involvement of doctors, nor does it provide any advantage to other powerful interest such as pharmaceutical industry and surgical equipment needed for invasive urodynamics. It emerged that behavior therapy should be the initial self-care based treatment for the vast majority of patients with UI.

This concept was further expanded to management of uterine prolapse (POP), since etiology (weakening of pelvic floor muscles) was similar. Thus, another RCT on impact of behavior therapy on POP was conducted as a part of MD thesis work of Dr Rashmi Kashyap. Similarly, Dr Aditi Chaudhuri conducted an RCT as a part of her MD thesis work on impact of behavior therapy / exercises on dysmenorrhea. Results of both these theses were very encouraging.

Based on this idea, a DBT project on behaviour therapy for UI among women was sanctioned to us (2010-12). It was quite successful. To expand this concept a separate MPBT room was established in Gyne. OPD in in December 2012 through another DBT project. Besides UI / POP this room also catered to the cases of dysmenorrhea, menopause, infertility, polycystic ovarian syndrome (PCOD), low back pain, ante-natal and post-natal cases.

In all these ventures active support from the Obstetrics & Gynecology department of PGIMER, Chandigarh was the main catalyst. A fruitful collaboration was established under the leadership of Dr LK Dhaliwal (erstwhile head of department)and Dr Vanita Suri(present head of department) was also crucial. Other faculty from department, viz. Drs. Vanita Jain, Seema Chopra, Neelam Aggarwal, Shalini Gainder also collaborated in these projects. Dr AK Mandal, head Urology was a co-investigator in our first project on UI.

Actually, the idea of MPBT room was based on the Family Clinic concept Implemented successfully by Dr Prema Bali, Professor, Centre for Community Medicine, AIIMS, New Delhi.

Faculty and co-investigators from National Institute of Nursing Education (NINE), PGIMER, Chandigarh were also involved in implementing these projects esp. Dr. Avinash Rana & Dr. Sukhpal Kaur. An ICMR project on maternity preparedness training was sanctioned to Dr. Avinash Rana and implemented in MPBT room successfully. Another DBT funded RCT was done in Surgery OPD with Dr. Gurpreet Singh on "Impact of two educational interventions on the shoulder dysfunction, lymphedema and quality of life among the breast surgery patients". Thus, it was an inter-disciplinary effort in the real sense (Obstetrics & Gynecology, Surgery, Public Health experts & Nursing Faculty).

Since all this involved physiotherapy related interventions another PhD work was initiated on fitness level of pregnant & lactating women wherein Mr. Pradeep Sarkar, senior physiotherapist of the institute has successfully completed the RCT in 2018 with demonstration of beneficial effect of the training given to women. Dr Paramveer Singh, from Sports department of, Panjabi University, Patiala was the chief guide & Dr MS Dhillon, Head, Orthopedics, PGIMER, Chandigarh was the co-guide. Another PhD work based RCT was conducted by Dr Meenakshi Sharma with Dr MS Dhillon. She also demonstrated improvement in the quality of life of knee osteoarthritis cases through lifestyle modifications, dietary counselling, exercise training etc.

Above all sincere efforts of our PhD students and DBT/ICMR research workers are worth mentioning. This book essentially is a compilation of the published modules used them as a part of educational interventions delivered to patients and their caregivers. We attribute the success of all these projects to the tireless and patient efforts of these girls. Dr. Purnima Kaushal, Dr. Ruchi Sharma, Ms Neha Pankaj, Ms Kamalpreet Kaur, Ms. Isha Bajaj, Ms Prerna John, Ms Rajni Amit Koli deserve special mention. PhD students included Ms Ishwarpreet Kaur (A Woman's Guide to Deal with PCOS), Dr Risha Gupta(adolescent girls' puberty related changes ; Dr AK Sinha is her co-guide), Dr Neha Chanana (Prevention and management of low back pain; Drs RK Kanojia & Babita Ghai were her co-guides), Dr. Amudeep Singh (Dealing with therapy related issues of cervical cancer; Dr. Sushmita Ghoshal is her co-guide), Dr Alka Rani (How to Deal With Congenital Malformations & Genetic Disorders ; Dr Inusha Panigrahi, Dr Abhik Ghosh & Dr Neelam Aggarwal are her co-guides), Dr Davinder Kaur (Infertility Management in OPD Setting).

I, on behalf of the editors thank all the contributors, the publishers and above all our subjects – the patients and their family caregivers. Partial financial support from Unique Biotech, a probiotic manufacturing company is duly acknowledged.

Amarjeet Singh

List of Abbreviations

AID	:	Artificial Insemination of Donor
AIH	:	Artificial Insemination of Husband's sperm
ART	:	Assisted Reproductive Technology
BBT	:	Basal Body Temperature
BMI	:	Body Mass Index
CARA	:	Central Adoption Resource Authority
CBC	:	Complete Blood Count
CC	:	Clomiphene Citrate
CDC	:	Centers for Disease Control
COH	:	Controlled Ovarian Hyperstimulation
CVS	:	Cardio Vascular System
FNAC	:	Fine Needle Aspiration Cytology
FSH	:	Follicle Stimulating Hormone
GnRH	:	Gonadotrophin-Releasing Hormone
GIFT	:	Gamete Intra Fallopian tube Transfer
GPP	:	Good Practice Point
HCG	:	Human Chorionic Gonadotropin
HIV	:	Human Immunodeficiency Virus
HSG	:	Hysterosalpingography
ICMR	:	Indian Council of Medical Research
ICSI	:	Intra Cytoplasmic Sperm Injection
IUI	:	Intra Uterine Insemination
IVF	:	In Vitro Fertilization
LAPA	:	Licensed Adoption Placement Agency
LH	:	Luteinizing Hormone
LUF	:	Luteinized Unruptured Follicles

NFHS	:	National Family Health Survey
NICE	:	National Institute for Clinical Excellence
NRHM	:	National Rural Health Mission
NSAID	:	Non Steroidal Anti-Inflammatory Drug
OATS	:	Oligoasthenoteratospermia
OD	:	Once a Day
OHSS	:	Ovarian Hyper Stimulation Syndrome
PCOS	:	Poly Cystic Ovary Syndrome
PCR	:	Polymerase Chain Reaction
PHC	:	Primary Health Centre
PID	:	Pelvic Inflammatory Disease
POF	:	Premature Ovarian Failure
RCH	:	Reproductive and Child Health Services
RCOG	:	Royal College of Obstetricians and Gynaecologists
RIPA	:	Registered Adoption Placement Agencies
RS	:	Respiratory system
SAA	:	Special Adoption Agency
SHG	:	Saline Hysterogram
SOGC	:	Society of Obstetrician and Gynaecologists of Canada
STI	:	Sexually transmitted infections
TAS	:	Trans Abdominal Sonography
TESA	:	Testicular Sperm Aspiration
TSH	:	Thyroid Stimulating Hormone
TVS	:	Trans Vaginal Sonography
WHO	:	World Health Organization

Chapter - 1

Introduction

—Amarjeet Singh

BMJ reported in 2018 that doctors in India see patients for barely 2 minutes. Such a short consultation adversely affects patient care, workload and stress of doctors. In western countries, consultation crosses 20 minutes. Over last 15 years, globally, new concepts have emerged about doctor-patient interaction, viz., Patient and family-centered care, patient-as-person, social prescription, information therapy etc. There is focus upon active collaboration and shared decision-making between patients, families, and providers. Aim is to design and manage a customized and comprehensive care plan, giving more emphasis on the patients' problems than on their diagnoses. Person-centred care is underpinned by values of respect for persons, individual right to self-determination, understanding, empathy, two-way communication and eye-to-eye contact.

Doctors generally prescribe pills to make people feel better. Social prescribing is a relatively new holistic approach to wellness in which patients are encouraged to fit their lifestyle, interests, and special needs in ways that complement any pharmaceutical prescriptions. This highlights the concept of patient self-care with 'information prescriptions' supporting them to take greater control of their own health. All this become more crucial when we discuss women's health.

It is matter of coincidence that the abovementioned newer concepts in patient care were already being implemented in the MPBT (multi-purpose behavior therapy) room project @ PGIMER, Chandigarh, where we proved that many of the problems of women reporting at Gyne.OPD can be resolved by non-medicinal interventions, e.g., appropriate behavior therapy, exercises and counselling. Our results proved that they can be weaned off their dependence on medicinal cure. Human body's power of self-healing was strongly emphasized. Concept of salutogenesis was also popularized. Because of the enormous patient load in hospitals the doctors in overcrowded Gynecology OPD usually have no time to explain these things to the patients. Much of their time is wasted on routine queries of patients. This can be avoided if we stress upon conservative management of health problems of women through decentralized counselling in OPDs. MPBT room project did exactly that. When such a concept is propagated through an apex institution like PGIMER, it carries a lot of weight.

Our earlier studies had proved that behavior therapy along with pelvic floor exercises can easily provide relief to women having urinary incontinence or uterine prolapse (UI / POP) without using any medicine or surgery. Based on this idea, a DBT project on "Hospital Based BT of UI among Women: A Feasibility Study" was successfully completed during 2010-12.To expand this concept of health promotion and de-medicalization, a separate MPBT room was established in Gyne. OPD in PGIMER, in December 2012 through another DBT project. Besides UI / POP this room also catered to the cases of dysmenorrhoea, menopause, infertility, polycystic ovarian syndrome (PCOD), low back pain, ante-natal and post-natal cases. Overall, > 8000 women in Gyne. OPD have been successfully managed through this approach in last 5 yrs. Favorable results of non-medicinal interventions were reported. menopausal patients(> 300), patients UI and POP(> 1500) ANC patients (~ 4500), infertility (400 +),dysmenorrhea(100 +) and others(>1000) patients also benefitted.

This project was successfully completed in May 2016. Now, the MPBT room concept is being maintained & nurtured by PhD research scholars through their thesis based activities with full support from Gyne.OPD. An RCT on use of Furocyst (A fenugreek based product) in PCOD patients is also being conducted in the MPBT room.

Thus, modality of delivering a health promotion orientation package of services through a MPBT room has been developed & implemented in Gyne. OPD, which is replicable in similar settings. In this model, after referral from main OPD, staff in MPBT room provide counselling including behaviour therapy and exercises to antenatal women or those with dysmenorrhea, urinary incontinence, uterine prolapse, menopause or infertility. Concept of healthy diet-healthy lifestyle is explained to them. In MPBT room women are counselled together with their family members. This way the husbands, the mothers in law and other relatives can also understand her problems, especially in cases of infertility. Even adoption services were linked with MPBT room for those who cannot conceive. Queries of patients are resolved at leisurely pace. Sufficient time is devoted to each patient. Exercises and lifestyle changes (simple exercises/yoga) are also explained to the cases of POP, UI & dysmenorrhoea. Pregnant women are counseled on self – care about minor disorders such as morning sickness, backache, cramps, fainting spells, heart-burn, constipation, etc.

The demedicalization philosophy inherent in the MPBT room approach helps in empowering the women in self-care of their reproductive and other health problems. The latest addition is the use of mobile phone / laptops for video-based counselling. In effect, MPBT room concept is operationalization of a multi-disciplinary team work in OPDs.

The unique features of MPBT room approach is a family-centered individualized as well as group counselling sessions; adoption of 'demedicalization' approach for tackling the routine OBG problems of women + integrated training strategies are used:

- Couples are counselled together in MPBT room. Thus, they can understand each other better and express their concerns without any hesitation.
- Patients are counselled along with their family members.
- Queries are resolved at leisurely pace. Sufficient time (15-20 min) is devoted to each patient.
- Efforts are made to improve adherence to dietary counselling and weight reduction regime.
- Exercises are demonstrated individually in the room. Patients repeat them (Return demonstration). A special set of floor as well as bed based exercises have been developed.
- Videos are shown regarding ante natal and post-natal care
- Easy to understand IEC materials like- charts, flip cards, posters are displayed in the room
- Laptop based IEC material is also given
- Yoga and meditation related counselling is also given as per the need.
- Every patient is given booklet on relevant management aspect of her problem free of cost (Hindi/ English/Punjabi)
- Patient are followed up on mobile phone to ensure compliance. WhatsApp groups have been used successfully.

Impact: Our data indicates that it is feasible to impart health promotion orientation in Gyne., Orthopedics and Surgery OPDs through counselling of women for de-medicalization of management of their routine health problems. Doctors also reported reduced workload since they did not have to spend time on routine cases. Burden on family care givers also reduced. Simultaneously, this also helped to instill a sense of confidence among patients and their caregivers when they observed the positive results of their taking charge of their own health. Their concept of self-efficacy also improved.

Use of mobile phone / laptops for video-based counselling also eliminated the need of repeating the same set of instructions by doctors / nurses to patients with similar complaints. Exercises were demonstrated individually in the MPBT room. Easy to understand IEC materials like- charts, flip cards, posters were displayed in the room. Booklets on Menopause, Dysmenorrhoea, Prolapse and Urinary Incontinence in 3 different languages (Hindi, Punjabi and English) have been published; UI booklets are posted on PGIMER website. These are given to the patients free of cost. Mobile phone based follow up was also done to ensure compliance. Propagation of the Idea of MPBT Room through Women's Health Kitty Party has been initiated.

This room has enhanced the level of satisfaction of patients and their relatives. Women are also happy that they are being listened to patiently.

The demedicalization philosophy inherent in the use of behavior therapy/ counselling in MPBT room provides relief to them without resorting to any medication. This also has a potential to improve the socio-medical environment of 'pill for every ill' kind of medicalised life & mindset of citizens.

Problems & Constraints faced and solutions achieved: OBG junior doctors kept on changing every few months. Fresh batches had to be reoriented towards the idea of MPBT room through meetings / seminars.

Details of viable economic/social model developed having multiplier impact: MPBT room idea has been propagated through >20 national and international conferences, social networking sites; newspaper coverage; Seminars/CME, Jyotirgamaya 91.2 FM Radio Station Panjab University, All India Radio FM Channel, Chandigarh, @ PGIMER, Chandigarh website.

MPBT room set-up has even been replicated at Military Hospital, Nasirabad, Ajmer and at Military Hospital, Jodhpur. Four ICMR seminars on MPBT room related topics were organized (low back pain /Menopause / Disability /ANC).

Our room has also become a suitable training (and research) place for MD, MPH, PhD & nursing students of PGIMER, Chandigarh. Similar approach has been introduced in Orthopaedics and Surgery OPDs@ PGIMER, Chandigarh. An RCT funded by UT-DST (Chandigarh) was completed in Orthopedics OPD, on mild to moderate knee osteoarthritis (KOA) patients. They were counselled on lifestyle intervention (a set of exercises, weight reduction, meditation, dietary modifications, posture correction etc.). Another DBT funded RCT was done in Surgery OPD on "Impact of two educational interventions on the shoulder dysfunction, lymphedema and quality of life among the breast surgery patients". In all these OPDs, laptop was also used for video-based counselling. Patients were also trained through one to one demonstration. Four separate educational video CDs (~40-50 minutes each), 10 booklets and other IEC material have been developed on these issues. Hindi /English/ Punjabi versions are available. These are distributed free of cost to the patients. Mobile phone based feedbacks are regularly taken. An ICMR sponsored project on "maternity preparedness" was also successfully completed in December 2015 in MPBT room, OBG OPD.

This concept can be expanded to harness the potential of IT to empower the women in self-care. A smart mobile phone / computer based counselling system can be developed to educate and train women and their caregivers in OPD setting regarding management of OBG problems. For this, SOPs (Standard Operating Procedure) may be developed in the form of a booklet + posters + handouts+ soft copy versions for managing the listed cases. Smartphone App may be developed in order to make the SOPs (as problem based text/PDF/audio/videos on OBG related problems) accessible to the users by clicking on the phone. Similar service may also be sought to be provided through establishment of kiosk based computer aided information counters (with counsellors in attendance) in OBG OPD. Here drop down menu approach can be used to provide customized multilingual guidance to women. Husbands / mothers in law and other escorts can be actively involved in such training to ensure that optimal care is received at home by the cases. Given the profile of Chandigarh as a model smart planned city it will be quite feasible to implement the information technology based approach to tackle OBG cases @ PGIMER, Chandigarh to nurture it as a smart hospital

Publications based on the project work

1. Kaur T, Dudeja P, Sharma M, Jain V, Singh A. Impact of Running a Behavior Therapy Room for Various Categories of Urinary Incontinence Cases in Different Age Groups in Obstetrics-Gynecology Outpatient Department of a Tertiary Care Hospital.JPMER.2014; 48:159-163
2. Sharma R, Dhaliwal LK, Suri V, Kaushal P, Singhal N, Rana AK & Singh AJ. Implementing a Life Cycle Approach through Establishment of a Multipurpose Behavior Therapy Room in PGIMER, Chandigarh for Enhancing the Fitness Level of Women. JPMER, 2017; 51: 115-122
3. Kaushal P et al."Rajoneevriti-Menopause se sambhandhit samasyaon k samadhan ka ek naya drishtikon" in Punjabi & Hindi, New Delhi, New Era International Imprints, 2013
4. Kaushal P et al "Menopause- A new approach to deal with menopause related problems" New Delhi, New Era International Imprints, 2013

5. Sharma R et al. "Bacchedani Bahar Ana-Prolapse Uterus",New Delhi, New Era International Imprints 2013.
6. Sharma et al."Bacchedani Bahar Ana-Prolapse Uterus" in Hindi & in Punjabi. New Delhi, New Era International Imprints, 2013.
7. Sharma R et al "Mahawari da dard- Bachaav atey elaaj" New Delhi, New Era International Imprints 2013.
8. Sharma R et al. " "Mahilaon mein peshab leakage"(Hindi) New Delhi, New Era International Imprints 2013
9. Sharma R, et al."Auratan vich pishab leakage"(Punjabi) New Delhi, New Era International Imprints 2013.
10. Neha and Singh A.J. "Promoting Empowerment of Adolescent girls by Demedicalizing Management of Dysmenorrhea." Ind.J.Youth Adol. Health 2015; 2(4)
11. Sharma, M., Singh, A.J. and Dhillion, M.S. spending time with patients significantly influences outcome of non-operative treatment of knee osteoarthritis. JPMER, 2015;49: v-vi.
12. Gupta R, et al. Managing common problems at puberty- A guide for adolescent girls, New Delhi, Century Publications, 2017
13. Kaur I, Suri V, Rana SV Singh, A, Sachdeva N, Sahni N. Impact of Lifestyle Intervention for Management of the Modern Life Scourge of Polycystic Ovarian Syndrome among Girls – A Case Series. Ind J Youth Adol Health 2017; 4(3): 21-24.
14. Singhal N and Singh AJ. Promoting Empowerment of Adolescent Girls by Demedicalizing Management of Dysmenorrhea. Ind. J. Youth Adol. Health 2015; 2(4): 1-3
15. Sharma M, Singh AJ and Dhillon MS. (Editorial) Spending time with patients significantly influences outcomes of non-operative treatment of knee osteoarthritis. JPMER, 2016; 50:v-vi
16. Kaur I, Singh A. Empowering Adolescent Girls to Manage the Impending Epidemic of PCOS. Ind J Youth Adol Health 2016; 3(2): 1-3.
17. Sharma M, Singh A, Dhillon MS et al. Conservative Therapy through Adequate Doctor Patient Interaction Improves outcomes in Patients Suffering from Mild and Moderate Knee Osteoarthritis. Int J Health Care Edu & Med Inform 2017;4(3&4): 1-2
18. Neha et al ' garbhavastha se sambandhit sankaye ve unka samadhan'. New Delhi, New Era International Imprints; 2015.

Theses guided by PI on MPBT Room approach (PhD; MPH) during & after the project

(i) "Impact of an intervention package on selected health fitness problems of antenatal and postnatal women"

(ii) "Efficacy of probiotic based dietary and lifestyle regime in management of PCOS"

(iii) "Impact of two interventions on the postural and ergonomical health and fitness of Antenatal and postnatal women: A randomized controlled trial"

(iv) "Development of information booklet for infertile couple: An exploratory Study"

(v) "Evaluation of posture in postnatal women having Low back pain"

vi) "Comparative efficacy of two IT based educational approaches promoting the concept of self-care for conservative non- medicinal management of selected OBG health problems among women reporting at OBG OPD PGIMER Chandigarh."

(vii) "Devising and validating a counseling protocol for couples reporting at OBG Department of PGI, Chandigarh with problems related to congenital disorders in their children."

(viii) "Impact of lifestyle modification and educational interventions on the information needs and satisfaction level of infertile cases reporting at OBG OPD, PGIMER, Chandigarh."

(vii) "Comparative impact of two educational intervention strategies for improving Quality of Life of cervical cancer patients reporting at PGIMER, Chandigarh: A two group RCT".

Besides these, new academic initiatives have been taken. PhD theses on infertility and ovarian cancer have been initiated. Booklets on cervical cancer and congenital malformations & genetic disorders have been published. Seminars on these topics sponsored by ICMR & MCI have been organized at PGIMER, Chandigarh. Best oral as well as poster presentation awards based on these works have been received by Ms Ishwarpreet (on PCOS in 2017) & by Dr. Amudeep Singh (on cervical cancer in 2018) in Malaysia and Thailand respectively.

Oration / health talk on topics related to MPBT Room approach delivered by the PI

1. "Proposing a Settings Based Approach of Quaternary Prevention to Cultivate a new Health Culture in Chandigarh – Potential for a joint

venture between Panjab University & PGIMER" @ at Anthropology Deptt., Panjab University on 13.2.18 @National Science Congress

2. Dhanwantri Oration in Kolkata@ 44th IAPSM conference (10th Feb 2017),"I Also Practiced Quaternary Prevention through MPBT Room by Default (& Still Continuing with it)"
3. "How to Address Reproductive Health Issues of Girls in Gynec OPDs? : Some Experiences from PGIMER Chandigarh"- @ ICMR-DST-SERB sponsored Symposium: "Adolescent and Youth Friendly Health Initiative Through Mentoring Programs for Students" at GMCH Chandigarh (2015)
4. "Introducing Quaternary Prevention through Health Promotion and De-Medicalization Approach in OPDs- Experiences from PGIMER, Chandigarh". @ Indo-Global Summit & Expo on Novel Approaches and Recent Practices on Health Care on Oct 5, 2015, New Delhi
5. "Integrating the Concepts of Health Promotion, De-Medicalization, Salutogenesis, Social Iatrogenesis & Quaternary Prevention "@ National Conference on 'Innovative Approaches in Public Health', AFMC, Pune (2015)
6. AIR FM Lifeline programme on 26.08.2015 "Avoiding harmful effects of drugs by treating diseases without medicine - some experiences from Gyne and Orthopedics OPD based projects in PGIMER Chandigarh
7. Jyotirgamaya 91.2 FM, Radio Station, Panjab University "Empowerment of women through self-care training on non-medicinal/ non- surgical approach for management of common gyne problems faced by them".
8. "Demedicalising Women's Health: Health Promoting Approach-Problems in Gynecology OPDs" at SRMS,Bareilly. March 20, 2014
9. "Reducing the burden of doctors in OPDs by adopting a Health Promoting Hospital Approach for De-Medicalization of Routine Health Problems of Women – Potential of introducing mobile phone / laptops for video-based counselling",10th International Telemedicon, AIIMS Bhopal, Nov.7-9, 2014.
10. "Going Beyond MDG Rhetoric; Need to Focus on Routine Gynecological Problems of Women Through Health Promotion Approach in Hospitals". @ Pune Public Health conference 2014; Feb 25, 2014
11. "Promoting Demedicalisation of Women's Health Problems in Gynecology OPDs: Creating Evidence Base for Nonmedicinal

treatment of Urinary Incontinence in a Hospital of North India" at ICGO conference, Dalian, China, Oct. 12-14, 2013

12. "Why urinary incontinence is ignored by patients / doctors?" Paper presented at 13th World Congress on Menopause, Italy, June 8, 2011

Seminar / CME organized on topics related to MPBT Room approach

1. ICSSR seminar, "Developing and standardizing the modalities of college level interventions for in situ management of the modern life scourge of PCOS among girl students". 15th Feb 2018
2. MCI CME,"A capacity building seminar for strengthening communication skills of doctors for counselling of parents regarding birth defects" 8.2.2018.
3. MCI CME "Evolving a consensus for training the doctors and nurses regarding development of a communication protocol for dealing with the sexual and reproductive health care needs of adolescent girls in the OPD setting".28th September, 2017
4. MCI seminar, "Standardizing modalities of effective doctor-patient communication for training doctors in implementing a multipurpose behavior therapy room based approach in Gyne OPDs of medical colleges to manage PCOS cases." on 21st Sept.2017
5. ICMR seminar "Evolving a standardized protocol for management of Low Back Pain through Pain Clinic" 24th March, 2017.
6. ICMR Seminar "Orientation training of Gynaecology experts for adopting health promotion and de-medicalization approach in OPDs for addressing health issues of menopausal women" 5th February, 2015
7. ICMR seminar, "Strengthening of training & counselling expertise among nurses & other health care providers in 3 apex government hospitals of Chandigarh for imparting maternity preparedness skills to ante- & post-natal mothers reporting in Obstet & Gynaec OPDs" on 15th Jan 2015.
8. ICMR Seminar On 24th October 2015,"Evolving a consensus among various stakeholders for developing a model for making Gynaecology OPD and ward services in hospitals disabled friendly"
9. On 27th March, 2014, ICMR Seminar, "Orientation Training of Obstetrics & Gynecology Experts for Adopting Health Promotion

Approach in a Teaching Hospital for Reducing Patient Load in OPDs".

MPBT room team @ International Women's day 2014 on invitation by CDPO Mohali

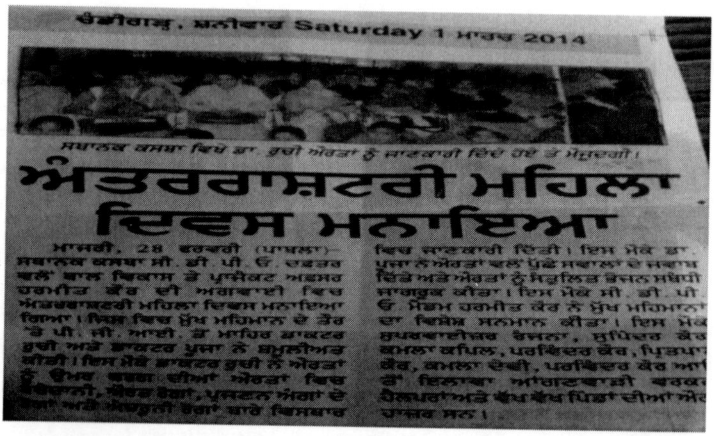

ਚੰਡੀਗੜ੍ਹ, ਸ਼ਨੀਵਾਰ Saturday 1 ਮਾਰਚ 2014

ਅੰਤਰਰਾਸ਼ਟਰੀ ਮਹਿਲਾ ਦਿਵਸ ਮਨਾਇਆ

MPBT Roomhas also figured in—

(i) a Documentary Film on **Biotechnology Based Programme for Societal Development** produced by DBT with the support of NFDC. The link on DBT website under video gallery section http://www.dbtindia.nic.in/videos/

https://www.youtube.com/watch?v=ZDEVbEUylU4

(ii) MPBT related interview is live on the following link:https://www.docplexus.in/#/app/infocenters/FDTD4/posts/457636b8-f203-4515-8403-0c205da3004e

Following photographs reflect the ambience in MPBT room.

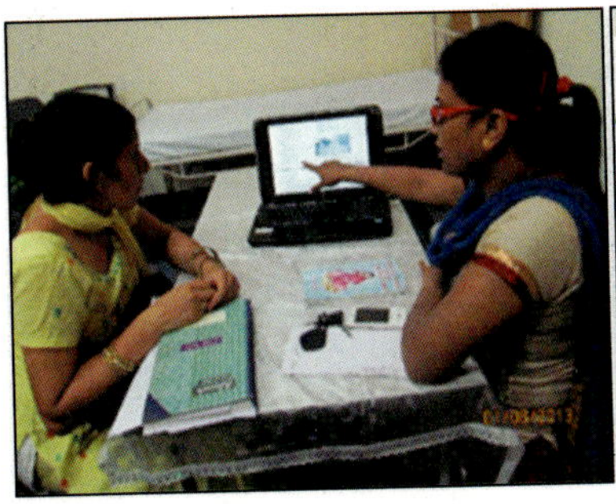

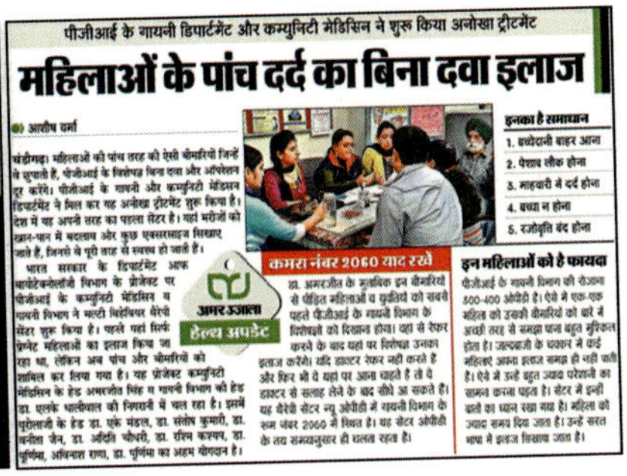

पीजीआई के गायनी डिपार्टमेंट और कम्युनिटी मेडिसिन ने शुरू किया अनोखा ट्रीटमेंट

महिलाओं के पांच दर्द का बिना दवा इलाज

आशीष वर्मा

चंडीगढ़। महिलाओं की पांच तरह की ऐसी बीमारियों जिन्हें वे छुपाती हैं, पीजीआई के विशेषज्ञ बिना दवा और ऑपरेशन दूर करेंगे। पीजीआई के गायनी और कम्युनिटी मेडिसन डिपार्टमेंट ने मिल कर यह अनोखा ट्रीटमेंट शुरू किया है। देश में यह अपनी तरह का पहला सेंटर है। यहां मरीजों को खान-पान में बदलाव और कुछ एक्सरसाइज सिखाए जाते हैं, जिनसे वे पूरी तरह से स्वस्थ हो जाती हैं।

भारत सरकार के डिपार्टमेंट आफ बायोटेक्नोलॉजी विभाग के प्रोजेक्ट पर पीजीआई के कम्युनिटी मेडिसिन व गायनी विभाग ने मल्टी बिहेवियर थेरेपी सेंटर शुरू किया है। पहले यहां सिर्फ प्रेग्नेंट महिलाओं का इलाज किया जा रहा था, लेकिन अब पांच और बीमारियों को शामिल कर लिया गया है। यह प्रोजेक्ट कम्युनिटी मेडिसिन के हेड अमरजीत सिंह व गायनी विभाग की हेड डा. एलके धालीवाल की निगरानी में चल रहा है। इसमें यूरोलाजी के हेड डा. एके मंडल, डा. संतोष कुमारी, डा. वनीता जैन, डा. अदिति चौधरी, डा. रश्मि कश्यप, डा. पूर्णिमा, अविनाश राणा, डा. पूर्णिमा का अहम योगदान है।

अमर उजाला हेल्थ अपडेट

इनका है समाधान

1. बच्चेदानी बाहर आना
2. पेशाब लीक होना
3. माहवारी में दर्द होना
4. बच्चा न होना
5. रजोवृत्ति बंद होना

कमरा नंबर 2060 याद रखें

डा. अमरजीत के मुताबिक इन बीमारियों से पीड़ित महिलाओं व युवतियों को सबसे पहले पीजीआई के गायनी विभाग के विशेषज्ञों को दिखाना होगा। वहां से रेफर करने के बाद यहां पर विशेषज्ञ उनका इलाज करेंगे। यदि डाक्टर रेफर नहीं करते हैं और फिर भी वे यहां पर आना चाहते हैं तो वे डाक्टर से सलाह लेने के बाद सीधे आ सकते हैं। यह थेरेपी सेंटर न्यू ओपीडी में गायनी विभाग के रूम नंबर 2060 में स्थित है। यह सेंटर ओपीडी के तय समयानुसार ही चलता रहता है।

इन महिलाओं को है फायदा

पीजीआई के गायनी विभाग की रोजाना 300-400 ओपीडी है। ऐसे में एक-एक महिला को उनकी बीमारियों के बारे में अच्छी तरह से समझा पाना बहुत मुश्किल होता है। जल्दबाजी के चक्कर में कई महिलाएं अपना इलाज समझ ही नहीं पाती हैं। ऐसे में उन्हें बहुत ज्यादा परेशानी का सामना करना पड़ता है। सेंटर में इन्हीं बातों का ध्यान रखा गया है। महिला को ज्यादा समय दिया जाता है। उन्हें सरल भाषा में इलाज सिखाया जाता है।

Laptop based counselling MPBT room.

Coverage of MPBT room concept in media.

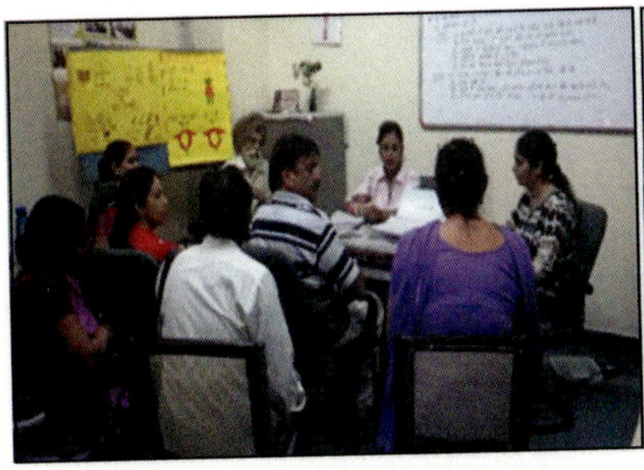

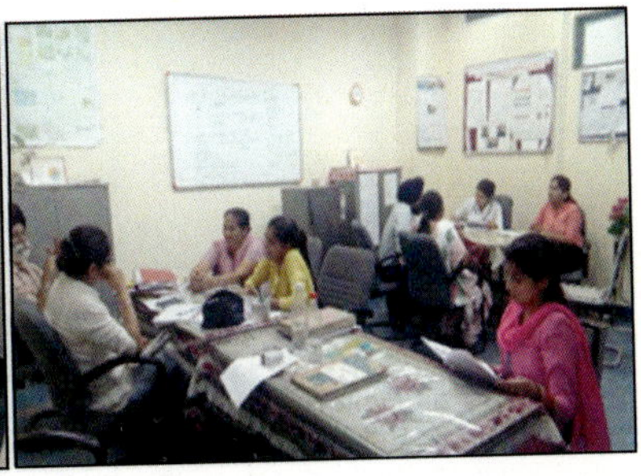

Group counselling @ MPBT room.

Multi-station counselling in MPBT room.

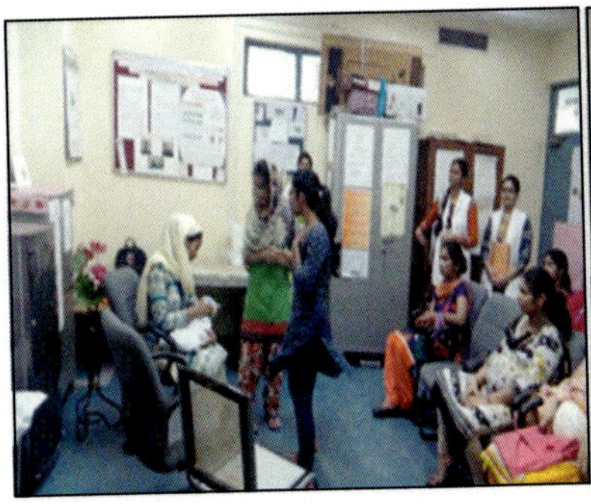

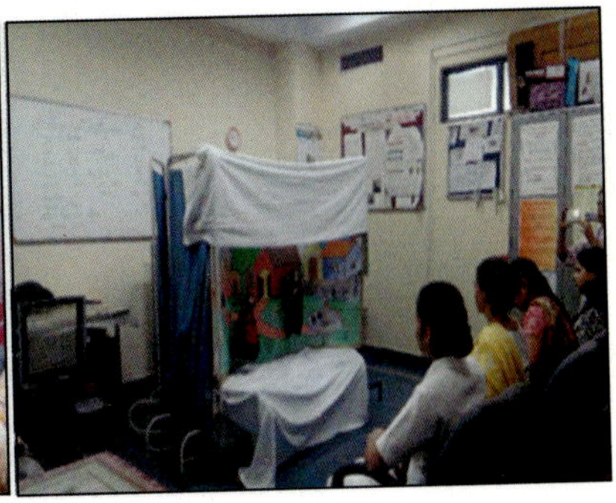

Training of nurses in MPBT room through role play & puppet show.

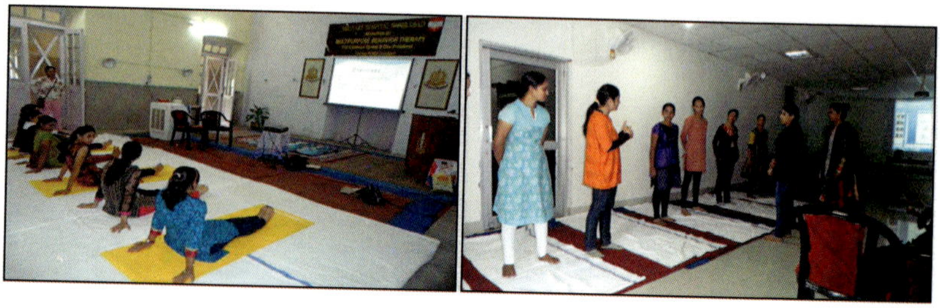

Team MPBT training nurses in this concept @ Nasirabad & Jodhpur Military Hospitals

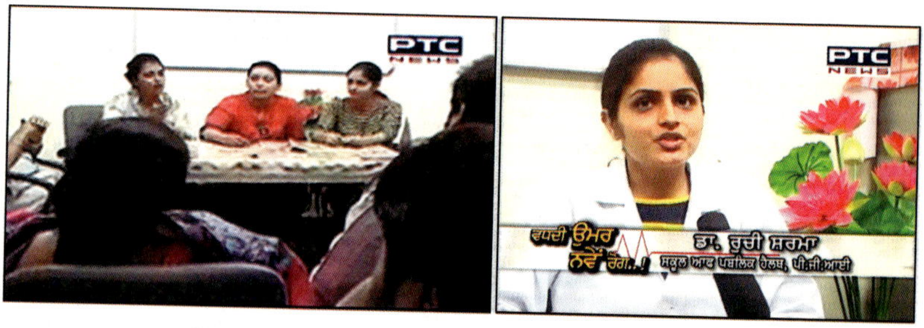

Screenshots of PTC news coverage of MPBT room

MPBT room related booklets / CD published through DBT grant

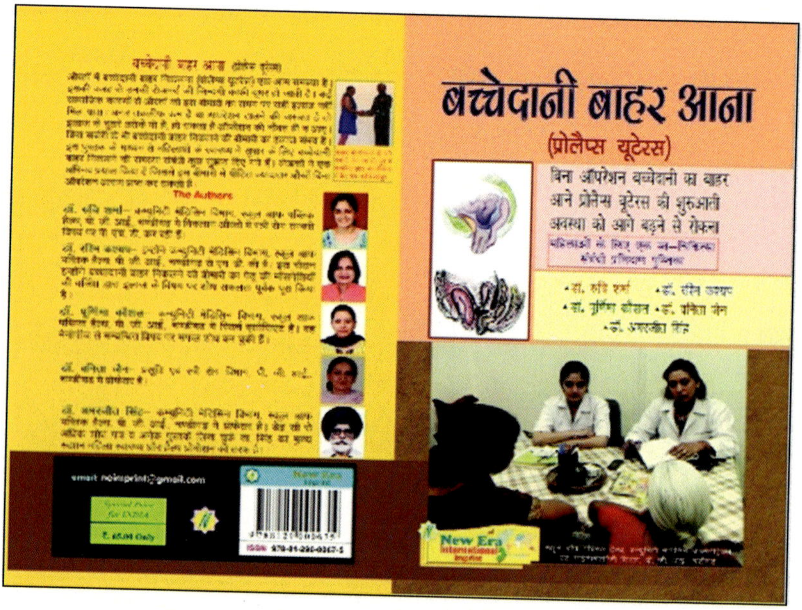

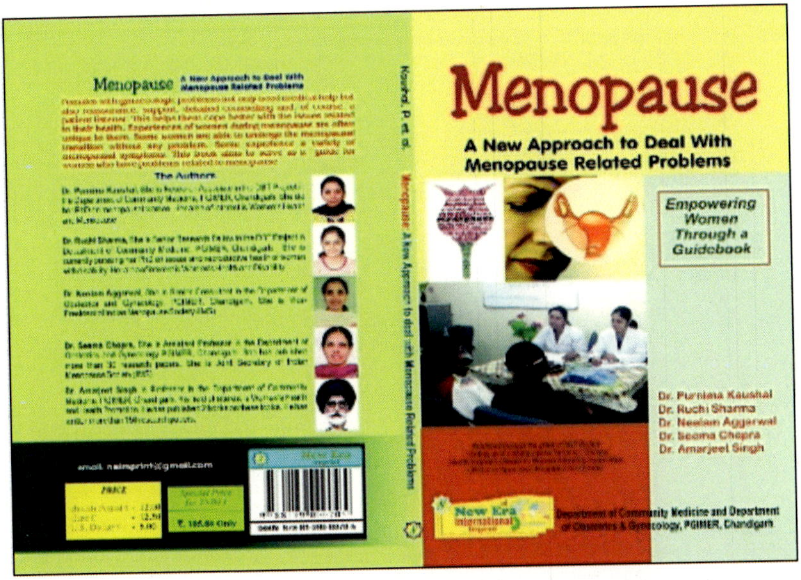
Menopause
A New Approach to Deal With Menopause Related Problems
Empowering Women Through a Guidebook
Dr. Purnima Kaushal
Dr. Ruchi Sharma
Dr. Neelam Aggarwal
Dr. Seema Chopra
Dr. Amarjeet Singh
New Era International Imprint
Department of Community Medicine and Department of Obstetrics & Gynecology, PGIMER, Chandigarh
Menopause A New Approach to deal with Menopause Related Problems
The Authors
email: neimprint@gmail.com
PRICE
Special Price for INDIA
New Era Imprint

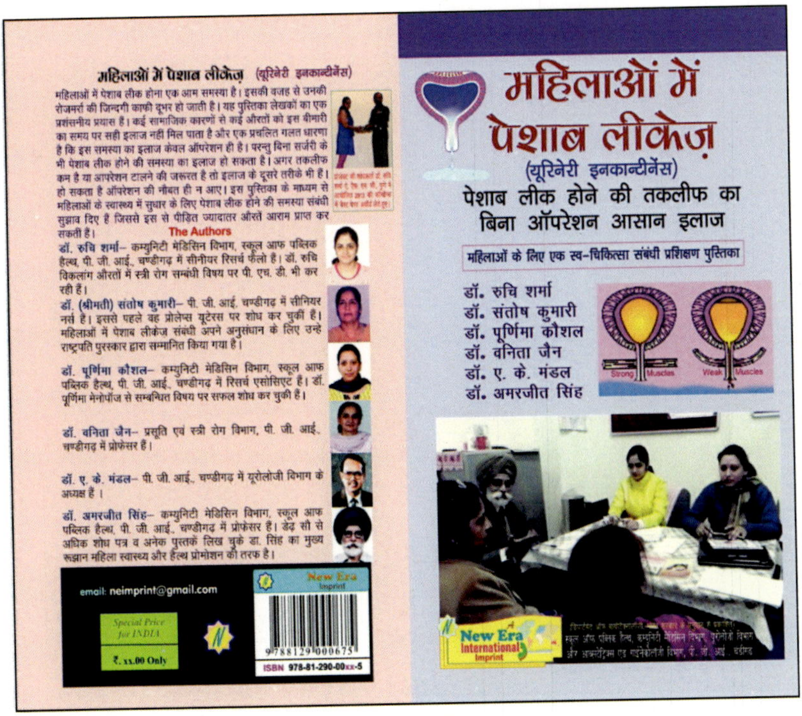
महिलाओं में पेशाब लीकेज़
(यूरिनेरी इनकान्टीनेंस)
पेशाब लीक होने की तकलीफ का बिना ऑपरेशन आसान इलाज
महिलाओं के लिए एक स्व-चिकित्सा संबंधी प्रशिक्षण पुस्तिका
डॉ. रुचि शर्मा
डॉ. संतोष कुमारी
डॉ. पूर्णिमा कौशल
डॉ. वनिता जैन
डॉ. ए. के. मंडल
डॉ. अमरजीत सिंह
Strong Muscles
Weak Muscles
New Era International Imprint
महिलाओं में पेशाब लीकेज़ (यूरिनेरी इनकान्टीनेंस)
महिलाओं में पेशाब लीक होना एक आम समस्या है। इसकी वजह से उनकी रोजमर्रा की जिन्दगी काफी दूभर हो जाती है। यह पुस्तिका लेखकों का एक प्रशंसनीय प्रयास है। कई सामाजिक कारणों से कई औरतों को इस बीमारी का समय पर सही इलाज नहीं मिल पाता है और एक प्रचलित गलत धारणा है कि इस समस्या का इलाज केवल ऑपरेशन ही है। परन्तु बिना सर्जरी के भी पेशाब लीक होने की समस्या का इलाज हो सकता है। अगर तकलीफ कम है या आपरेशन टालने की जरूरत है तो इलाज के दूसरे तरीके भी हैं। हो सकता है ऑपरेशन की नौबत ही न आए। इस पुस्तिका के माध्यम से महिलाओं के स्वास्थ्य में सुधार के लिए पेशाब लीक होने की समस्या संबंधी सुझाव दिए हैं जिससे इस से पीड़ित ज्यादातर औरतें आराम प्राप्त कर सकती हैं।
The Authors
डॉ. रुचि शर्मा– कम्युनिटी मेडिसिन विभाग, स्कूल आफ पब्लिक हैल्थ, पी. जी. आई., चण्डीगढ़ में सीनीयर रिसर्च फैलो हैं। डॉ. रुचि विकलांग औरतों में स्त्री रोग सम्बंधी विषय पर पी. एच. डी. भी कर रही हैं।
डॉ. (श्रीमती) संतोष कुमारी– पी. जी. आई. चण्डीगढ़ में सीनियर नर्स हैं। इससे पहले वह प्रोलेप्स यूटेरस पर शोध कर चुकी हैं। महिलाओं में पेशाब लीकेज़ संबंधी अपने अनुसंधान के लिए उन्हे राष्ट्रपति पुरस्कार द्वारा सम्मानित किया गया है।
डॉ. पूर्णिमा कौशल– कम्युनिटी मेडिसिन विभाग, स्कूल आफ पब्लिक हैल्थ, पी. जी. आई. चण्डीगढ़ में रिसर्च एसोसिएट हैं। डॉ. पूर्णिमा मेनोपॉज से सम्बन्धित विषय पर सफल शोध कर चुकी हैं।
डॉ. वनिता जैन– प्रसूति एवं स्त्री रोग विभाग, पी. जी. आई., चण्डीगढ़ में प्रोफेसर हैं।
डॉ. ए. के. मंडल– पी. जी. आई., चण्डीगढ़ में यूरोलोजी विभाग के अध्यक्ष हैं।
डॉ. अमरजीत सिंह– कम्युनिटी मेडिसिन विभाग, स्कूल आफ पब्लिक हैल्थ, पी. जी. आई., चण्डीगढ़ में प्रोफेसर हैं। डेढ़ सौ से अधिक शोध पत्र व अनेक पुस्तकें लिख चुके डा. सिंह का मुख्य रूझान महिला स्वास्थ्य और हैल्थ प्रोमोशन की तरफ है।
email: neimprint@gmail.com
Special Price for INDIA
₹. xx.00 Only
New Era Imprint
ISBN 978-81-290-00xx-5

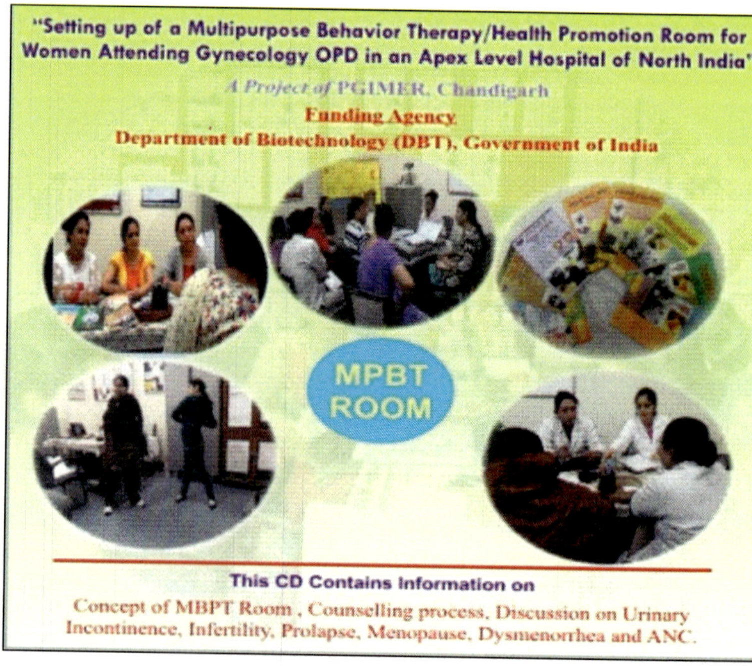
"Setting up of a Multipurpose Behavior Therapy/Health Promotion Room for Women Attending Gynecology OPD in an Apex Level Hospital of North India"
A Project of PGIMER, Chandigarh
Funding Agency
Department of Biotechnology (DBT), Government of India
MPBT ROOM
This CD Contains Information on
Concept of MBPT Room, Counselling process, Discussion on Urinary Incontinence, Infertility, Prolapse, Menopause, Dysmenorrhea and ANC.

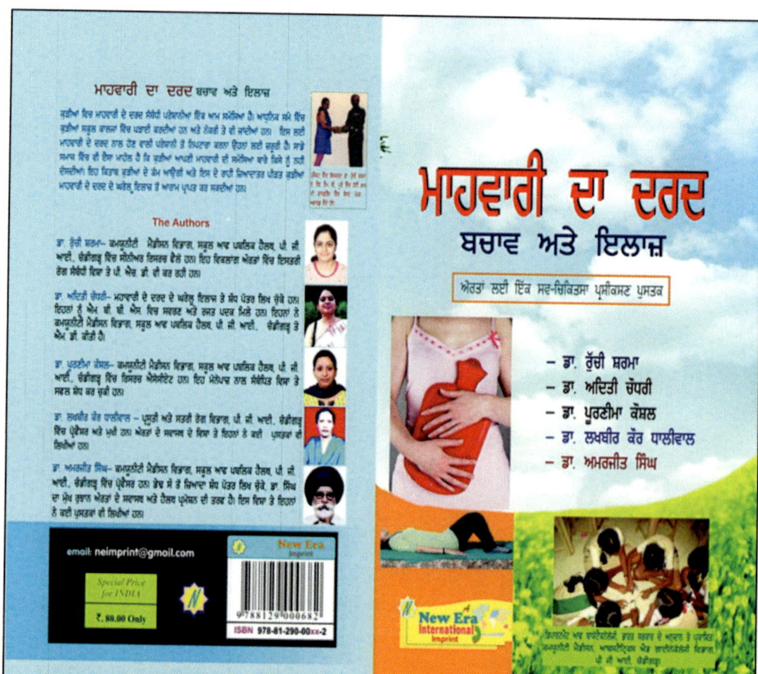
ਮਾਹਵਾਰੀ ਦਾ ਦਰਦ ਬਚਾਵ ਅਤੇ ਇਲਾਜ
The Authors
email: neimprint@gmail.com
Special Price for INDIA
New Era Imprint
ISBN 978-81-290-00xx-2
ਮਾਹਵਾਰੀ ਦਾ ਦਰਦ
ਬਚਾਵ ਅਤੇ ਇਲਾਜ਼
ਔਰਤਾਂ ਲਈ ਇੱਕ ਸਵ-ਚਿਕਿਤਸਾ ਪ੍ਰਸ਼ਿਕਸ਼ਣ ਪੁਸਤਕ
– ਡਾ. ਰੁੱਚੀ ਸ਼ਰਮਾ
– ਡਾ. ਅਦਿਤੀ ਚੌਧਰੀ
– ਡਾ. ਪੂਰਣੀਮਾ ਕੋਸ਼ਲ
– ਡਾ. ਲਖਬੀਰ ਕੌਰ ਧਾਲੀਵਾਲ
– ਡਾ. ਅਮਰਜੀਤ ਸਿੰਘ
New Era International Imprint

Chapter - 2

Project Completion Report

Setting up of a Multipurpose Behaviour Therapy/Health Promotion Room for Women Attending Gynaecology OPD in an Apex Level Hospital of North India

—Amarjeet Singh, Vanita Suri, Vanita Jain, Avinash Rana, AK Mandal

Objectives wise Achievements

S. No	*Objectives*	*Achievements*
1.	To set up a multipurpose behaviour therapy (MPBT) room for various reproductive health problems of women attending gynaecology OPD in PGIMER, Chandigarh.	MPBT Room has been set up in Gynaecology Department of New OPD First floor, PGIMER Chandigarh (Room No.2060) and is functioning well since Dec. 2012.
2.	To assess its benefits to the women patients for their various reproductive health problems.	Overall, > 6500 patients have been counselled here till May 2016. (Urinary incontinence / prolapse uterus= 1600; Menopause= 200; Infertility= 250; Dysmenorrhoea=100; Polycystic ovarian disease= 350; pregnant / lactating women= 3600; Women with Disability=150; others= 300). Most of them reported relief in symptoms
3.	To sensitize Medical Council of India & Nursing Council of India, about the need to include MPBT room concept in medical/nursing curriculum.	To be done later

(Contd...)

4.	To evaluate outcome / cost effectiveness of operating such a room.	To be done later
5.	To propagate the idea of MPBT room through Federation of Obstetricians and Gynaecologists of India and Indian Medical Association to include this concept in government as well as private hospitals / clinics.	Idea of MPBT room has been propagated by through > 20 National and Regional conference presentations including FOGSI (Annex IV). (Oral and Poster); through social networking sites (Face book); Newspaper Coverage; 1 Seminars/CME; through All India Radio, Chandigarh FM Channel's 'Life Line Phone in Program' and Panjab University Community Radio 91.2 MHz *Jyotirgamaya Padho aur Padhao* program ;through women's health kitty party. Military hospitals, Nasirabad, Ajmer and Jodhpur have already introduced MPBT room concept.
6.	Bring out popular booklets on antenatal/postnatal care, dysmenorrhoea, menopause and infertility in Hindi, English & Punjabi.	Booklets on Menopause, Dysmenorrhoea, Prolapse and Urinary Incontinence are being given to the patients free of cost in MPBT Room during counselling. Books on Booklets on ANC (in Hindi) was published in Oct. 2015.

Establishment of MPBT Room- 2060- in OBG OPD

The MPBT room has been set up in OBG OPD in PGIMER. Patients are regularly being referred here from the OPD. Utility of such a room has been demonstrated by the fact that apart from the patients of UI/Prolapse, menopause, infertility, ANC and dysmenorrhea, other patients with problems like PCOD, PID, cervicitis, preconception counselling, women with disability (WWDs), patients with low back pain are also regularly referred here in MPBT room from the main OBG OPD. Patients' family members (for ANC) and specially the husbands' involvement (for Infertility and menopause) during the counselling session has been an integrated part of MPBT room approach. This helps them to understand the women's predicament better. Our room has now also become a suitable / favorite place for training and research for Public health, physiotherapy, nursing students of PGIMER and Master of Public health students from Panjab University, Chandigarh.

Various activities / interventions being done through the MPBT room

(A) IEC material on display: Posters/Display/Notices have been put on PGIMER website as well as on the walls/doors/rooms of OBG OPD to inform the public about MPBT room. The posters displayed outside the room are changed from time to time to make patients aware about the MPBT room. A new component of care of Women with Disability (WWDs) has been added in the MPBT room. The display material for this has also been put on the doors/ walls/rooms of OBG OPD.

(B) Visitors in MPBT room

(i) Mr. Rakesh Aggarwal, Regional Passport Officer visited the room on 4 th April, 2015.

(ii) Dr. L.K. Dhaliwal, Ex- Professor and Head, OBG, PGIMER, Chandigarh, visited the room with the team of Concept Foundation which works on the various projects including the one on MTP in collaboration with PGIMER. Dr. Ruchi briefed them about the MPBT room.

(iii) Visit of DBT Experts- Dr. Jatinder Kaur Arora, Director, Punjab State Council Science and Technology, Chandigarh along with Dr. Suneela Garg, DBT Expert, Ministry of Home affairs, Govt of India visited MPBT room. Both experts were impressed by the set-up of MPBT room and its functioning of dealing with patients.

(iv) Mr. M.R. Chawla, Retd Assistant Director, BSNL, Ambala. He is currently a Volunteer Promotor and Member of Baba Ram Dev Yoga Team. He visited the room with his wife. She is having problem of prolapse. After the counselling provided by the MPBT staff to his wife, Mr Sharma told us about various yoga and meditation techniques. He appreciated our efforts and the counselling services provided to the patients.

(v) Dr. Arun Bansal, Assistant Professor, Department of Paediatrics, PGIMER came to MPBT room with her mother and Wife. His mother was referred from OBGOPD to MPBT room for Kegal exercises as she had UI. Dr. Bansal's wife appreciated the effort of MPBT staff. She was really impressed by OBG deptt having such room in PGI.

(C) Male involvement in Women's health: the MPBT room sets an example: Male involvement in reproductive health is a complex process in terms of social and behavioral perception of the society. In most societies, family members and the neighborhood usually frown upon the husbands who tend to attend to their wives reproductive health needs. It is not considered OK for men to accompany women to a gynecologist. Most men do not co-operate with their wives when they are also advised treatment along with their wives, e.g. in cases of infertility, sexually transmitted infections. Even in OBG OPDs doctors are not tuned to welcome husbands during consultation/ examination of their wives. It is not uncommon to see, "GENTS ARE NOT ALLOWED" signboard on the doors of OBG OPDs .However but the MPBT team propagated the idea of male involvement and spread the awareness through seminars, conferences, etc. As a result of which, such signboards have been removed from the doors of OBG OPD.

Surely, results are good if male are involved in women's health issues. For example, men who are educated about reproductive health issues are more likely to support their partners in decisions on contraceptive use, pregnancy and family planning. They can also communicate with their partners and health providers in a more effective manner. This way they can ensure that their partner receives requisite obstetric services when needed. MPBT room approach goes even a step further. The idea is to go for full family involvement. We invite husbands, mothers, mothers in law, sisters, sisters in law, fathers, fathers in law, children etc. in t he MPBT room. This gives an opportunity to the women to discuss their reproductive health issues in a familiar family atmosphere in a relaxed manner at a leisurely pace. Results have been very encouraging.

(D) Newspaper coverage: This endeavor has also paid rich dividends as after the press coverage, attendance always increased in succeeding weeks (and people brought newspaper cuttings to MPBT room)

—चंडीगढ़ सवेरा

विकलांग महिलाओं को उनके अधिकार से वंचित न किया जाए : प्रो. वनीता

चंडीगढ़, 28 सितंबर (राकेश): विकलांगता होना वैसे ही अभिशाप होता है और इसकी शिकार महिलाएं हो जाएं तो पूरा परिवार प्रभावित हो जाता है। ऐसे में महिलाओं में विकलांगता आने पर परिवार के लोग उसके स्वास्थ्य की और ठीक से ध्यान नहीं दे पाते हैं। विकलांग महिलाओं को अपने जीवन को जीने के लिए कई चुनौतियों का सामना करना पड़ता है। विश्व स्वास्थ्य संगठन की रिपोर्ट के अनुसार भारत एवं दूसरे देशों में महिलाओं की बढ़ती विकलांगता ही नहीं एक्सीडेंट के शिकार होने पर युवा भी विकलांग बड़ी संख्या में होने से देश के आर्थिक विकास पर प्रतिकूल प्रभाव पड़ रहा है।

इस विषय पर पी.जी.आई. के गायनीकोलॉजी विभाग की ओर से सम्मेलन करवाया गया। इसमें विशेषज्ञों ने कहा कि महिलाओं में किसी कारणवश विकलांकता आने पर उसकी सेहत के प्रति रुचि कम होना स्वाभिक है और इससे बाहर निकालने के लिए परिवार के लोगों को उसके साथ भावनात्मक तरीके से पेश आना चाहिए।

सम्मेलन में गायनी विभाग की प्रो. वनीता सूरी ने कहा कि ऐसी महिलाओं को समाज की मुख्य धारा से पुनः जोड़ने के लिए चिकित्सा सिस्टम एवं पारिवारिक सहयोग से संभव किया जा सकता है। उन्होंने कहा कि विकलांग होने पर महिला गर्भ धारण करने के योग्य होती है लेकिन परिवार के लोगों की गलत सोच के कारण वह अपने इस अधिकार से वंचित रह जाती हैं। ऐसे में गायनी विशेषज्ञों एवं अन्य क्षेत्रों के विशेषज्ञों को एक मंच पर आकर महिलाओं के अधिकारों के बारे में विचार करना होगा। वहीं विकलांग महिलाओं को अस्पतालों में विशेष सुविधाएं प्रदान करनी होगी। ऐसी महिलाओं को सुविधाएं मिलेगी तो उनके प्रति परिवार की सोच भी बदलेगी।

पंजाब केसरी

विकलांग महिला पेशैंट्स की स्थिति पर मंथन

चंडीगढ़, 28 सितम्बर (अर्चना सेठी): शहर के अस्पताल डिसेबल पेशैंट्स फैंडली नहीं हैं। विकलांग महिलाओं के साथ-साथ गर्भवती और बुजुर्ग महिलाओं की स्थिति के मद्देनजर न तो ओ.पी.डी. डिजाइन की गई है और न ही वाईस तैयार किए गए हैं। यह बात आज पी.जी.आई के नेहरू अस्पताल में आयोजित चिकित्सीय संगोष्ठी के दौरान विशेषज्ञों ने कही। गाइनीकोलॉजी विशेषज्ञ डा. वनिता सूरी, पी.जी.आई कम्युनिटी हैल्थ विशेषज्ञ डा. अमरजीत सिंह, रिसर्च स्कोलर रुचि शर्मा ने संगोष्ठी में गाइनीकोलॉजी विभाग से जुड़े मुद्दों पर विचार विमर्श किया। सैंट्रल सोशल वैल्फेयर बोर्ड के डिप्टी डायरैक्टर ए.के. दुआ, नैशनल इंस्टीच्यूट ऑफ टैक्नीकल टीचर्स ट्रेनिंग के प्रोफैसर डा.जे.एस.सैनी, नैशनल इंस्टीच्यूट ऑफ नर्सिंग एजुकेशन (नाइन) की लैक्चरार डा. सुखपाल कौर, डा. नेहा ने इस अवसर पर एक प्रश्नोतरी का आयोजन भी किया। पी.जी.आई., जी.एम.सी.एच.-32, जी.एम.एस.एच.-16 के गाइनीकोलॉजी विभाग से 100 प्रतिभागियों ने प्रश्नोतरी में भाग लिया।

—चंडीगढ़ भास्कर H.T. CHANDIGARH

डिसेबल फ्रेंडली नहीं हैं हॉस्पिटल

चंडीगढ़ | चंडीगढ़ के हॉस्पिटल पूरी तरह से डिसेबल फ्रेंडली नहीं हैं।इन हॉस्पिटल की ओपीडी और वार्ड विकलांग महिलाओं और गर्भवती की हालात को ध्यान में रखकर डिजाइन नहीं किए गए हैं। ये बात पीजीआई में हुई वर्कशॉप में सामने आई। इस वर्कशॉप में शामिल सभी डॉक्टरों का मानना था कि हॉस्पिटल में विकलांगों की सुविधा के मुताबिक भी पेशेंट केअर देने की सुविधा होनी चाहिए।

Workshop on making gynaecology OPD patient-friendly held

CHANDIGARH: A meet on 'how to make gynaecology OPD and ward services in hospitals disabled-friendly' was held at the PGIMER on Monday. Dr Vanita Suri from obstetrics and gynaecology, inaugurated the session, followed by several lectures by experts. Around 100 participants from the PGIMER, GMSH, Sector 16, GMCH, Sector 32 attended meet.

CHANDIGARH TRIBUNE

Seminar at PGI

Chandigarh: Women with disabilities encounter a range of barriers when they attempt to access healthcare. Especially women with disabilities (WWDs) are marginalised from Sexual and Reproductive Health (SRH) issues. They face numerous challenges in accessing optimum SRH services. These challenges include socio-cultural, political, economic and structural factors. Prohibitive costs, lack of availability of appropriate services (and equipment), attitude of health service providers and physical access to health facilities are other issues that need solution. It has been documented in World Report on Disability 2011 that inaccessible environments create disability by creating barriers to participation and inclusion. To bring together various experts in field of disability, a seminar, "evolving a consensus among various stakeholders for developing a model for making gynaecology OPD and ward services in hospitals disabled friendly", was organised at PGI on Monday. The initiative will help work towards removing barriers and making existing healthcare systems more inclusive and accessible to people with disabilities. Opinions of target group i.e. person with disabilities/WWDs will help identify gaps and priorities to reduce health inequalities and plan improvement for access and inclusion. — TNS

(E) Seminars: Seminar on Disability: On 24th September, 2015, Department of Obstetrics & Gynaecology, PGIMER, Chandigarh hosted an ICMR sponsored Seminar entitled "Evolving a consensus among various stakeholders for developing a model for making Gynaecology OPD and ward services in hospitals disabled friendly"

(a) Objectives of the Seminar :To evolve a consensus among various stakeholders for developing a model for making Gynaecology OPD and ward services in hospitals disabled friendly.

(F) SPECIAL MENTION: Urinary Incontinence And Prolapse Patients' Feed Back Maximum benefit of MPBT room has been seen among women having urinary incontinence and xxxv pelvic organ prolapse. During OPD visits, patients in the counselling are taught skills and strategies for preventing incontinence. They are also asked to do 40-60 pelvic muscle exercises sets every day (10-15 times exercises, 4 times per day). Duration of individual contraction and relaxation advised is individualized for each patient. Gradually it is increased across sessions to a maximum of 10 seconds each. Patients are advised to practice in various positions, including lying, sitting, and standing. During counselling, we focus on helping patients to identify pelvic floor muscles. We teach them how to contract and relax these muscles selectively while keeping abdominal muscles relaxed. They are also taught how to respond adaptively to the sensation of urgency. Instead of rushing to the toilet, which increases intra-abdominal pressure and exposure to visual cues that can trigger incontinence, subjects are encouraged to p ause, sit down if possible, relax the entire body, and contract pelvic muscles repeatedly to diminish urgency, inhibit detrusor contraction, and prevent urine loss. When urgency subsides, they are advised to proceed to the toilet at a normal pace. In follow up, we review the progress and compliance of patient. We also encourage their persistence with the exercise and life style modifications.

(G) Management of menopause patients in MPBT room: When menopausal patients visit the MPBT room after the Gynae OPD referral they have lots of queries in their mind as how to deal with menopause and its symptoms. Behaviour therapy along with counselling, exercises and lifestyle changes are advised to menopausal patients in MPBT room by the research staff. Patient handling approach in MPBT room lays stress on de-medicalization and patient empowerment. Patients are counselled here at leisurely pace and their queries are duly solved. Unlike OBG OPDs, here patients are attended along with their husband/family members. Thus, they can share their queries without hesitation. Patients are also given booklets on menopause (available in Hindi, English and Punjabi) and other IEC material related to their menopause related problems.

Verbatim responses of the patients before and after counselling

Patient A: Before counseling: *"I have become very sensitive these days. Baat baat par ro padhti hoon. Mere colleguaes bhi kehte hai ki aap mein thoda change hai. Bahut gussa aata hai, aur baachon par bahut gussa karti hoon".*

After Counseling: *I am trying meditation these days. I see change in me after doing meditation. I am very much relaxed these days. I am following your diet plan, included more of fruits and juices in my diet. Overall, I am following many things which u told. I am better now".*

Patient B: Before counseling *"Depression rehta hai. Ghar par akeli rehti hoon. TV dekhti rehti hoon. Sir bhi bahut bhari bhari rehta hai. Neend bhi theek se nahi aati". Aaj toh sirf 3 ghante he neend aayi"*

After Counseling: *"Book padhi aap ki usko padh ke routine follow kiya. Aap ki batayi baaton se aur book se farak padh raha hai. Husband bhi keh rahe hai ki tujhe medicine se itna farak nahin pada par kitab padh kar aur madamji ki baatein follow karke kafi farak padha hai. Khane mein kafi changes kiye hai. Weight bhi reduce hua hai. Paet ki exercises se bhi farak padha hai"*

(I) Management of infertility patients in MPBT room: Queries of infertility patients are resolved in a relaxed atmosphere in MPBT room. Sufficient time (15-20 min) is devoted to each patient. For those who cannot conceive despite treatment, adoption services have been linked up with MPBT room. Most couples ask about available options for treatment like IUI, IVF, GIFT, ICSI etc.

Patients Queries before coming to MPBT Room

Wife Said *"Andar husband ko aane nahi diya infertility clinic mein"* (My husband was not allowed inside)

Husband Said *"Main andar nahin gaya, mujhe jane hi nahi diya. Wife ne mujhe thoda bataya ki andar kya bola. Phir humein bola 2060 mein chale jana."*. (I did not go inside. Wife told me what happened inside)

After counselling: *"Aapki batayi baton se kuch dimag ka bhoj toh halk a hua. Kafi cheezon k bare mein maloom nahi tha ab pata chala iss kamre mein aakar""* (The things told by you have helped us...lifted burden off our head...feel relieved now...many things were learnt by us in this room)

Patient satisfaction has been the main beneficial result as revealed through verbatim response of the patient-

"GMCH mein dikhaya wahan kisi ne hamari baat thek se suni nahin...kam se kam aap sun aur samjh toh rahe ho hamari baat" (We went to GMCH. Nobody listened to our problems properly. At lea st you understand our issues patiently)

"Bahar likha hua padha toh socha aap se Salah le lun.. andar toh koi puri baat hi nahin sunta" (I read your poster outside and came to consult you...In OPD nobody listens).

(J) Management of ante - and post-natal patients in the MPBT room: In MPBT room RA / SRF also counsel women on self – care during pregnancy and labor, e.g., diet, clothing, posture, exercises, rest, warning signals of labor, drugs, vaccines and weight gain. They are taught about anatomy & physiology of labor; what to do during labor; warning signals during labor ;anatomy & physiology of breast; self-care of mothers during puerperium; care of the baby, breast care, breast feeding, skin care, perineal care, diet, bonding, clothing, rest, exercises, family planning, coitus; immunization, complementary feeding after delivery.They are also told how to deal with pregnancy related minor disorders such as morning sickness, backache, cramps, varicose veins, fainting spells, heart-burn, constipation, piles, swelling on feet, hands & ankles, insomnia, craving, skin changes etc. The respondents are be encouraged for regular follow-up & to contact the investigator any time during antenatal clinics. More than 500 ante-, intra- and post- natal patients have been seen so far during the reporting period in MPBT Room.

(K) Dysmenorrhoea patients' management @ MPBT room: So far, we have registered 28 patients of dysmenorrhoea. The patients are demonstrated exercises in the room and are counselled about the lifestyle changes, dietary modification and menstrual hygiene.

(L) PCOD (polycystic ovarian syndrome) management in MPBT room: So far, 176 patients with PCOD were referred in the MPBT Room for lifestyle, weight reduction and dietary modification. Services of a dietician have also been added.

(M) Women with disability (WWD) management through MPBT room: To overcome the issues of disabled patients a humble attempt has been made by MPBT team to provide assistance to WWDs visiting OBG OPD. Dr. Ruchi Sharma, (Ex-SRF in MPBT Project) is doing her PhD research on Sexual & Reproductive Health of WWD. Checkup of WWDs in OBG OPD is facilitated by the research team. They are seen in OPD on priority basis. Their opinion is also sought on making OBG services disabled friendly. Banners have been displayed outside the room so that they can access hospital services easily. Referral of such patients into the room has also been requested. Newspaper coverage is being done so that more WWDs approach hospitals with their problems. So far, 120 WWDs patients attended the MPBT room.

(N) MPBT team gets invited by the School for the Blind of Chandigarh: Drs Ruchi and Neha educated the students of the school on 21st Nov. 2015 on Gyne problem management, including dysmenorrhea (invitation letter enclosed)

Field Demonstrations and Propagation of the Idea of MPBT Room Through -

(H) Women's Health Kitty Party

(Please see photographs at the end of the chapter)

Usually people associate kitty parties with a favourite past time of housewives. A common impression is the women get together to dress-up, eat display and enjoy tambola. Even working women has such groups. But all of this is set to change, as the forum is now being used to spread awareness among women on various gynaecological health-related problems. Under this venture the team of Multipurpose Behaviour Therapy (MPBT) room

Project staff Dr. Purnima, Research Associate, Dr. Neha SRF, Dr. Ruchi, JRF from the Department of Community Medicine were invited to visit one such kitty group in Panchkula. The MPBT room got popular through word of mouth by the patients who visited this room. Most of the patients have benefited through the counselling provided by the staff in this room.

They have now started using the forum of kitty parties for this purpose. The project staff of MPBT room got an invite from a patient to address women in her kitty group. The purpose of the visit to such kitty group was that ladies often can't come to PGI. They face various constraint e.g., distance and lack of time. So the concept of outreach counselling through this health kitty has been initiated. First such session was held on 6th Oct., 2015 in a kitty group of Panchkula at Sagar Ratna rcstaurant. A total group of 15 ladies participated in the kitty. They were counselled on various gynaecological problems faced by women. They were given a brief presentation about the various problems on Prolapse, Urinary Incontinence, Dysmenorrhoea (painful periods), infertility, ANC/PNC and menopause. They were also given booklets free of cost (published xlviii through the DBT, Govt of India grant) related to their problems. For Urinary leakage and Prolapse problems Kegel exercises were taught. Simple lifestyle modifications were also advised. Ladies also enquired about the dysmenorrhoea exercises for their daughters.

One lady said that "she was going through the phase of menopause". Her husband said, "All of us should go to Himalayas when our wives are going through this phase. When this phase is over we may come back. "I cannot

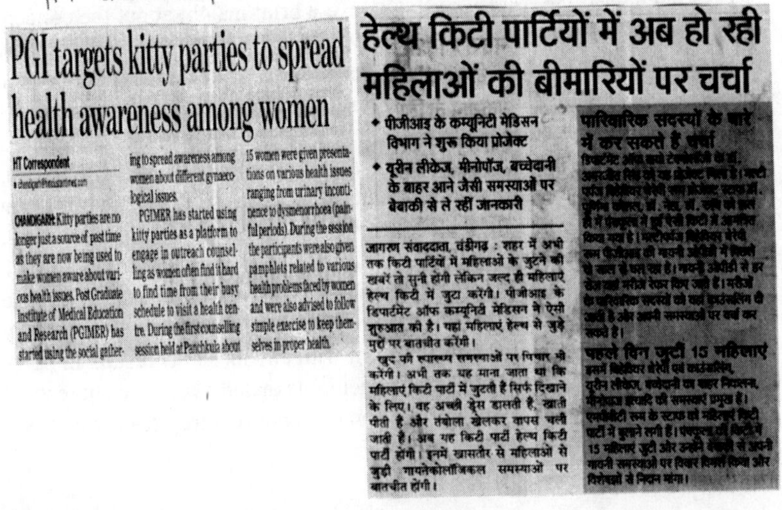

H.T. CHANDIGARH, 14-10-15

PGI targets kitty parties to spread health awareness among women

HT Correspondent

CHANDIGARH: Kitty parties are no longer just a source of past time as they are now being used to make women aware about various health issues. Post Graduate Institute of Medical Education and Research (PGIMER) has started using the social gathering to spread awareness among women about different gynaecological issues.

PGIMER has started using kitty parties as a platform to engage in outreach counselling as women often find it hard to find time from their busy schedule to visit a health centre. During the first counselling session held at Panchkula about 15 women were given presentations on various health issues ranging from urinary incontinence to dysmenorrhoea (painful periods). During the session the participants were also given pamphlets related to various health problems faced by women and were also advised to follow simple exercise to keep themselves in proper health.

चंडीगढ़ जागरण

हेल्थ किटी पार्टियों में अब हो रही महिलाओं की बीमारियों पर चर्चा

- पीजीआइ के कम्यूनिटी मेडिसन विभाग ने शुरू किया प्रोजेक्ट
- यूरीन लीकेज, मीनोपॉज, बच्चेदानी के बाहर आने जैसी समस्याओं पर बेबाकी से ले रहीं जानकारी

जागरण संवाददाता, चंडीगढ़ : शहर में अभी तक किटी पार्टियों में महिलाओं के जुटने की खबरें तो सुनी होंगी लेकिन जल्द ही महिलाएं हेल्थ किटी में जुटा करेंगी। पीजीआइ के डिपार्टमेंट ऑफ कम्यूनिटी मेडिसन ने ऐसी शुरुआत की है। यहां महिलाएं हेल्थ से जुड़े मुद्दों पर बातचीत करेंगी।

खुद की स्वास्थ्य समस्याओं पर विचार भी करेंगी। अभी तक यह माना जाता था कि महिलाएं किटी पार्टी में जुटती हैं सिर्फ दिखाने के लिए। वह अच्छी ड्रेस डालती हैं, खाती पीती हैं और तंबोला खेलकर वापस चली जाती हैं। अब यह किटी पार्टी हेल्थ किटी पार्टी होगी। इनमें खासतौर से महिलाओं से जुड़ी गायनेकोलॉजिकल समस्याओं पर बातचीत होगी।

पारिवारिक सदस्यों के बारे में कर सकते हैं चर्चा

[illegible]

पहले दिन जुटीं 15 महिलाएं

[illegible]

handle my wife's mood swings problem and her irritated behaviour." So these ladies were counselled that how it is important to have a joint counselling session for both husband and wife. This way husbands would understand the phase of menopause better.

Overall response of these ladies was very positive. Their queries on various reproductive health issues were also solved on the spot by the MPBT team. These ladies were also invited by MPBT staff to visit the room no 2060 in gynae OPD for any further counselling related to gynaecological problems. The concept of this type of healthy kitty party was very much appreciated by these ladies from Panchkula. They advocated propagation of this idea to other groups also".

(B) Radio talk @ PU Community Radio 91.2 MHz(Jyotirgamaya Padho aur padhao) 16th Oct.'15

Even with the advent of technology and modernisation of the means of communication radio is still considered as an effective way for reaching out to masses i.e different age groups such as students, housewives, working women etc. In view of this it was thought worthwhile to use this medium to publicise MPBT room project of DBT,Govt. of India. PU Community Radio 91.2 MHz Jyotirgamaya Padho aur Padhao was selected as the appropriate forum for this purpose. So our staff from MPBT room Dr. Purnima, Dr. Neha, Dr. Ruchi along with Principle investigator of the project Dr. AJ Singh prepared a radio programme for helping women to become their own best health and wellness advocate. As a part of community development initiative, MPBT Staff introduced the listeners to the concept of MPBT room, the reason and need of establishing such rooms in the hospitals.

At the outset, Dr. Amarjeet Singh gave a brief insight about the concept of MPBT Room. He talked about many common illnesses of women; how these could be managed without using any medicine. He also introduced the listeners about demedicalisation and salutogenesis concepts (these terms describe an approach focusing on internal self-healing potential of humans and using simple measures like exercise, diet control, change in lifestyle, tackling constipation, meditation to maintain health rather than on factors that cause disease).The three musketeers of the proj ect Dr. Purnima, Dr. Neha, Dr. Ruchi then explained the listeners about the unique features of MPBT room. Dr Ruchi introduced the listeners about urinary incontinence (UI). She explained that females usually bear discomfort due to UI and prolapse. They a lso feel too shy to discuss this problem with anyone. This results in non - consultation. They accept that UI as an incurable malady. It is often perceived by the wider society that UI is normal and does not require treatment.

Dr Neha shared her experiences with the listeners about how they deal with patients and their family members in this room. She explained to the listeners why family involvement was important as a part of treatment. If female is passing through menopausal stage then what she mainly needs is attention and care, because in this phase of life she passes through loads of hormonal changes which are not in her own hands. So, family support can play an important role in her life.

Dr Purnima Kaushal enlightened the listeners why MBPT room plays an important role in OPD setting. She told about different women health related issues they deal with in MBPT room, viz., UI, dysmenorrhea, prolapse, infertility, PCOS and gynecology problems faced by women with disability. She explained that much of the time of specialist doctors is wasted in OPD. Consequently they hardly have any time to attend to the complicated cases. Apart from this there are many other issues which females wish to discuss with the gynecologists. But even this is not possible in crowd ed situation witnessed in OBG OPDs. Adopting a health promoting hospital approach can be useful in resolving these issue by having a separate multipurpose counselling room in gynae OPDs. This way females can feel free to ask the counselling staff anything regarding these issues in MPBT room.

(A) Presentations: (Conferences of Federation of Obstetricians and Gynaecologists of India, Indian Public health Association, Indian Association of Preventive and Social Medicine, Indian Menopausal Society and International Menopausal Society).

1. Title of the paper: Integrating the Concepts of Health Promotion De-Medicalization, Salutogenesis, Social iatrogenesis And Quaternary Prevention Through Our OPD Experiences From PGIMER, Chandigarh.

Name of Authors: Dr. AJ Singh, Dr. Ruchi Sharma, DrMeenakshi Sharma, Dr. PurnimaKaushal, Dr. Neha Singhal, Mrs Isha Bajaj, Mrs Rajni, Dr.L.K Dhaliwal, Dr VanitaSuri, Dr Vanita Jain, Dr MS Dhillon, Dr Gurpreet Singh, Dr AvinashRana, Dr Sukhpal Kaur and Dr AK Mandal PGIMER, Chandigarh

Venue: 3rd Indi-global Summit and Expo on healthcare, New Delhi, 5-7 October, 2015.

Introduction: Many problems of reporting to OPDs can be resolved by non-medicinal interventions. But doctors are too overworked to explain this to patients. This compromises the quality of care. Hence, a multipurpose behaviour therapy (MPBT) room was established in PGIMER OPD in Dec 2012.

Objective: To share the experiences of operating an MPBT room in OPDs

Methodology: Patients from Obstetrics &Gynaecology (OBG) OPD are referred to MPBT room where women with pregnancy, infertility, prolapse, urinary incontinence, menopause, PCOD or dysmenorrhoea are advised non-medicinal interventions (dietary modifications, lifestyle changes, exercises/ yoga). Patients are given related IEC material. In Orthopaedics OPD, mild to moderate knee osteoarthritis (KOA) patients are counselled on lifestyle intervention (a set of exercises, weight reduction, meditation, dietary modifications, posture correction) with the help of brochures. Patients are also trained through one to one demonstration. In Surgery OPD mastectomy patients are trained on lifestyle changes / exercises to control shoulder dysfunction, lymphedema.

Results: Out of >100 menopausal patients referred to the MPBT room, 64 were followed up. Many (40; 63%) benefited from counselling while >35 patients reported partial relief. Out of ~ 800 patients UI and POP patients 160 (20%) reported complete and 400 (50%) had partial relief .Around 3000 ANC patients reported relief in symptoms and satisfaction with counselling. In Orthopaedics OPD > 60 % KOA patients reported relief in symptoms .In Surgery OPD, > 50 % breast surgery patients reported relief.

Conclusion: Health promotion & demedicalization approach has a potential for enhancing patient welfare in OPDs.

Investing time and patience to counsel menopausal women pays rich dividends- A successful example from PGIMER Chandigarh.

Authors: Dr. Ruchi Sharma, Dr. Amarjeet Singh, Dr. Purnima Kaushal, Dr. Neha

Venue: IMS, Chandigarh 17-18th, October, 2015

Introduction-All women approaching the menopause should have the opportunity to learn about the selfcare of changes they experience. To promote this concept of health promotion and demedicalization, a multi-purpose behavior therapy room (MPBT) was established in OBG OPDs in PGIMER, in December 2012.

Objective- To share the experiences of operating a counseling room for menopausal women in OBG-OPD.

Methodology- After referral from main OPD, behaviour therapy along with counselling, exercises and lifestyle changes are advised to menopausal patients in MPBT room by the research team.Unlike OBG OPDs here patients are attended along with their husbands and other family members. Here patients can share their queries without hesitation. Patients are also given booklets (available in Hindi, English, Punjabi) and other IEC material on menopause related problems.

Results- A total of 142 menopause patients were enrolled in MPBT room in last 1 year. Out of these 81 patients were followed-up successfully. Among them 47 patients reported complete benefit from the counselling while 29 patients reported partial relief after the counselling.

Before counselling a patient said: Raat mein neend nahi aati kafi pareshan rehti hoon. Hotflashes bhi aate hai. Soye soye ekdum se garmi lagti hai.

After Counselling she said: aapki book toh bahut interesting lagi mujhe …. kafi knowledge hai usmein. Kuch kuch baatein toh mujhe pata bhi nahi thi…. Walk aur yoga shuru ki hai maine…. meri colleagues bhi padh rahi hain book ko.. aap ne jo mujhe samjhaya tha diet mein bhi waisie he changes kiye hain maine…. kafi farak hai mujhe…. hot flashes mein bhi…. calcium ke ilawa koi medicine nahi le rahi hoon."

Conclusion-MPBT room approach has immensely helped the women having menopausal symptoms. Such room should be established in all medical hospitals to emphasize upon effectiveness of non-medicinal management of menopausal problems.

(i) Papers presented in seminars

1. **Title:** "Integrating the Concepts of Health Promotion, De-Medicalization, Salutogenesis, Social Iatrogenesis and Quaternary Prevention"

   Author: Dr. Amarjeet Singh

   Venue & date: AFMC, Pune (Nov. 18-20, 2015)

Introduction: Primary prevention addresses broad determinants of health. It includes all action taken before disease onset to maintain and promote our health. It aims to reduce the chances of disease occurrence. This involves actions at both individual level as well as society level.

Health Promotion is a part of primary prevention. It is visualized as a set of activities which are not directed at any particular disease but are intended to improve the general health and well-being of the individual and the community, viz.,safe water supply, safe disposal of excreta and other wastes, clean air, provision of adequate health services, adequate nutrition, healthful housing, control of insects and rodents, safe working conditions, recreation facilities, health education, marriage / genetic counselling; sex education, physical education, periodic health screening, improvement of standard of living of people and other such actions. In fact, health promotion is essentially GOOD LIVING. Simply put, health promotion at individual level will imply strengthening the mind and body of people. In individual approach, health education is a crucial strategy. This approach is dependent on compliance of the individuals with the advice or education given, i.e., it is behavior dependent. As a part of primary prevention **primordial prevention** seeks to prevent the onset of specific diseases via risk reduction by altering behaviors or exposures that can lead to disease. **Secondary prevention** includes procedures that detect and treat preclinical pathological changes and thereby lvi control disease progression. Once the disease has developed and has been treated in its acute clinical phase, **tertiary prevention** seeks to soften the impact caused by the disease on the patient's function, longevity, and quality-of-life by focusing on rehabilitation. **Quaternary prevention** has also now been added to the list. It is defined as "action taken to identify patient at risk of over-medicalization, to protect him from new medical invasion. It involves a set of health activities to mitigate or avoid the consequences of unnecessary or excessive intervention of the health system. It counters the phenomenon called disease mongering, which could be translated as commercialization of disease. This needs to be promoted as an essential component of prevention. It aims to avoid iatrogenesis. Main idea is to avoid patient over diagnosis and overtreatment. The intent is not to eliminate but to moderate the medicalization of the daily life.

Social iatrogenesis sponsors sickness by reinforcing a morbid society. Here the disease is socially created, i.e., people expect and demand a medical diagnostic label. Structural iatrogenesis destroys the potential of the people for a healthy response to suffering and disease. It makes people dependent on medical profession for even those things which they could have managed themselves. This can be reversed only through **self-care** by people. This belief of people that they cannot cope with illness without modern medicines reinforces and lays the ground for iatrogenesis by surrendering themselves to the doctors, i.e., **'a pill for every ill'** concept. This is **medicalization** of the society. **Demedicalisation** implies a process of reversing the trend of medicalization of society i.e. emphasizing non-medicinal/non-medical solution of our health problems, thus **empowering the lay public**. In the present medicalised world the professional and physician-based health care system takes away the power of the individual of self-healing. Medicalization forces all of us to think that we are ill, impotent and in need of technical repair. The medicalization of life encourages our dependence on professional care, and also on medical drugs. In such a scenario, people expect and accept routine medical intervention at each stage of their lives. When this happens, life turns from a succession of different stages of health into a series of periods each requiring different therapies. There are many medical interventions which are simple, cheap and often without any need of medicine yet are quite effective. However, such simple remedies are often neglected or altogether ignored. It is well known that **859 or more of the diseases are largely self-limiting.**

Many diseases make the best progress when these are treated least. So in majority of illnesses medical treatment is not required. We need to bring back self-care and family support in the management of common illnesses. This will help in building a society which can reduce professional medical intervention in routine life and thus provide the best conditions for health. In traditional pathogenic model of health, the focus is on causes of disease and on risk factors involved in disease generation. External healing devices and interventions are resorted to for eliminating the disease. **Salutogenic model** focuses on creation and maintenance of good health. Emphasis is on our internal healing resources. In this context it is worthwhile to share our experiences from PGIMER, Chandigarh. Many problems of reporting to OPDs can be resolved by non-medicinal interventions. But doctors are too overworked to explain this to patients. This compromises the quality of care. Hence, a multipurpose behaviour therapy (MPBT) room was established in PGIMER OBG OPD in Dec 2012.Patients from Obstetrics &Gynaecology (OBG) OPD are referred to MPBT room where women with pregnancy, infertility, prolapse, urinary incontinence, menopause, PCOD or dysmenorrhoea are advised non-medicinal interventions (dietary modifications, lifestyle changes, exercises/ yoga). Patients are given related IEC material. Similarly, in Orthopaedics OPD, knee osteoarthritis patients are counselled on lifestyle intervention (a set of exercises, weight reduction, meditation, dietary modifications, posture correction). Patients are also trained through one to one demonstration. In Surgery OPD mastectomy patients are trained on lifestyle changes / exercises to control shoulder dysfunction, lymphedema. **Results:** Out of >100 menopausal patients in MPBT room, 64 were followed up. Many (40; 63%) benefited from counselling while >35 patients reported partial relief. Out of ~ 800 patients UI and POP patients 160 (20%) reported complete and 400 (50%) had partial relief; ~ 3000 ANC patients reported relief in symptoms. In Orthopaedics OPD > 60 % KOA patients reported relief in symptoms .In Surgery OPD, more than 50 % breast surgery patients reported relief.

Conclusion: There is need for replicating such concept in OPDs of all medical colleges. This venture has a potential to be a trendsetter in demonstrating a workable collaborative mechanism between OBG, Orthopaedics, Surgery and Community Medicine departments for enhancing patient welfare in OPD as well as home care settings. The demedicalization philosophy inherent in the MPBT room approach will help in empowering the women in self-care of their reproductive and other health problems. The hallmark of MPBT room approach is the integration of the concepts of health promotion, de-medicalization, salutogenesis, iatrogenesis and quaternary prevention for tackling a significant share of health problems of women.

2. **Title:** Barriers Faced by Women with Disabilities in Access to Sexual and Reproductive Health Care- Experiences from North India

   Authors: Dr. Ruchi, Dr. AJ Singh, Dr. Vanita Suri, Dr. Sukhpal Kaur PGIMER, Chandigarh

   Venue: 1st Mysore International Conference on Medical and Social Sciences, Mysore

Introduction-Women with disabilities (WWDs) face numerous challenges in accessing sexual and reproductive (SRH) related services. These barriers include socio-cultural, political, economic and structural factors, prohibitive costs, lack of availability of appropriate services (and equipment) and attitude of family/ health service providers. **Objectives-**To explore the opinion of WWDs regarding barriers faced in access to sexual and reproductive health care services. **Methodology-** 50 WWDs with age 15+ were enlisted from various sources viz- Hospitals, Colleges, banks etc. Their in-depth interview was done to gather information regarding socio-demographic details, self-reported symptoms suggestive of gynecological morbidity. Their treatment seeking behavior and barriers they faced pertaining to SRH care were also explored. **Results-** Average age of respondents was 29.84 yrs. 78% females had loco motor disability followed by blindness (8%). 36% respondents reported that access was major problem faced when they visited hospitals e.g. transportation, lack of ramps, inappropriate examination tables etc. Long waiting hours (22%) and inaccessible toilets (20%) also impedes disabled women's access to reproductive health services. 8% women referred to attitude of Health care providers as barrier to health care. Their verbatim responses reflected a range of such barriers to SRH -*"Lift operator did not allow us to use lift and my husband took me through ramp to fourth floor". "We are not considered part of society. People think we are useless and burden to society". "Attendants and clerks use abusive language for us". "I did not go for check-up because nobody gives us priority and I can't wait for that long. Govt. should make some special arrangements for us"*

Conclusion-WWDs continues to experience 'health disadvantage' with respect to SRH in terms of lack of physical access, hostile attitude of providers and discrimination in the society.

3. **Title:** Spreading the Good Word about Self Care Intervention for Selected Health Problems of Women: Evidence Base from PGIMER Chandigarh

   Authors: Dr. Ruchi Sharma, Dr. Neha, Dr. Purnima Kaushal Dr. Vanita Suri, Dr. Amarjeet Singh PGIMER, Chandigarh

   Venue: All India Congress of OBG: Women's Health – Conception to Senescence, Agra.

Background: Often the results of the research done on women's health remains confined to files that too of the implementing centre or the funding agency. Conversion of research results to tangible benefits for women themselves is even rarer. One of the duties of the researchers is to disseminate their results. This presentation shares our experience of propagating the results of research done by the authors in PGIMER Chandigarh as was one of the objectives of project. **Objective:** To trace the efforts of staff of a DBT sponsored project, "Setting up of a Multipurpose Behaviour Therapy/Health Promotion (MPBT) Room for Women Attending Gynaecology OPD in an Apex Level Hospital of North India" at PGIMER Chandigarh in propagating concept of MPBT room across India. **Methodology:** The project involved referral of cases of pregnancy, infertility, prolapse, urinary incontinence, menopause and dysmenorrhoea from OBG OPD to MPBT Room for non-medicinal interventions like dietary modifications, lifestyle changes and simple exercises/yoga. Results are publicised through lectures, seminar, conferences, reports and media (including Facebook).Booklets on these interventions are also distributed to patients and other interested people. Research by the nurses and doctors is also encouraged on related topics. **Results:** In MPBT room > 5000 patients have been successfully counselled. Most patients (e.g. >75% urinary incontinence/ prolapse) have reported relief in symptoms after kegel exercises and behavior therapy. This has been disseminated through 23 presentations (5 regional; 12 national; 6 international). MPBT model has been successfully replicated by research team in Military Hospitals in Ajmer and Jodhpur. More than 10 dissertations / new projects have been initiated on related issues. **Conclusion:** Dissemination of our results has been successful in changing the mind set of patients, doctors and researchers. Replication of this model in medical colleges will help in reducing the load on doctor while simultaneously enhancing patient satisfaction.

4. **Title:** Stigma and discrimination associated with sexual reproductive health problems of Women with Disabilities (WWD)

   Authors: Dr. Ruchi Sharma, Dr. AJ Singh, Dr. Vanita Suri, Dr. Sukhpal Kaur PGI, Chandigarh

   Venue: 26th annual meeting - Indian Society for the Study of Reproductive and Fertility, Ahmedabad

Introduction- In recent past, there has been a lot of discussion about disability and related issues among the medical fraternity. Still, the sexual and reproductive health (SRH) rights of the WWD has remained on the paper. Disabled women tend to postpone or ignore their SRH problems till these progresses to unbearable severity because of stigma and discrimination faced by them. This compromises their opportunity of unrestrained participation in various spheres of life. **Objective-**To ascertain the status of stigma and discrimination associated with SRH problems among WWDs. **Methodology-** 50 WWDs with age above 15 years were enlisted from various sources viz- Hospitals, Colleges, banks etc. They were interviewed to gather information regarding socio-demographic details, self-reported symptoms suggestive of SRH morbidity. Stigma and discrimination pertaining to SRH problem was also explored. **Results**-Average age of respondents was 29.84 yrs. Majority (78%) females had loco motor disability, blindness (8%) and hearing impairment (6%).Majority (58%)of respondents said that their SRH problem were ascribed by people to disability-***"2 baar abortion hua to sabhi ne kaha ki iss polio ki dikkat ki vjah se baccha kharab hua hai, sara din bethi jo rehti hai".*** Many WWD (47%) told that people embarrassed them because of their SRH problem. Majority (65%) of WWD told that people's reaction forced them to hide their problems. Most of them (76%) felt that their health problems made them feel that life was unfair to them. Furthermore, the negative attitudes health professionals and family member to disabled women's sexuality resulted in their own views of their sexual selves becoming negative. Some of them (21%) felt they were discriminated against by health professionals: "2 abortion k baad yahan ayi to doctors ne kaha ki- *"Tumhe baccha karne ki kya zarurat hai. Adopt nahin kar sakti thi..baccha kaise paida karegi. Koi tang karta hai kya bachhe k liye??" "Meri bed wetting ki problems ko doctors ne kabhi seriously liya hi nahin".* **Conclusion-** Stigma and discrimination impede disabled women's ability to access quality health services that respect the dignity of all users. Many disabled women have poor experiences in gynae OPDs with misinformed or insensitive health professionals.

5. 60th National Annual Conference Indian Public Health Association, 2016, Dehradun

10. List of publications / patents filed / extension manuals/ monographs

* Following 5 chapters in the book. "*Health Promotion: Need for Public Health Activism Vol I,* AJ Singh, S Goel and J Kathiresan (editors) *Germany,* LAP LAMBERT Academic Publishing, 2013.

  1. Kumari S, Jain V and Singh AJ. Health Promotion Efforts are Biased against Women: Why Behavior Therapy for Urinary Incontinence has been Ignored in Hospitals?
  2. Promoting Health of School Girls—Empowering them by Training them in Non-Pharmacological Management of Primary Dysmenorrhea -A Chaudhuri, A J Singh, L K Dhaliwal lxii
  3. Promoting Health of Recently Married Working Women- J Kaur, Jayanti D Roy, AJ Singh
  4. Health Promotion Approach for Enhancing Maternity Care Preparedness of Primigravida Women through Self Care Training -Avinash Rana, Vanita Suri, Indarjit Walia, Amarjeet Singh

5. Promoting Health of Women: Conservative Management of Pelvic Organ Prolapse - Rashmi Kashyap, Vanita Jain, Amarjeet Singh

* Following chapters in the book, "Singh AJ, Kaur S and Kishore J(editors).' Comprehensive Textbook of Elderly Care', New Delhi, Century Publications, 2014."

1. Kaur S, Dudeja P, Singh AJ and Walia I. Special needs of Elderly Postmenopausal Women: 188-193

* Following books related to MPBT room –

1. Sharma R, Kashyap R, Kaushal P, Jain V, Singh A." "Bacchedani Bahar Ana-Prolapse Uterus",New Delhi, New Era International Imprints 2013.ISBN No-978-81-290-0067-5
3. Sharma R, Chaudhary A, Kaushal P, Jain V, Singh A "Mahawari da dard- Bachaav atey elaaj"New Delhi, New Era International Imprints 2013. ISBN No-978-81-290-0075-0
4. Sharma R, Kumari S, Kaushal P, Jain V, Mandal A.K Singh A." "Mahilaon mein peshab leakage"(Urinary Incontinence) New Delhi, New Era International Imprints 2013.ISBN No-978-81-290-0074-3
5. Sharma R, Kumari S, Kaushal P,Jain V,Mandal A.K Singh A." "Auratan vich pishab leakage" (Urinary Incontinence) New Delhi, New Era International Imprints 2013.ISBN No-978-81-290-0074-3
6. Sharma R, Kashyap R, Kaushal P, Jain V, Singh A. "Bacchedani Bahar Ana-Prolapse Uterus" (Punjabi) New Delhi New Era International Imprints,2013 vide ISBN No-978-81-290-0068
7. Kaushal P, Sharma R, Aggarwal N, Chopra S, Singh AJ "Menopause- A new approach to deal with menopause related problems" (English) New Delhi, New Era International Imprints, ISBN No-978-81-290-0070-5
8. Kaushal P, Sharma R, Aggarwal N, Chopra S, Singh AJ "Rajoneevriti-Menopause se sambhandhit samasyaon k samadhan ka ek naya drishtikon" (Hindi), New Delhi, New Era International Imprints; ISBN No-978-81-290-0081-1.
9. Kaushal P, Sharma R, Aggarwal N, Chopra S, Singh AJ." Rajoneevriti-Menopause se sambhandhit samasyaon k samadhan ka ek naya drishtikon" (Punjabi), New Delhi, New Era International Imprints vide ISBN No-978-81-290-0083-5.
10. Neha, Sharma R, Rana A, Suri V, Singh AJ and Kaushal P, '*garbhavastha se sambandhit sankaye ve unka samadhan'*.

New Delhi, New Era International Imprints; 2015; ISBN 978-81-290-0121-4

*** Paper published**

1. Kashyap R, Jain V and Singh AJ.Comparative effect of 2 packages of pelvic floor muscle training on the clinical course of stage I–III pelvic organ prolapse. International Journal of Gynecology & Obstetrics, 2013; 121: 69-73
2. Kaur T, Dudeja P, Sharma M, Jain V, Singh A. Impact of Running a Behavior Therapy Room for Various Categories of Urinary Incontinence Cases in Different Age Groups in Obstetrics-Gynecology Outpatient Department of a Tertiary Care Hospi-tal.JPMER.2014;48 :159-163
3. Singhal N and Singh AJ. Promoting Empowerment of Adolescent Girls by Demedicalizing Management of Dysmenorrhea. Ind. J. Youth Adol. Health 2015; 2(4): 1-3
4. Kaur I, Singh A. Empowering Adolescent Girls to Manage the Impending Epidemic of PCOS. Ind J Youth Adol Health 2016; 3(2): 1-3.

Technology developed / transferred

* **Steps taken to sustain the activities after the DBT funding is over:** Discussions have been held with Head OBG deptt. / Institute authorities. They have assured to continue the MPBT room format in OBG OPD. A 6 month extension of the project is being sought for the transition and transfer phase ,i.e., from project to service mode. Scanned copies of letters of support from the HOD OBG and our Dean are enclosed.

* Military hospitals, Nasirabad, Ajmer and Jodhpur have already introduced MPBT room concept. They invited our team for this purpose (pl. see details in 2014-15 report).

Special features of the approach adopted in the MPBT room

- Unlike OBG OPDs couples are counselled together in MPBT room. Thus, they can understand each other better and express their concerns without any hesitation
- Exercises are demonstrated individually in the room. Patients repeat them (Return demonstration). A special set of floor as well as bed based exercises have been developed.
- Videos are shown regarding ante natal and post-natal care

- Easy to understand IEC material (charts, flip cards, posters are displayed in the room)
- Laptop based IEC material is also given
- Every patient is given booklet on relevant management aspect of her problem free of cost (Hindi/ English/Punjabi)
- Patient are followed up on phone to ensure compliance
- Queries are resolved at leisurely pace. Sufficient time (15-20 min) is devoted to each patient
- Yoga and meditation related counselling is also given as per the need.

Recommendation- There is a need to develop, pre-test and pilot this approach in OBG OPD of other medical colleges of India. There is need for establishing such room and also for extending such concept of demedicalization in in OPDs of all medical colleges. Suitable modification may also be done in this strategy as per local culture and requirements.

Setting up of MPBT room will help in enhancing the image of reproductive health care services in India by targeting the client satisfaction of women availing the services of OBG OPD/wards and also stress upon conservative management of various diseases.

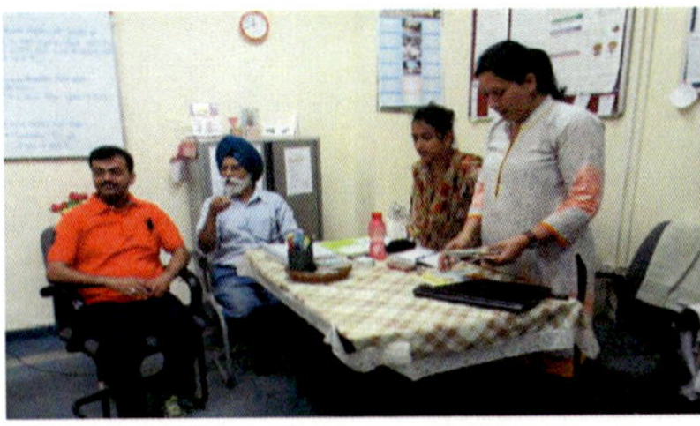

Pix 1: PI briefing Mr. Aggarwal about the activities done in the room

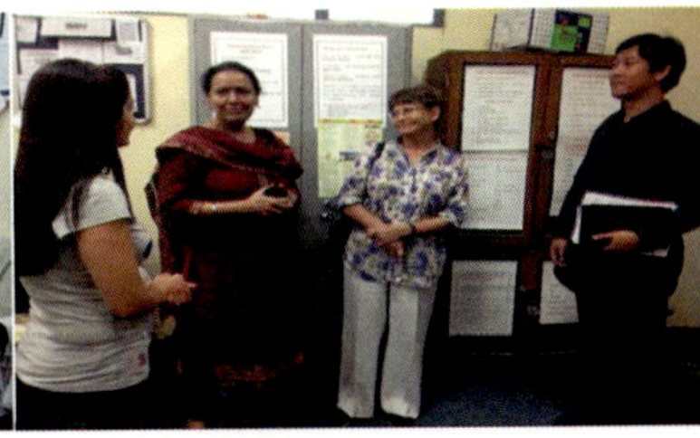

Pix 2: Dr. Ruchi with the team of Concept Foundation

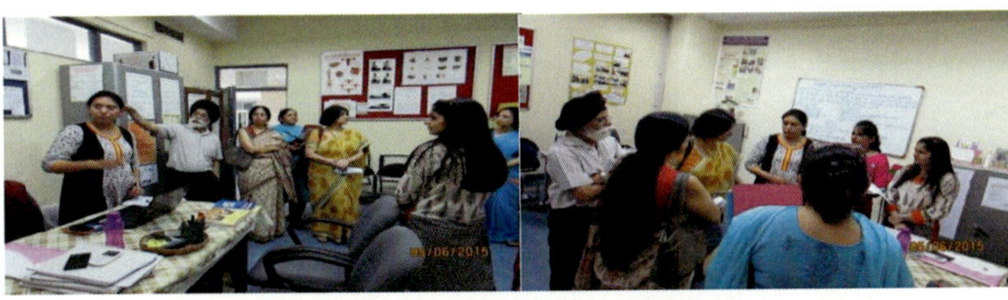

Pix 3: Dr. AJ Singh briefing Dr. Jatinder Kaur Arora & Dr. Suneela Garg about the project

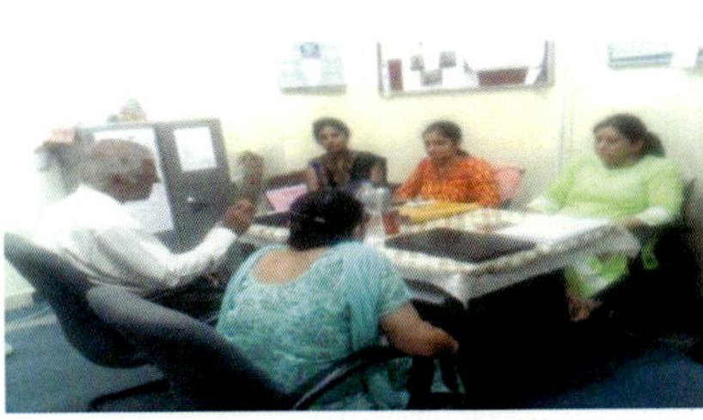

Pix 4: Mr. Sharma telling about various yoga / meditation techniques

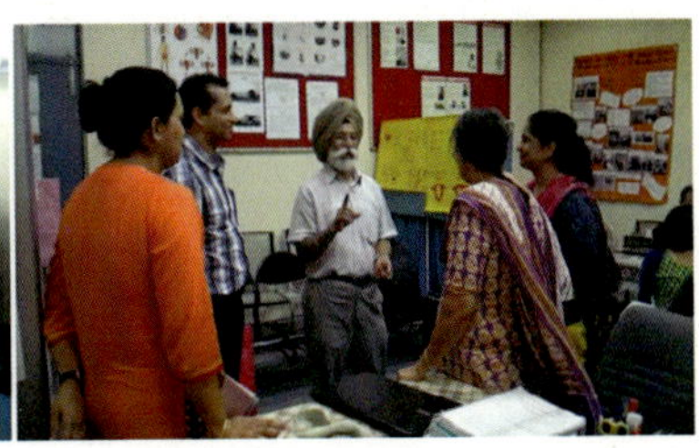

Pix 5: Dr. Bansal visits MPBT room with wife

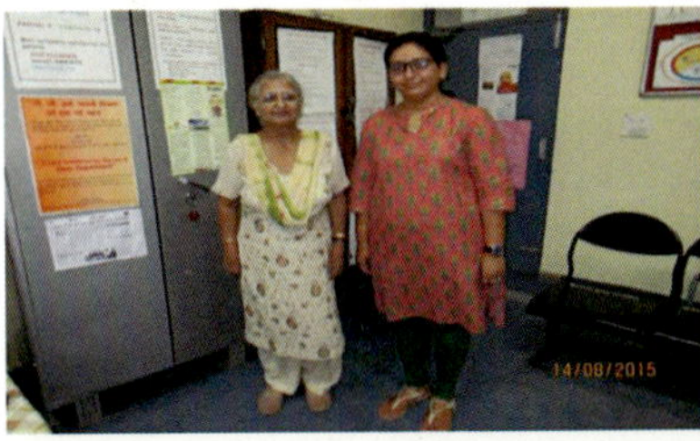

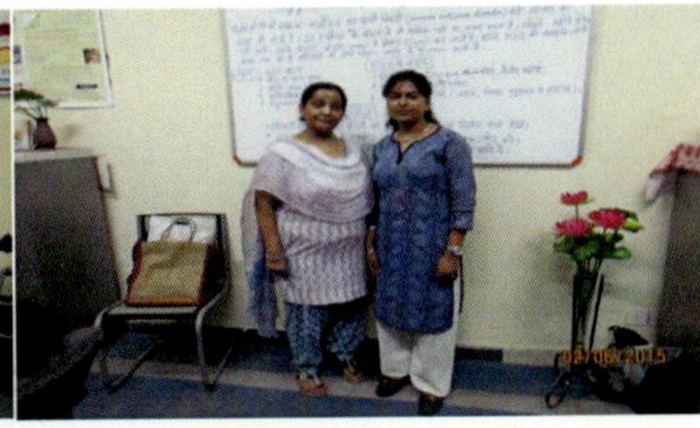

Pix 6-7: Patients who benefited with Kegal exercises.

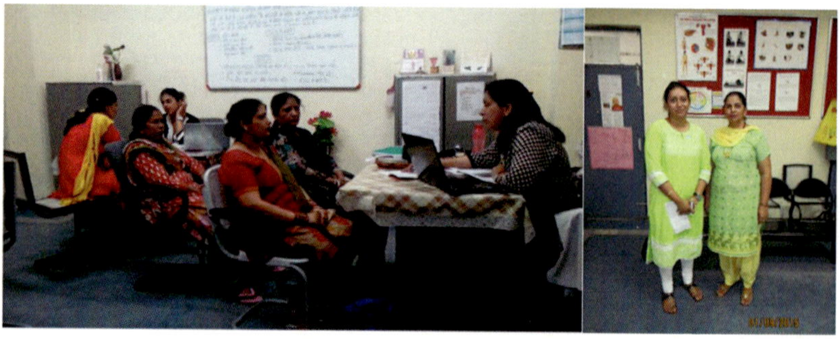

Pix 8-9: Successful menopausal patient @ follow up after counselling.

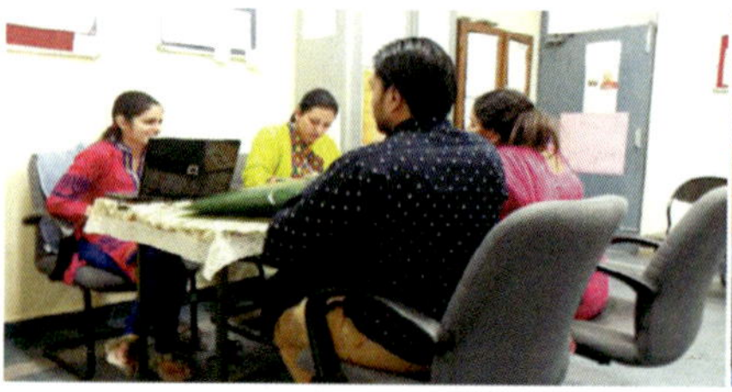

Pix 10: Male involvement in MPBT room – Infertility Counselling.

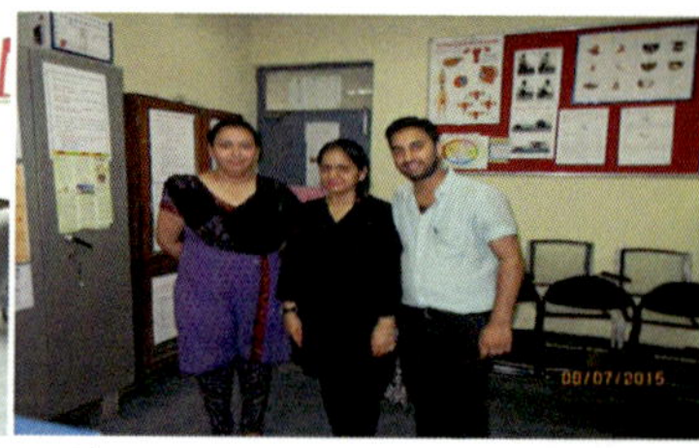

Pix 11: Successful infertility patient who conceived after counselling.

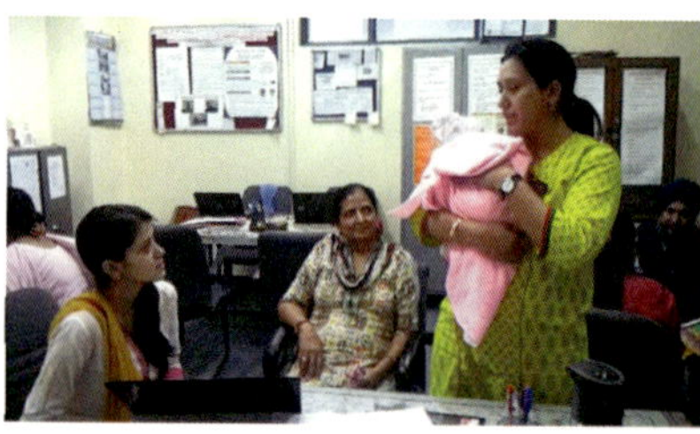

Pix. 12: Baby care counselling.

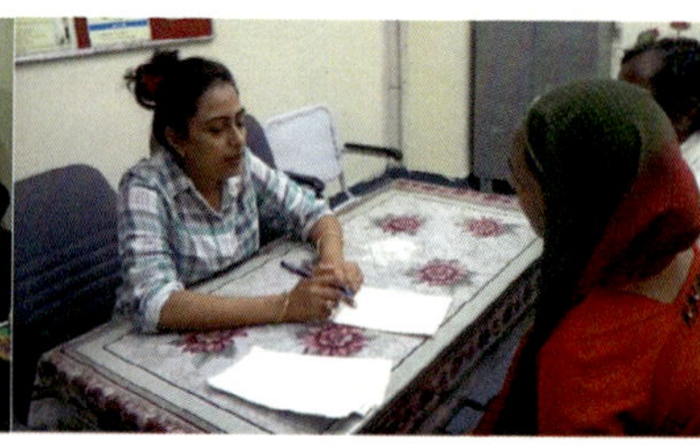

Pix. 13: DFMC Chart explained to antenatal female.

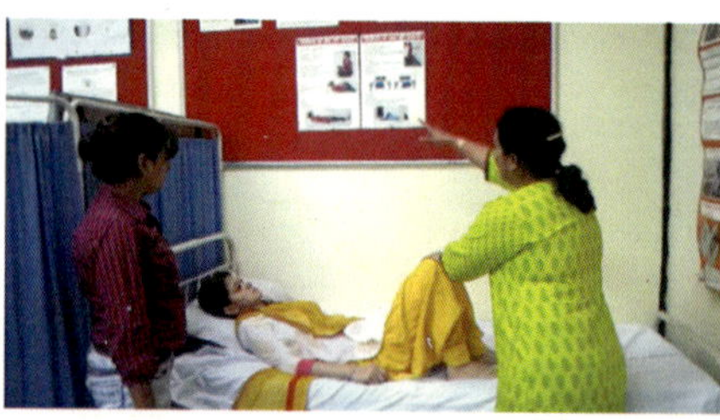

Pix. 14: Explaining exercises with charts.

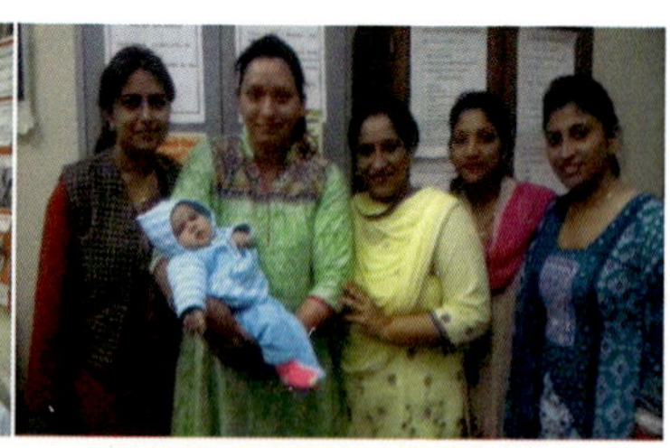

Pix. 15: Patient visit MPBT room after delivery.

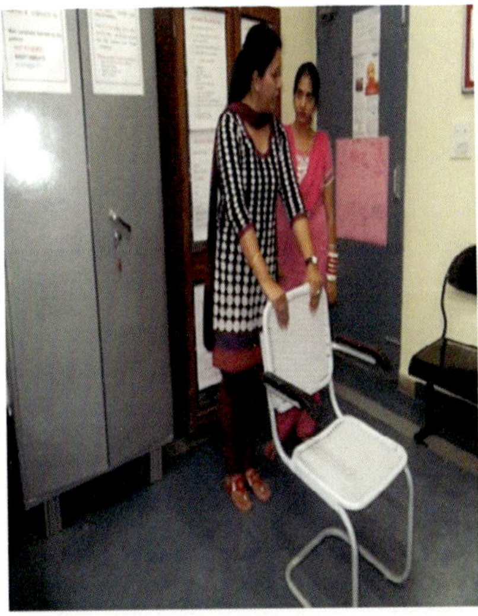
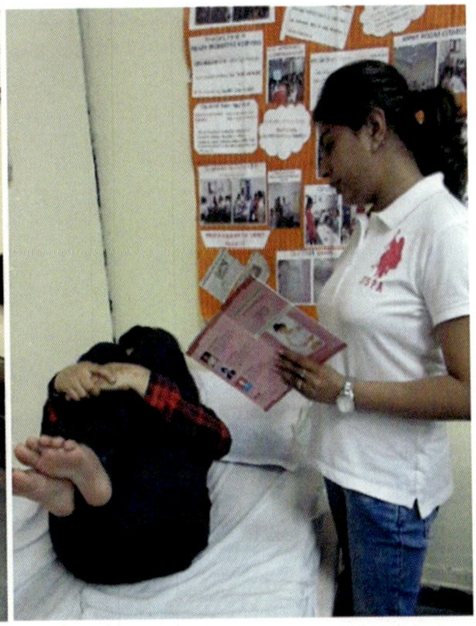

Pix. 16-17: Dr. Neha & Dr. Purnima demonstrating exercises for Dysmenorrhea.

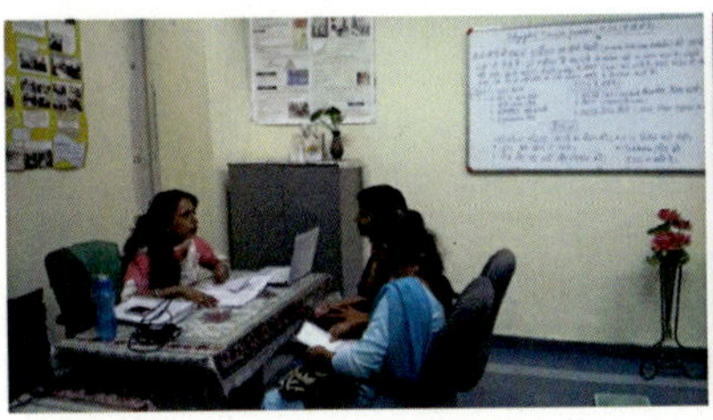
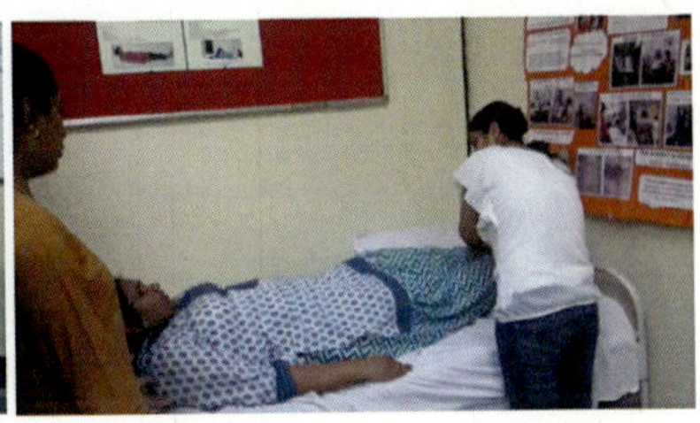

Pix. 18-19: Dr. Neha & Dr Ruchi counselling a sister duo on PCOD + exercises.

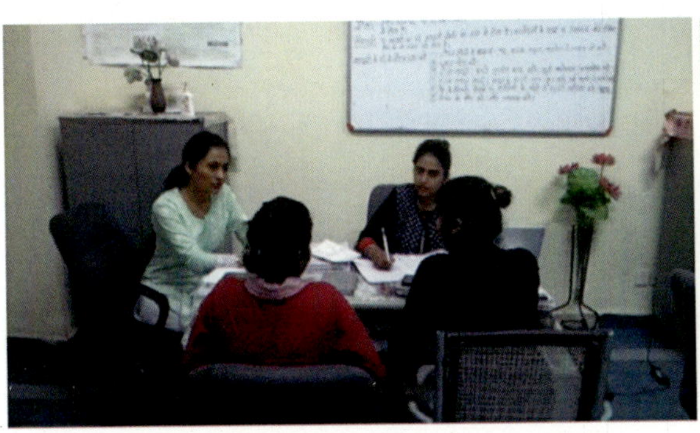

Pix. 20: A dietician counselling a PCOD case.

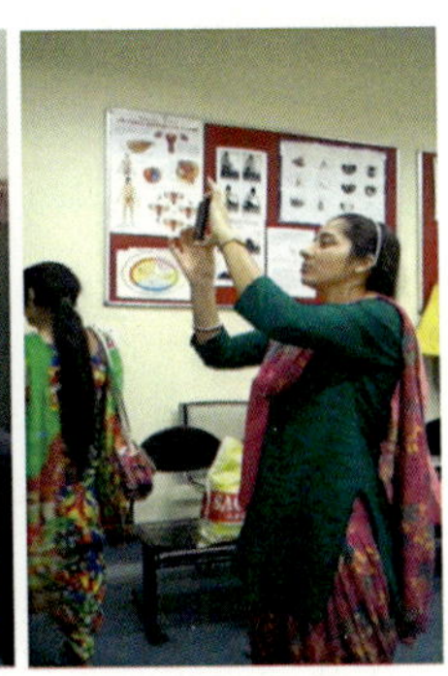

Pix. 21: Patient use display board matter on PCOD.

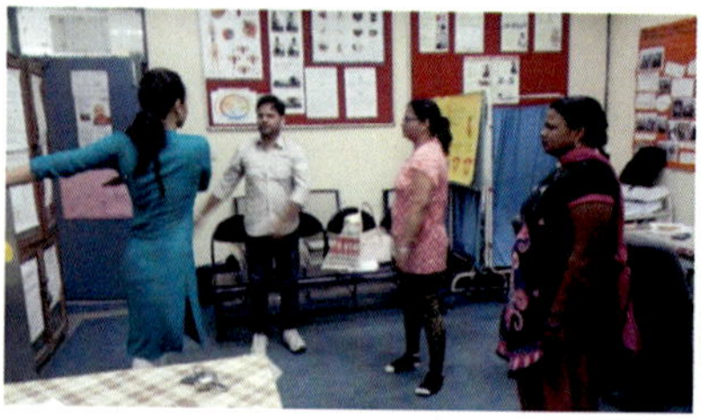

Pix. 22: Exercise demonstration in MPBT room.

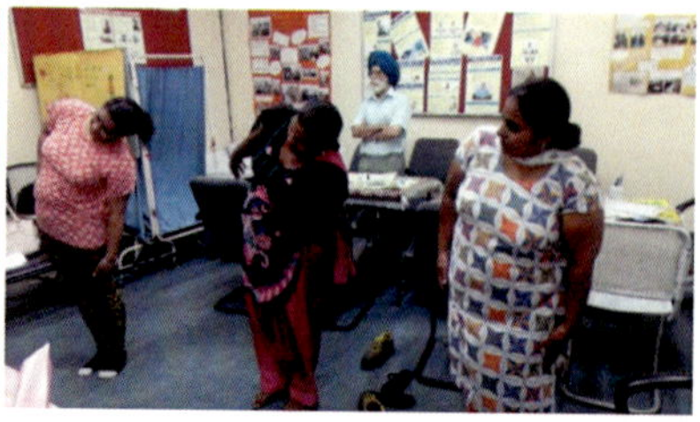

Pix. 23: Group exercise session.

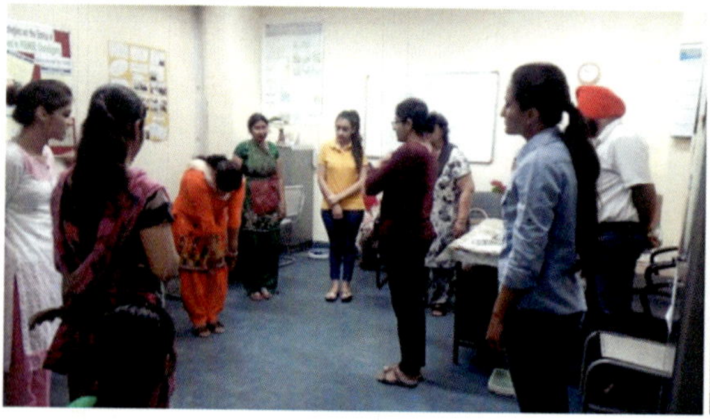

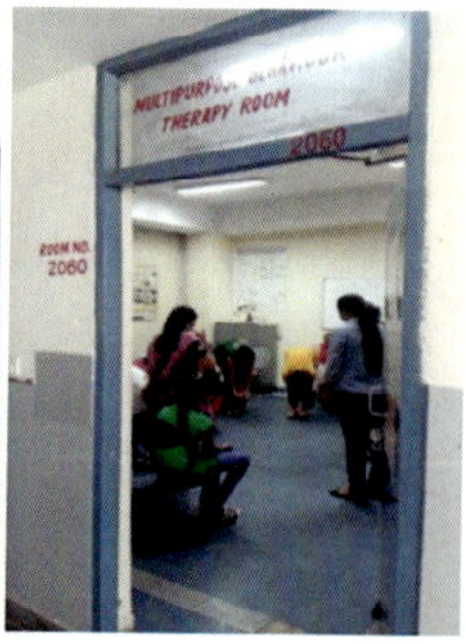

Pix. 24-25: Group exercise session.

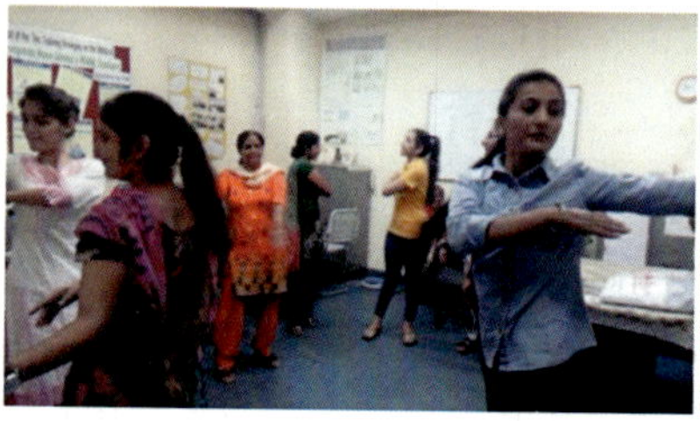

Pix. 26: Group exercise session in MPBT room.

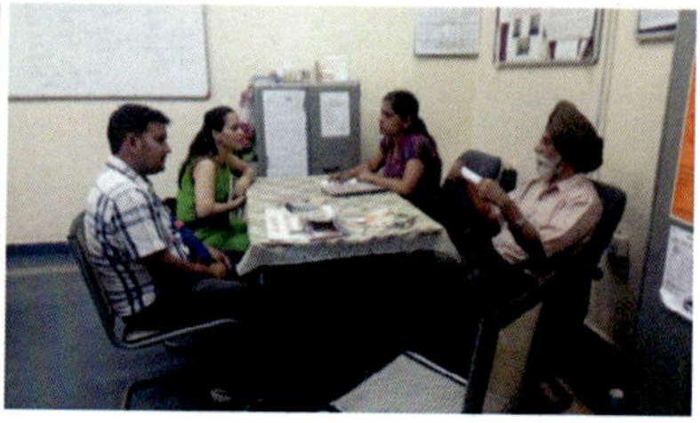

Pix 27: Couple counselling in MPBT room.

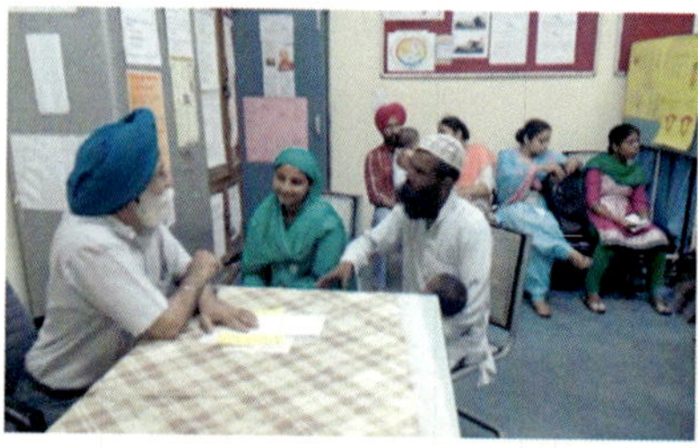

Pix. 28: Couple counselling in MPBT room

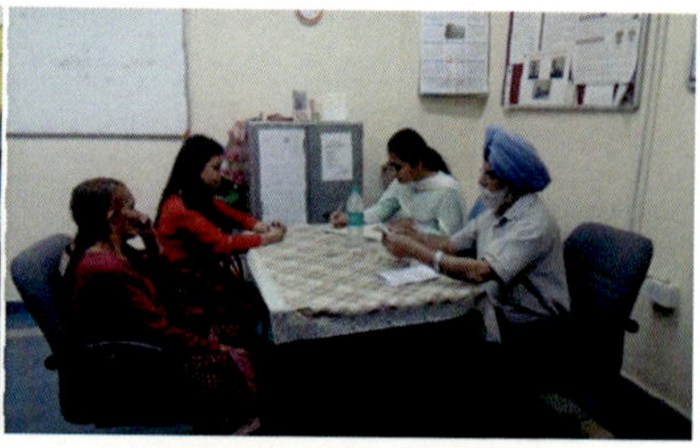

Pix. 29: Mother daughter counselling in MPBT room

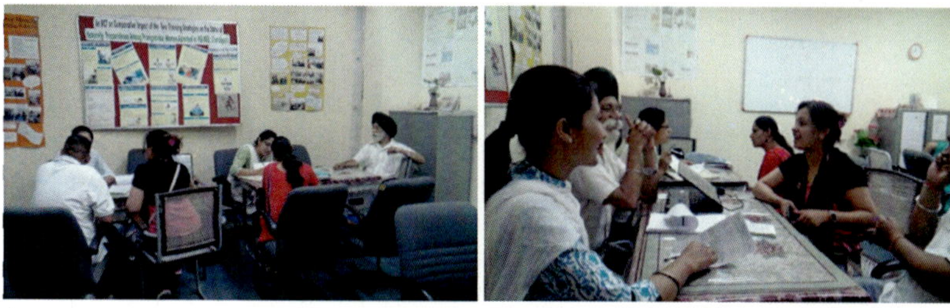

Pix. 30: Couple counselling session in progress in MPBT room.

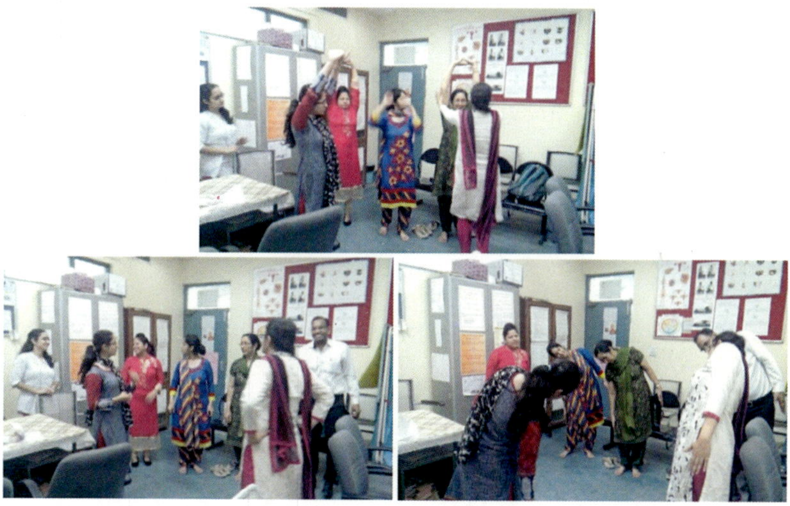

Pix. 31: Group exercise session in progress in MPBT room.

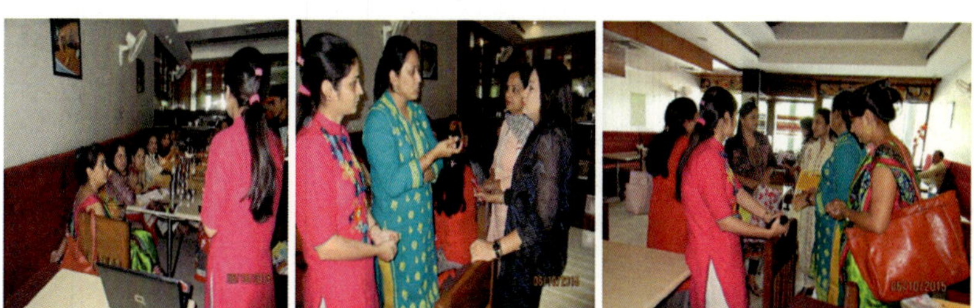

Pix. 32: Drs. Purnima &Ruchi addressing the ladies @kitty party about MPBT Room.

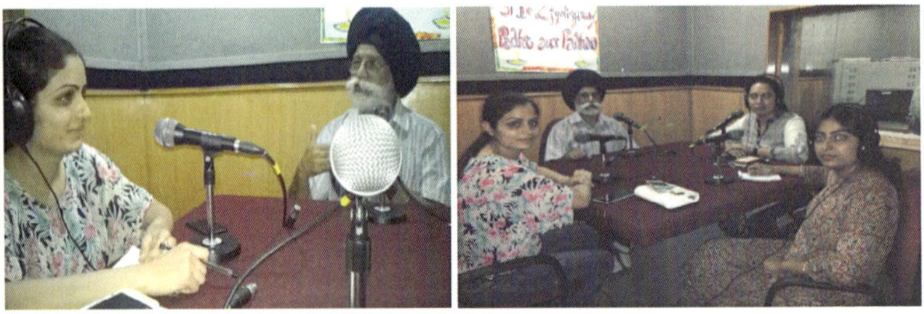

Pix. 33: MPBT team at PU **Jyotirgamaya** *Radio station.*

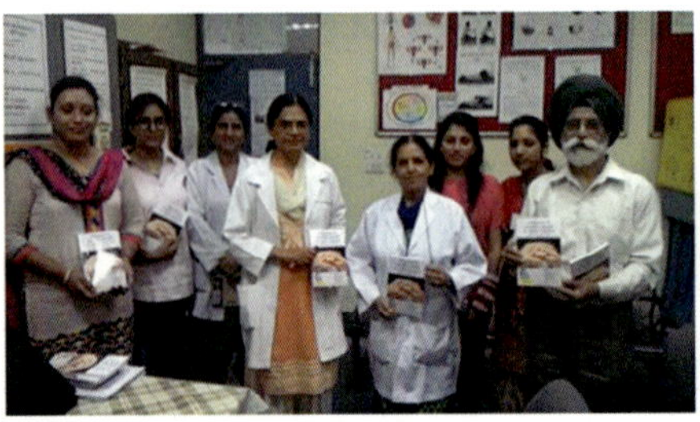

Pix. 34: Release of book on ANC By Dr Vanita Suri.

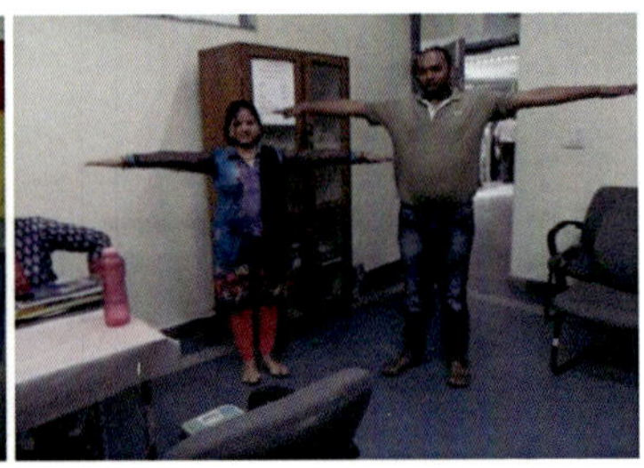

Pix. 35: Male involvement in MPBT room.

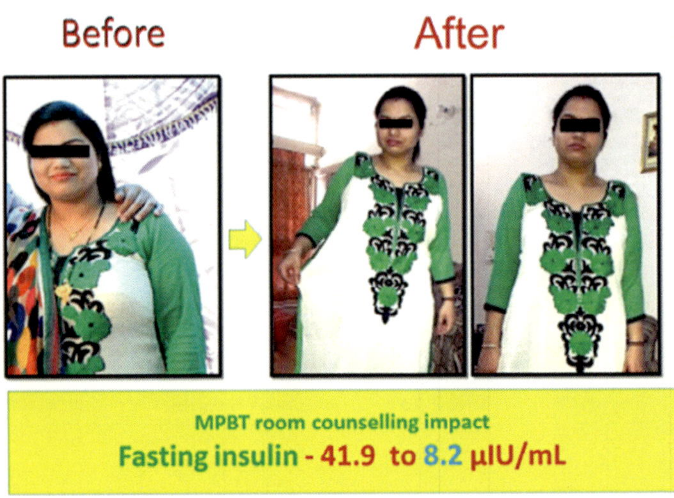
Before
After
MPBT room counselling impact
Fasting insulin - 41.9 to 8.2 µIU/mL

Impact of MPBT room counselling in a PCOD patient.

Chapter - 3

Prevention and Management of Low Back Pain in Women through Exercise and Posture Correction

—Dr. Neha Chanana, Dr. Babita Ghai, Dr. R.K. Kanojia, Dr. Sukhpal Kaur, Dr. Amarjeet Singh

Woman or superwoman-*Kahani Ghar Ghar ki*

"Haye meri kamar.....iodex maliyie kaam pe chaliye"!!!!

For more than 20 years, we have been watching these television commercials of gels and balms that claim to relieve low back pain. The brand names of these products may be different but have a common brand ambassador "THE OVERWORKED MODERN DAY WOMEN." They showcase women are busy with office as well as household chores like washing, ironing, kitchen chores, cleaning cupboards, looking after children, etc. In the rush to perform these daily activities/pre-set duties are shown to over exert themselves. Moreover, in this hustle bustle, they unknowingly adopt wrong posture and suffer from low back pain (LBP).

Changing the frame from reel world to this real world, we would find no difference in the life of a woman. For centuries, women have experienced a similar life almost every day. Woman fulfilling the roles of a wife, mother, daughter in law, daughter or sister encounter the well-known morning rush hour. She single handedly works in the kitchen- prepares breakfast; packs lunch; get kids ready for school; drops them to bus stop; helps her husband get ready for office; cleans the house; supervises maids; wash clothes and utensils; looks after in-laws; and only then she gets a chance of getting ready for her own day at work. Finishing all this in just 2 hours after getting up in the morning is surely over burdening and exhausting.

Moreover, the day does not end here. They commute to work in overcrowded buses sometimes even standing/ drives car or two- wheelers for long hours. After slogging in the office for 8-9 hours, they come back and again indulge in household activities. They keep working even when all the other members are fast asleep. During my coursework of Master in Public Health, I got the opportunity to know what working women feel about their daily life. I would like to share a few of them:

> *"Humein sab super woman samajhte hain, ghar bhi sambahlo aur office bhi. Apne liye to time hi nahin milta" (Everyone thinks we are kind of some superwoman!! We are so busy looking after work in offices as well as look after the family. We do not get any time for ourselves.!!!)*
>
> *"Itna zyaada kaam hota hai ki even when the physical body is at rest, the mind is still calculating what next to do. The list of 'things to do' is never ending for us." (We are overloaded with work so much that even when the physical body is at rest, the mind is still calculating what next to do. The list of 'things to do' is never ending for us.)*
>
> *"Every day coping up with the pressure to juggle work and family responsibilities is like wining Padma shree but the only difference is there is no one to acknowledge this win."*
>
> *"I try to finish everything as quickly as possible especially in the morning so that I can relax. But how much hard I try; I get no time for myself".*

This is another trait where in women have a forceful habit of finishing everything at one go. If they have to lift heavy things or shift furniture or say flower pots they will not wait or ask for help in the family. They will do it on their own with a mindset of finishing the work as soon as possible. This is surely very tiring for them.

In this kind of set up, they are not cautious and often commonly suffer from sudden jerks; falls or injury; bathroom slippage hurting the lower back which often causes or precipitates low back pain (LBP).

Other contributing factors which may precipitate LBP among women are wrong/ incorrect postures, lack of physical activity and many more. These are discussed in further chapters.

The story does not end here. A typical woman will not mention about her suffering to anyone. She neglects the pain and continues with her daily routine. A woman suffering from LBP for 20 years shared her experience saying, *"I consulted a doctor 2 years back for the first time for LBP. He had asked me to take rest and not over exert. But!!! if I take rest, who will look after my family."* This is a popular belief among women when it comes to their own health.

Hence, to get rid of the pain she resorts to self-medication and gels/balms, etc. but never consults a doctor. Even if she is asked to seek advice from the physician, she ignores it by saying, "*kuch nahi hua, bus thoda dard hai, theek ho jayega" (It is nothing, just little pain, I will be fine)*Therefore, she neglects her LBP keeping family priorities first.

Woman is an incredible creature. She is the first one to satisfy the needs of her family in every aspect of life. On the contrary, when it comes to fulfilling her own needs she puts it on a back burner. For example, women,

- are the last one to get ready for office when everyone has left;
- are the last to have dinner after she has served everyone;
- are last to sleep in the house after she is done with all her work.

Moreover, any Indian woman is expected to take health decisions for her family but is expected to be the last one to think about her own health issues!!! She is expected to suffer from her ailments quietly. Women avoid seeking proper treatment because of other factors also like distance, time constraints, shyness, overloading of hospitals, costly and inaccessible treatment, etc. All these factors force women to tolerate their suffering. This is known as 'culture of silence', which often leads to delay in diagnosis and worsens the condition. Similarly, LBP is no different.

Understanding the anatomy of lower back

In order to understand and manage low back pain we need to first understand the anatomical structure related to the lower back. Like all joints the lower back is made of bones, muscles, ligaments, tendons and cartilage.

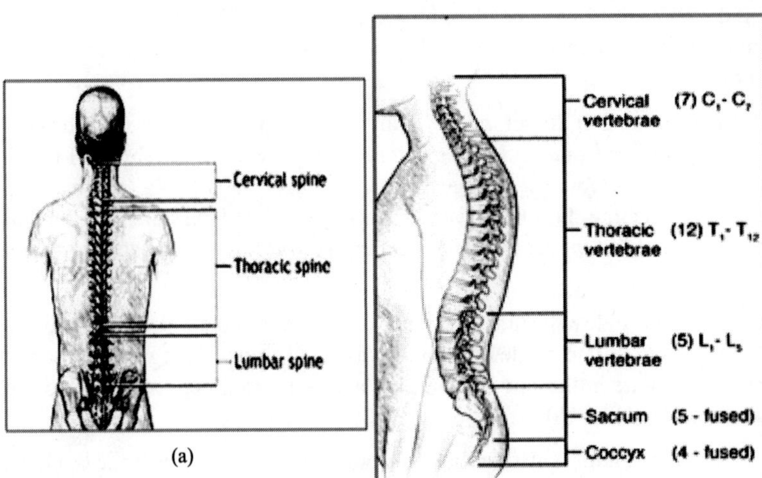

(b)

Fig. 1: Spine as viewed from back and side.

Damage (due to injury, fall, sudden jerk, disease, age-related wear and tear, tumour, etc) to these structures can cause low back pain. Thus, the basic information about various structures of the low back will help us know how our lower back works and what can go wrong with it. This understanding will also help us to better communicate with the doctor.

Our spine, also known as vertebral column or spinal column (in Hindi called as *reerh ki haddi*) when viewed from the back (rear or posterior) appears straight from the neck to the tailbone. However, looking at the spine from the side, it has a natural front-back curve that resembles 'S' shape. The curve in the neck and low back balance each other. This helps us to stand up straight with minimum effort and minimum usage of our energy.

The spine is made up of series of bones, known as vertebrae (called *manake* in Hindi) arranged one above the other. We have 33 vertebrae extending from the neck to the tailbone. These are divided into 5 main regions: cervical, thoracic, lumbar, sacral and coccyx (Fig. 1. a, b).

Cervical: The neck region of the spine is known as cervical spine. This consists of 7 vertebrae, viz. C1 to C7. These vertebrae support the head and allow various head movements.

Thoracic: Beneath the cervical spine, in the chest/trunk (*chhati* in Hindi) region we have the thoracic spine. This consists of 12 thoracic vertebrae viz. T1-T12 (top to bottom). The vertebrae increase in size as we go down the thoracic spine i.e. T1 is the smallest and T12 the largest thoracic vertebrae. Each thoracic vertebra is attached to a pair of ribs-referred to as *pasliyan* in Hindi (we have 12 pairs of ribs) to form the rib cage. This makes the thoracic spine more stable than the cervical spine and also protects many vital organs of the body.

Lumbar: Our lower back region of the spine is known as lumbar spine (known as *kamar* in Hindi). Our lumbar spine has 5 vertebrae L1 to L5. The lumbar vertebrae are bigger, wider and broader than the cervical and thoracic vertebrae. This is the weight bearing portion of the spine. The lumbar vertebrae help in movements like bending forward, bending backwards and side bending.

Sacrum: Below the lumbar spine, we have 5 vertebrae which are combined together to form one single bone known as the sacrum (hip region). It is a flat triangular bone in the low back region and is located between our two hip bones (*kulhe ki haddi*).

Coccyx: People call it tailbone in common language. This is the last bone in the vertebral column. The coccyx bears our body weight when we sit and also provides attachment to the hips and lower abdomen muscles.

Within the spinal canal, which is looped with vertebral bodies, is a bundle of nerves called the spinal cord. The spinal cord stretches from the brain and ends at L2. After L2, it forms a bundle of nerves called as *cauda equina* which in Latin means "horse's tail". From the neck area to the coccyx there are 31 pairs of spinal nerve roots that exit the spinal canal and reach the various parts of the body (through a hole in the vertebra known as foramina) which control various body movements. The nerves of the cervical spine go to the upper chest and arms. The nerves of the thoracic spine go to the chest and abdomen. The nerves of the lumbar spine go to the legs, pelvis, bowel, and bladder.

Now, coming to the anatomy of the lower back, our lumbar spine is made of series of joints. Like every joint, our lumbar spine has bones, ligaments, tendons, cartilage and muscles.

(a) Bones of the spine: These are known as vertebrae and as discussed, in the lumbar region we have 5 vertebrae. Each vertebra has the following parts (Fig. 2):

(i) Vertebral body is disc- shaped

(ii) Vertebral arch is composed of pedicles and laminae that surround the vertebral foramen.

(iii) Vertebral foramen (hole) – It is the central part of vertebrae. The vertebral foramina of all the vertebrae one above the other forms the vertebral column through which the spinal cord passes.

(iv) Bony processes: These are present on the back of the vertebral body. The **transverse processes** are located on the two sides and the **spinous**

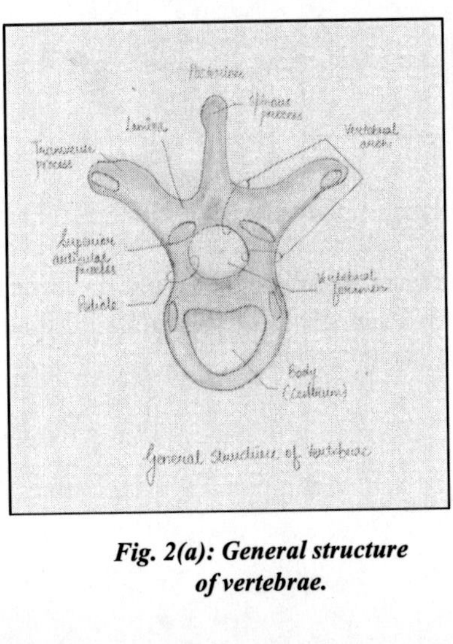

Fig. 2(a): General structure of vertebrae.

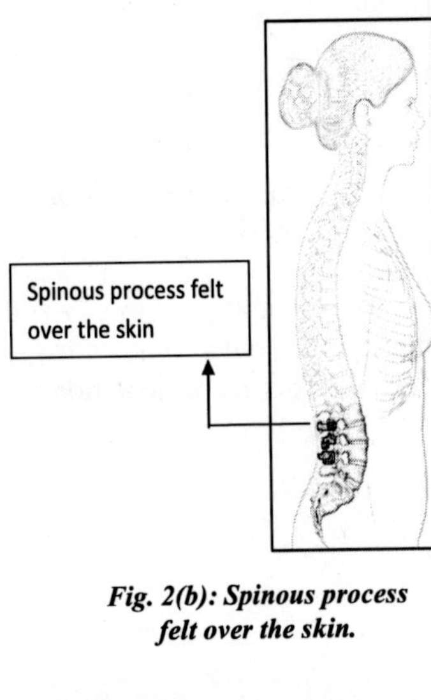

Fig. 2(b): Spinous process felt over the skin.

process appears in the centre. Spinous process is a bony portion present opposite to the vertebral body. This part can be felt by the finger as we slide down on the centre of the back. These are even visible over the skin (Fig. 2b). The **superior and inferior articular processes** are located above and below the meeting point of pedicle and lamina. These bony processes are the connection points for ligaments and tendons.

These vertebrae are arranged one above the other to form series of joints known as facet joints. These are formed by joining of the articular processes. The facet joints make our spine flexible and help us to bend forward, bend backwards and side to side. In between the vertebrae, there are intervertebral discs that act as cushions by keeping the vertebrae separated in case of forceful impact of any activity. It also protects the nerves that run down the middle of the spine (Fig. 3 a & 6). Each disc is designed like a jelly donut with a central softer component (nucleus pulposus) and a surrounding outer ring (annulus fibrosus) (Fig. 3 b). The annulus fibrosus can be divided into the outermost, middle, and innermost fibers.

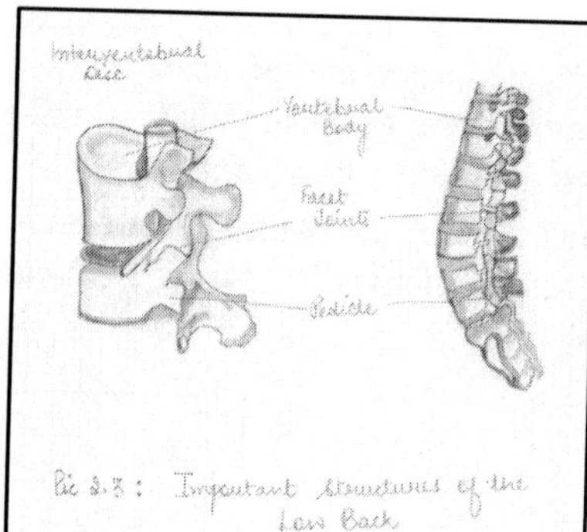

Fig. 3 (a): Important structures of the low back.

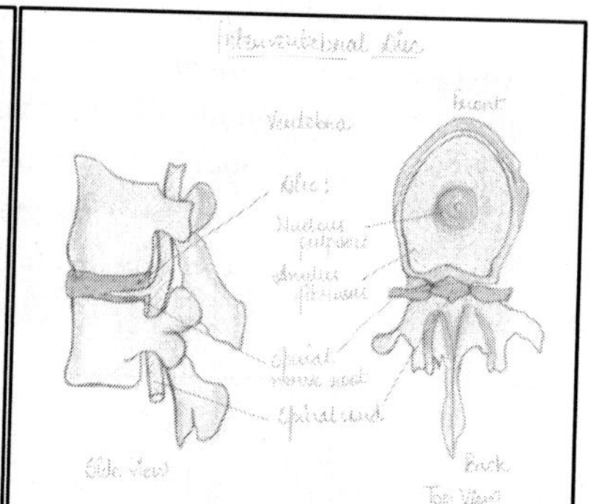

Fig. 3 (b): Structure of the intervertebral disc.

The central portion of the disc is capable of rupturing and projecting through the outer ring known as herniation of the disc (herniated disc) (Fig. 4). This causes irritation to the adjacent nerves.

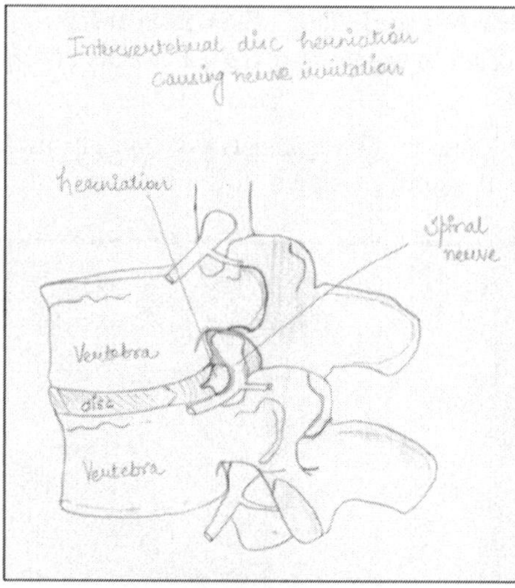

Fig. 4: Intervertebral disc herniation causing nerve irritation.

(b) Ligaments: They link the lumbar vertebrae to each other and provide stability to the spine and help prevent injury from excessive movements like excessive forward or backward bending. These are damaged most often because of exercise due to sudden jerk. Ligaments of the lumbar spine (Fig. 5 a) are:-

(i) Anterior longitudinal ligament (ALL): It covers the front of the vertebral body and the discs. It is attached to the outermost annulus disc fibers. It limits back bending of the spine.

(ii) Posterior longitudinal ligament (PLL): This is located within the vertebral canal over the posterior surface of the vertebral bodies and discs. It limits forward bending of the spine.

(iii) Supraspinous ligament: This joins the tips of the spinous processes of adjacent vertebrae from L1-L3.

(iv) Interspinous ligament: It interconnects the adjacent spinous processes from root to apex.

(v) Ligamentum flavum: This is the strongest ligament and runs in front of and between the lamina. It forms the posterior wall of the vertebral canal.

(vi) Intertransverse ligament: This ligament joins the transverse processes of the adjacent vertebrae.

(vii) Iliolumbar ligament: This arises from the tip of the transverse process of L5 and connects to the upper inner border of the hip bone (Fig. 5 b).

(c) Tendons: These are like ligaments but connect muscles to the lumbar vertebrae and guard against excessive movement in any one direction.

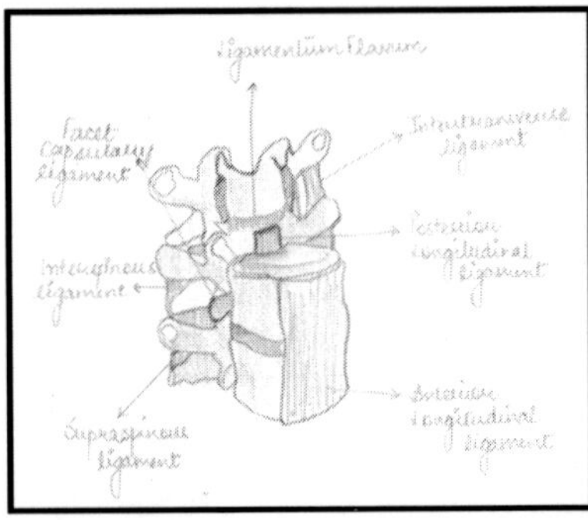

Fig. 5(a): Ligaments of the lumbar spine.

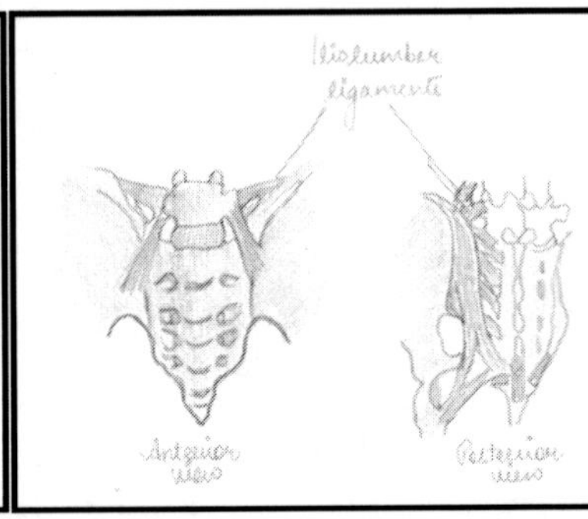

Fig. 5 (b): Iliolumbar ligaments.

(d) Cartilage: It is a firm rubbery material present in between the vertebrae on the outer edge of the intervertebral discs and also the facet joints. The cartilage helps to bend and twist our back and act as a 'shock absorber' (Fig. 6). Break down or degeneration of the cartilage causes pressure on the nerve (nerve compression) in the spinal column. This may cause acute or chronic back pain, tingling, numbness and muscle weakness can occur within

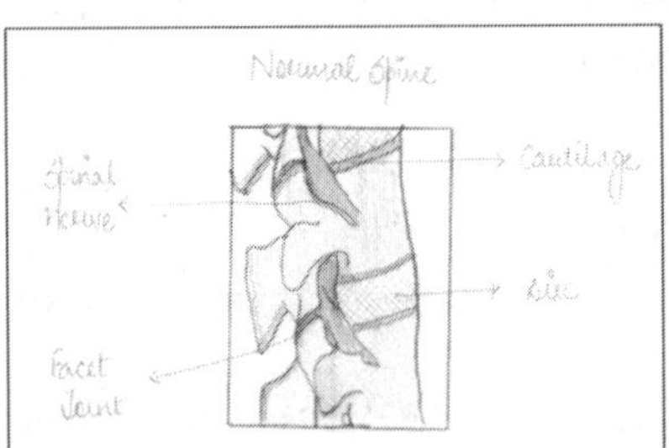

Fig. 6(a): Cartilage of the normal spine.

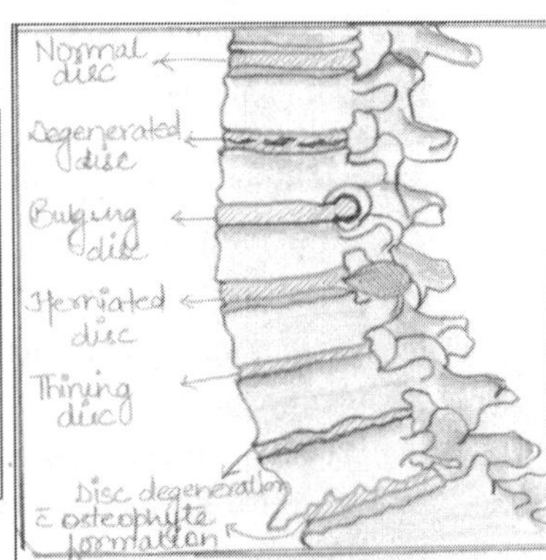

Fig. 6(b): Conditions caused by breakage of cartilage.

the shoulders, arms and legs. It may lead to conditions like osteoarthiritis, herniated disc, buldging disc, degenerative disc disease, etc. which are discussed in subsequent chapters.

(e) Muscles: Many groups of muscles are responsible for flexing, extending, and rotating the waist, as well as moving the lower extremities. These include the muscles of the low back and the posterior (back) abdominal wall muscles (Fig. 7).

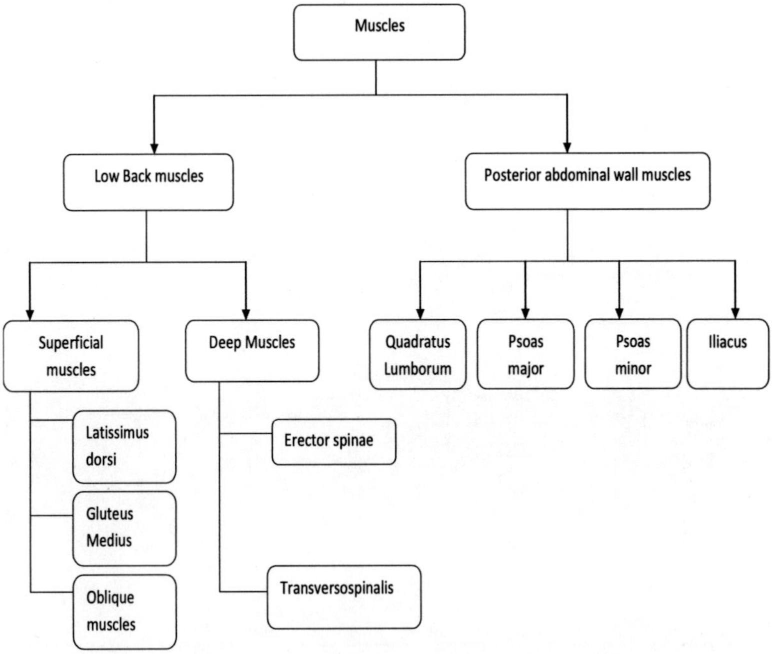

Fig. 7: Muscles of low back and posterior abdominal muscles.

I. Muscles of the low back: These can be divided into superficial and deep muscles.

- **(a) Superficial muscles:** There are 3 main superficial muscles of the lower back (Fig. 8)
  - (1) Latissimus Dorsi: This is the largest muscle of the lower back which is responsible for pulling the arm downwards and backwards. It plays a role in maintaining heathy lower back as it originates from the vertebrae of the lower spine (T6-T12, all lumbar and sacral vertebrae and the Iliac crest- upper border of the hip bone).

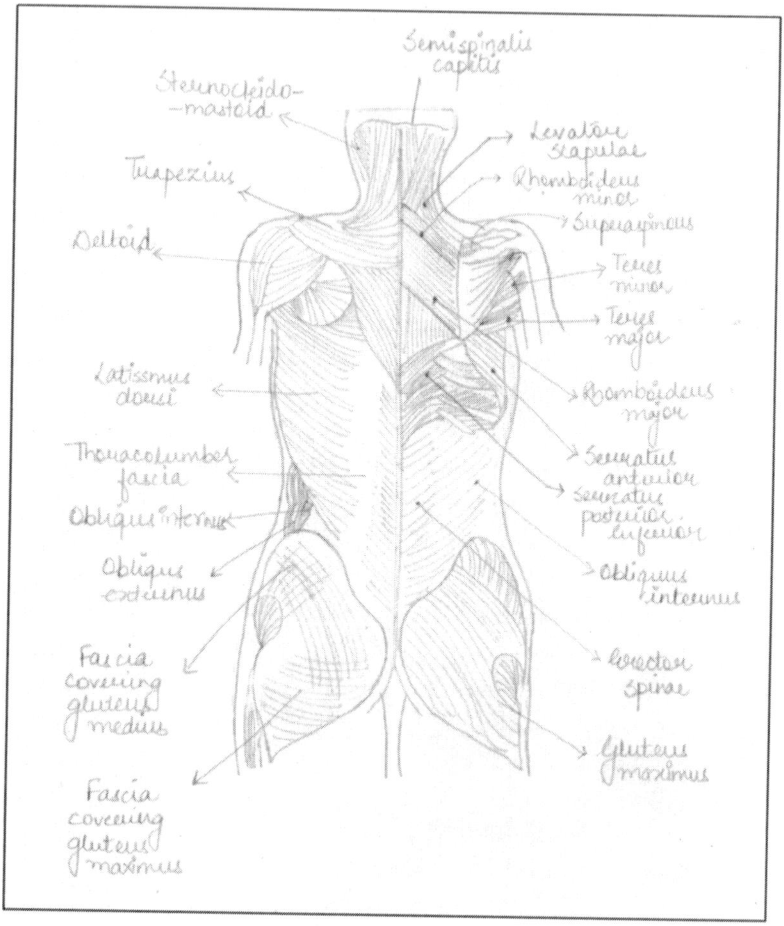

Fig. 8: Superficial muscles of lower back.

2. Gluteus Medius: Although strictly a hip muscle, it is often associated with low back pain. Its action is to turn the leg inwards and take the leg away from the centre of the body.
3. Internal and external oblique (Obliquus internus and Obliquus externus): These muscles help us in forward and side bending. It also aids in rotating the trunk.

(b) Deep muscles:There are 2 groups of deep muscles- Erector spinae and Transversospinalis muscles (Fig. 9).

(1) Erector spinae: These are the erector spinae and are attached to the back of the spine. These are present in pairs one on each side of the

vertebral column. The erector spinae consists of 3 muscles viz. spinalis, longissimus and iliocostalis from inside out. These help in backward & side bending, standing and lifting objects.

2. Transversospinalis: These are located deeper than the erector spinae. This group consists of three 'layers', semispinalis, multifidus and rotators from top to bottom.

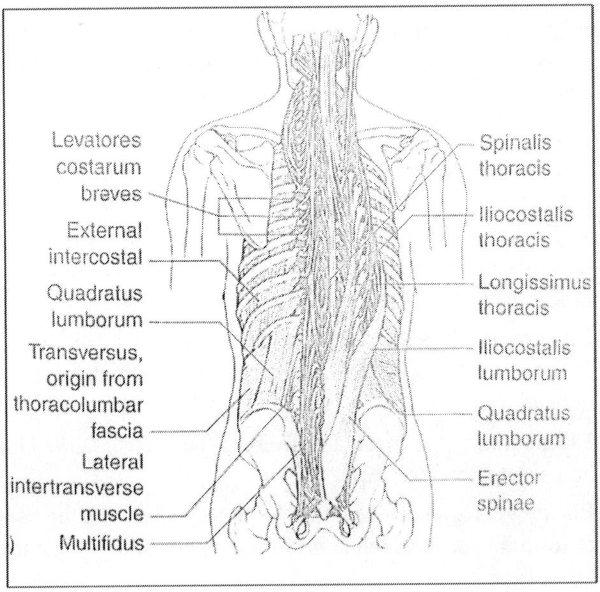

(a)

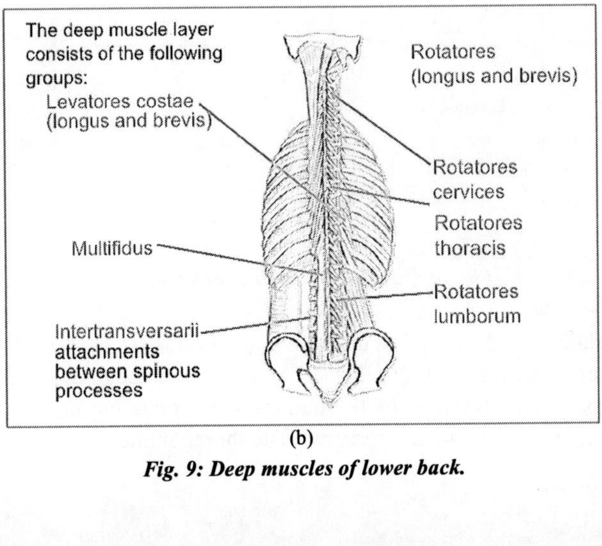

(b)

Fig. 9: Deep muscles of lower back.

(i) Semispinalis thoracis: These help us in back bending and rotating the trunk to the opposite side.

(ii) Multifidus: These help us in rotating and bending the trunk to the opposite side. It also aids in bending backwards.

(iii) Rotatores: These help in rotating the trunk to the opposite side.

II Posterior abdominal wall muscles: The muscles present in front of the spine i.e. posterior (back) wall of the abdomen are also the lower back's major support. These are attached to the lower back. These abdominal muscles support the lower back muscles which keep the lumbar curve and spine stable. These groups of muscles also help in activities such as lifting. The important muscles are as follows (Fig. 10):

1. Quadratus Lumborum: This muscle is responsible for side bending, backward bending and also fixes the 12th rib during inspiration. It originates at the Iliac crest (upper part of hip bone) and passes upwards to attach to the lowest rib (12th rib) and to the transverse processes of L1-L4 (Fig. 10).
2. Psoas major: It is located immediately near to the lumbar vertebrae. It originates from T12-L5 and attaches to the thigh bone. It helps us in bending sideways.
3. Psoas minor: It is located in front of the psoas major. This muscle helps us to bend forward.
4. Iliacus: It is a fan shaped muscle. It combines with the psoas major to form iliopsoas which helps in forward bending of the trunk.

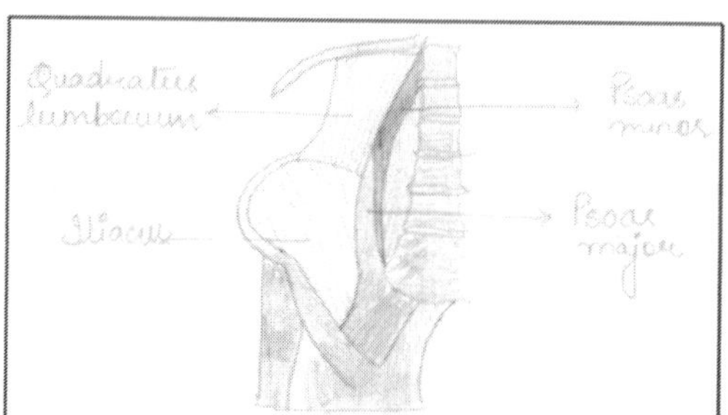

Fig. 10: Posterior abdominal wall muscles.

In addition to the muscles, thoracolumbar fascia is present in front of the lumbar vertebrae and 12th rib (Fig. 8). Fascia is a thin, tough connective tissue that wraps most structures of the human body including muscles. Fascia supports and protects these structures. The thoracolumbar fascia consists of the three layers; posterior (back), middle and anterior (front). Muscles are enclosed between these layers. The quadratus lumborum is present between the anterior and middle layers. The deep back muscles are located between the middle and posterior layers.The posterior layer extends between the 12th rib and the iliac crest on the back. On the sides, the fascia meets the internal oblique muscles. As it forms these attachments it covers the latisimus dorsi (Fig. 7).

Now, after an understanding of the structures of the spine, we must know about low back pain (LBP), its causes and impact. These are discussed in detail in the next chapter.

Low Back Pain- Its causes & impact

Low Back Pain (LBP) is a condition wherein pain is usually localized below the rib cage and above the lower part of the hips (Fig. 11). It may be with or without leg pain.

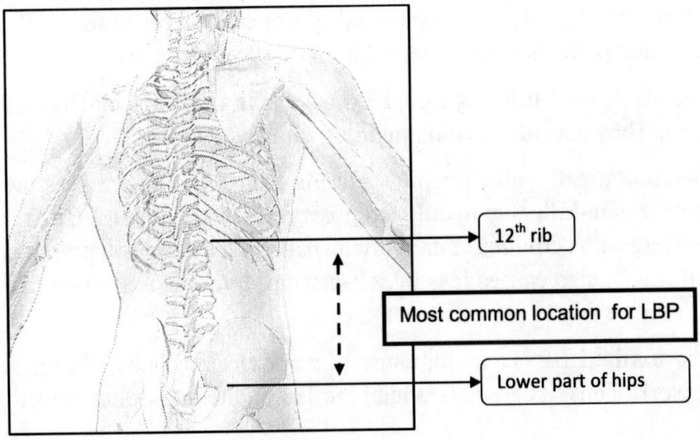

Fig. 11: Usual location of LBP.

Low back pain (LBP) is a common problem among adults. Both men and women are affected by LBP. However, it is seen to be higher among women. It is estimated that two out of three women suffer from LBP.

Classification of LBP

LBP can be classified according to different parameters like duration, cause, etc. According to duration of symptoms, LBP can be divided into:-

- *Acute*: low back pain lasting for less than one month.
- *Sub-acute*: is low back pain lasting between one and three months

- *Chronic*: is defined as low back pain persisting for more than 3 months. It includes recurring (repeated) back pain that off and on, affects an individual over a long period of time.

Another aspect of classifying LBP is Specific and Non Specific LBP.

- *Specific LBP*: is defined as that caused because of some specific defect in the body (pathology) such as injury, infection, inflammation, tumour, etc.
- *Non-specific LBP:* is defined as symptoms of unknown origin or without known pathology.

Impact of LBP

LBP affects the life of individuals in totality. All the following aspects of their health may be affected:-

Physical: Pain, stiffness and discomfort are the most commonly presenting physical symptoms among people suffering from LBP. They cannot sit or stand or perform any activity for long period of time. In severe cases LBP can be disabling and patients may be bedridden.

Social: People suffering from LBP have to limit their social lives to quite an extent. They may also avoid attending family functions.

Psychological: Some people suffering from LBP ignore it as they feel that routine pain-killers give only temporary relief. However, LBP, if severe, can interfere with activities of daily living making the patient depressive. They feel left out. It also causes loss of self-esteem. Even their sleep is disturbed (which may be due to pain/stiffness).

Economic: LBP is a major cause of work absenteeism and productivity loss at work. Thus, it causes financial burden on the individual as well as the family.

LBP is a symptom and not a disease. Therefore, for managing LBP, we need to have a clear understanding of the causes of LBP.

Initially, till some 50 years back, LBP was considered to be associated with degenerative (wear and tear) disorders among elderly. However, the changing trend suggests LBP to also be common among middle aged people (30-40 years) as well. This trend may be associated with lack of exercise/ physical activity, adoption of wrong posture, etc. To have a better understanding of this, we need to go back to the times of hunter-gatherers in the history of human civilization. The level of our physical activity and posture has changed significantly in comparison to the era of hunter-gatherers.

I. Physical activity

Evolutionary medicine suggests that hunter-gathers seldom complained of low back pain. During that era, the people were engaged in lot of physical activity in daily life. Walking for 9 to 15 km, climbing on trees, gathering plant foods, digging, hunting animals, lifting/carrying heavy stones or rocks, etc. were a part of their everyday routine. Thus, physical activity was not optional for them. With progress of time, the level of physical activity has declined. In present days, our lifestyle has almost become sedentary. In every sphere of life, viz. occupational, personal or housework, the level of physical activity has declined extraordinarily. With this the use of our muscles has also reduced.

For example, in older times around 100 years ago, warriors used a sword which involved physical activity of moving their hands. However, these are replaced by a revolver or rifle used by modern day cops, which does not involve even the moment of hands or arms. Walking or cycling was replaced by kick start scooters some 50 years back. Now in this mechanized world, the kick start of scooters/bikes has been replaced with push start button and now even cars have power steering.

Technology has also reduced the work load related to household activities among women. The vacuum cleaner has replaced the broom for cleaning the house. Mixer-grinder is used for cutting vegetables and food processor to

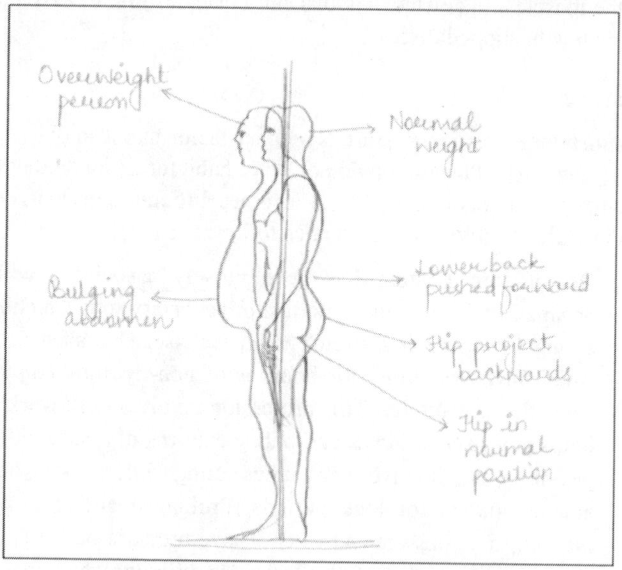

Fig. 12: Obesity putting the spine out of alignment.

dough the flour which was done earlier using hands. Moreover, use of automatic washing machines for washing clothes, etc. has certainly reduced the level of usage of our muscles and bodies. Owing to all these mechanized technologies our bodies have negatively adapted to being sedentary. These inactive adaptations have caused people to become overweight and obese.

Being obese means muscles of the body become weak and flabby (loose) especially those of abdomen. As the abdominal muscles become weak, the support to the spine decreases. This creates an imbalance in lumbar disc pressure which increases it chances of rupture. It also increases wear and tear of the facet joints. Moreover, weak abdominal muscles result in an expansion of the stomach wall (as is more evident in people who are overweight). This contributes to a posture where the low back is pushed forwardand hip backwards (Fig. 12).

This causes stress on the lower spine as it tries to maintain the balance posteriorly increasing the chances of LBP.The story does not end here. In today's scenario when lifestyle diseases like hypertension or diabetes are on the rise, weight reduction is needed. Often it happens that women in their 30's with the aim to lose weight join some fitness club or gym. Other reason for joining these clubs is to become physically attractive and have slim bodies.They may even fall for discount on membership of such clubs. In such a scenario, a lady who is not accustomed to regular exercise in routine is subjected to sudden overuse of the inactive muscles and bones. Sudden vigorous exercises often injure the muscles, ligaments, tendons and bones leading to LBP.They may also end up with slipped disc.

II. Posture

As mentioned earlier, posture is another factor that also plays a crucial role in causing LBP. Posture is habitual. Once habit forces our bodies to adopt a particular posture in our daily life, it becomes difficult to mend it. Posture is related to various activities which are as follows:

(a) Occupation: Posture has been closely associated with one's occupation. The trend of clerical or sedentary jobs which involves sitting for hours at a stretch is on the rise. One such occupation which involves sitting for hours is of non-teaching employees in educational institutes. This profession involves desk work for long hours at a stretch. Moreover, online entering of results, attendance, pay-slips, etc., involves continuous sitting while working on laptops and computers for long periods. Prolonged sitting in faulty or inappropriate posture causes excessive pressure on the spine. As a result the intervertebral disc loses its flexibility which may cause it to protrude from between the vertebrae (herniated disc). This increases the chances of developing LBP.

(b) Travel: Very often these women travel via 2-wheelers and cars. They habitually adopt wrong postures while driving and also if they are a passenger. While riding a two-wheeler, feet are wide apart in the same position for a long time which puts pressure on the low back and hips. While driving a car, in order to reach the clutch/ brake/ accelerator with feet, the lower back is brought forward creating a gap between the seat and the lower back (Fig. 13a). Similar posture is adopted, when we pull the seat too close to the steering (Fig. 13b). Travelling in buses involves standing for long periods in wrong postures which is also tiresome and puts pressure on the lower back. The baggage that women carry on their shoulders while travelling also puts pressure on the spine and cause LBP.

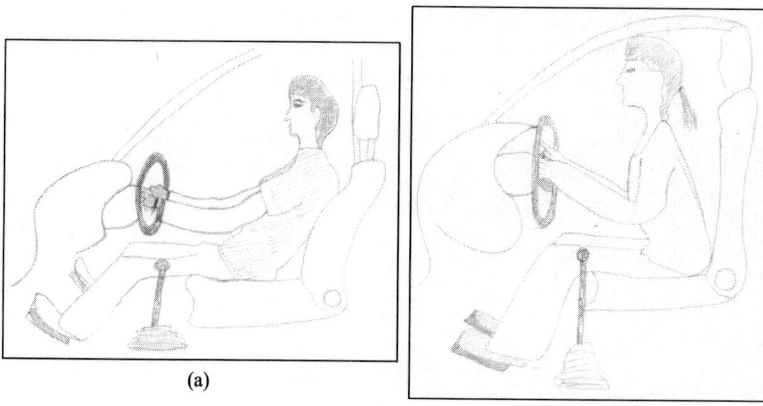

(a) (b)

Fig. 13: Wrong postures while driving car.

(c) Household activities: Non-teaching women employees bear a dual burden of work-office as well as household chores. This adds up as a contributing factor of LBP. While working in the modern day kitchens at home, women adopt standing posture for long hours. Using semi-automatic machines, while transferring clothes from the tub to the drier, women often adopt faulty posture that puts pressure on the back. Similarly, while using vacuum cleaners, standing with backs bent inappropriately also causes LBP. Thus, standing for long hours while at work or performing household work, often strains the back. Moreover, while watching TV for long hours we adopt incorrect postures which hurt the lower back and often aggravate it.

(d) Furniture: Another factor which influences posture is our furniture. Once bought any furniture is used for years. It is usually inherited. Thus, we are forced to use furniture which is either ancestral or that came as dowry say 20 years back. Many a times, such furniture, gifted by others is not favourable for a healthy posture. The ergonomic aspect is often ignored (i.e. it is not according to the individuals need) while ordering furniture. For example, in most cases the sofa used in the drawing room, does not support the lower back. Sometimes, the bottom seat portion of the sofa i.e. the width of the seat is too long. Thus, to sit comfortably, the individual will try to reach the floor with his feet. In order to adopt this posture, the individual has to drag his lower back parallel to the bottom portion of the seat leaving a gap between the lower back and the sofa (Fig. 14). As the lower spine has no support, this puts excessive pressure on the lower back causing LBP. Hence, the usual household furniture is not correct for the lower back.

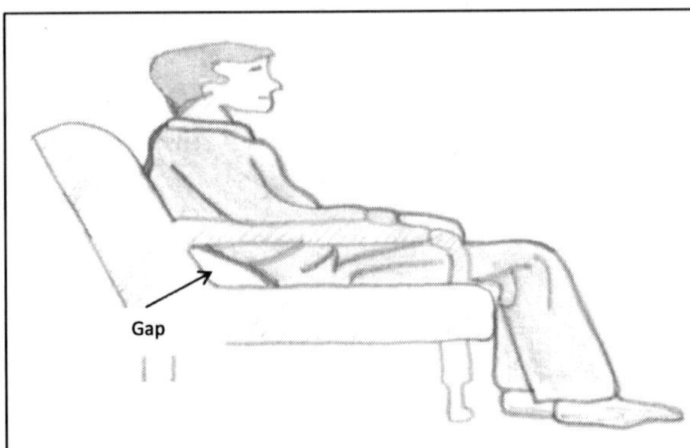

Fig. 14: Posture when the bottom portion of the sofa is too long (lower back has no support)

Similarly, the furniture used in offices is purchased in bulk. The chairs and tables used for working on computers, laptops or even writing tables are often incorrect and hurt the lower back. The details of the correct furniture are discussed in subsequent chapters.

(e) Footwear: Nowadays, trying to adopt the latest fashion, women wear high heels. Wearing high heels changes the posture considerably. This is because the leg goes into a position where the load is more on the forefoot (front part of the foot- known as *panja* in Hindi). The posture is shifted forwards. This puts pressure on the spine as it tries to maintain its normal position with respect to an unnatural height (changed platform) because of heels (Fig. 15).

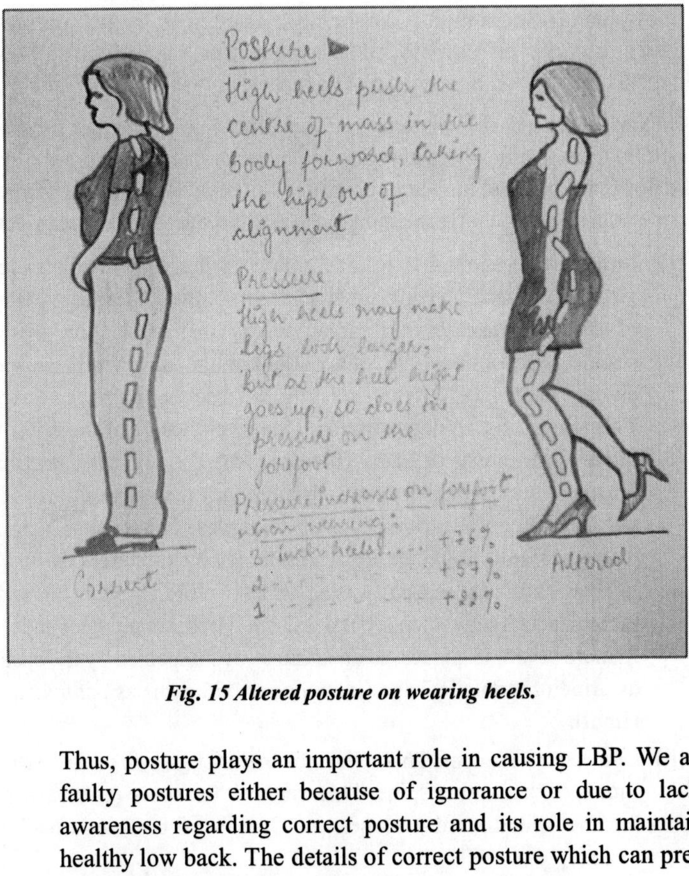

Fig. 15 Altered posture on wearing heels.

Thus, posture plays an important role in causing LBP. We adopt faulty postures either because of ignorance or due to lack of awareness regarding correct posture and its role in maintaining healthy low back. The details of correct posture which can prevent and treat LBP are discussed in subsequent chapters.

Other conditions that cause LBP

In addition to the above causes, there are other risk factors and conditions that cause LBP. However, discussion on these conditions is beyond the scope of this book but we are briefly describing them as in these **conditions you need to go to the doctor.**

1. Lumbar strain: Lumbar strain is considered one of the most common causes of low back pain. A lumbar strain is a stretching injury to the ligaments, tendons, and/or muscles of the low back. This can occur due to overuse, improper use, or (injury) trauma. In women it is caused because of the tendency to work at a stretch for hours trying to finish the household work as soon as possible. They also lift heavy things or shift furniture or say flower pots by themselves without any help. This causes sudden jerk in the lower back causing low back pain. The condition is commonly classified as "acute"(present for less than one month) or "chronic" (if lasts longer than three months). Lumbar strain most often occurs in people in their forties, but it can happen at any age.

2. Nerve irritation: The nerves of the lumbar spine can get pressed or irritated by disease any where along their paths i.e. their exit from the spinal cord till it reaches the skin. These conditions include lumbar radiculopathy, bony encroachment, and inflammation of the nerves caused by a viral infection.

(i) Lumbar radiculopathy: Radiculopathy is derived from latin terms viz "radix" meaning **root** and greek term "pathos" meaning **suffering** or **disease**.Thus, lumbar radiculopathy is irritation or pressing/ compression of the nerve roots of the lumbar spine that is caused by damage to the intervertebral discs i.e. the discs between the vertebrae. This occurs due to degeneration ("wear and tear") of the outer ring of the disc, injury, or both. Therefore, the central softer portion of the disc can rupture (herniated) through the outer ring of the disc and put pressure on the spinal cord or its nerves. This causes "sciatica" pain that shoots down the leg accompanied by numbness (*sunn hona* in Hindi) and tingling (*jhunjhunahat* in Hindi). The pain commonly increases with movements at the waist and with coughing or sneezing. In more severe instances, sciatica can be accompanied by the problem of urine or stools leakage (incontinence, knowns as *asanyamita* in Hindi).

(ii) Bony encroachment: This is the movement or growth of the vertebrae (bone) of the lumbar spine. This can limit the space (encroachment) for the spinal cord and nerves. Causes of bony encroachment include:

(a) Narrowing of the foramen through which spinal nerves pass out of the spinal canal to the body

(b) Slippage of one vertebra relative to another known as spondylolisthesis

(c) Spinal stenosis i.e. compression of the nerve roots or spinal cord by bony spurs or other soft tissues in the spinal canal. Spinal stenosis can cause lower-extremity pains that worsen with walking and are relieved by resting.

3. Bone and joint conditions: Bone and joint conditions existing from birth (congenital), due to wear and tear (degenerative) or injury, and inflammation of the joints (arthritis) can lead to low back pain.

(i) Congenital bone conditions—include scoliosis and spina bifida. Scoliosis is the sideways (lateral) curvature of the spine Spina bifida is a birth defect in the bony vertebral arch over the spinal canal, often with absence of the spinous process. This birth defect most commonly affects the lowest lumbar vertebra and the top of the sacrum.

(ii) Degenerative bone and joint conditions:As we age, the water and protein content of the body's cartilage changes. This change results in weaker, thinner, and more delicate cartilage. Because both the discs and the facet joints that stack the vertebrae are partly composed of cartilage, these areas are subject to wear and tear over time (degenerative changes). Degeneration of the disc is called spondylosis and degenerative arthritis (osteoarthritis) of the facet joints is also a cause of lumbar pain.

(iii) Injury to the bones and joints:Fractures (breakage of vertebral bone) of the lumbar spine and sacrum causes severe LBP. Vertebral fractures in younger patients occur only after severe trauma, such as from motor-vehicle accidents. In elderly, if bones are unhealthy, it can occur even on minimum stress on the spine e.g. bending to tie shoe laces.

(iv) Arthritis: The inflammatory types of arthritis e.g. ankylosing spondylitis can affect the lower back and sacroiliac joints. This causes low back pain and stiffness, which is typically worse in the morning. These conditions usually begin in the second and third decades of life.

4. Gynaecologic causes: It brings in a lot of discomfort to the ladies. LBP due to gynaecological causes are sacral and therefore felt below the region of L5 vertebra (below the level of the iliac crest). LBP can occur in physiological conditions like pregnancy and after child birth which recovers on its own after some time. However, if it does not, consultation with the doctor is needed. Pelvic inflammatory diseases (PID) i.e. infection of the female reproductive organs and Prolapse uterus (*bachhe dani bahar aana* in Hindi) are conditions very common in females. These often cause LBP.

5. Osteomalacia is also one of the causes of LBP in females. This occurs due to defeciency of vitamin D and calcium. The pain is felt in the lumbar spine, lower abdomen and both the thighs.

6. Psychological causes: Sometimes LBP can occur without any underlying pathology wherein emotional or psychological factors are involved. Stress, anxiety, negative mood can cause LBP.

All these factors may cause as well as aggravate LBP. Thus, the underlying pathology, if any, causing LBP should be treated appropriately. However, as discussed this book focuses on LBP caused by lack of physical activity and/or inappropriate body postures that can be reduced through simple measures taken by women. These are non-medicinal approaches and easy to follow. This can help in providing relief in LBP in majority of cases. The details are discussed in further chapters.

How healthy is our back: fitness test for different group of muscles

In the modern era, there have been significant changes in our lifestyle. We use power steering cars and two wheelers that start with a push button. We use lifts and escalators instead of the stairs. As for household work, we have access to automatic washing machines, food processors which have undoubtedly decreased our work load. However, all these facilities have greatly reduced the level of our physical activity. Moreover, when Indian women have come out of their houses to work, they have to bear the dual burden of work at office as well as home. They are occupied in office- meeting targets and deadlines. Simultaneously, at home in their families, they are busy looking after in-laws, husband and children. They end up sparing time for everyone but no time for themselves. As a result they do not take care of their health and rarely exercise. In Indian culture women usually do not do any exercise. This happens especially after marriage and is further reduced after they bear children. When women are asked to exercise they say, "*time hi kahan hai exercise ka. Office ke baad ghar mein bachhe and baki kaam hi itne hota hai, exercise kab karein*?" (We don't have time. After office we need to look after children and other household work, where do we get time to exercise?) This kind of lifestyle and daily routine is a major cause of low back pain in females.

Due to insufficient exercise and low level of physical activity, the muscles of the back and abdomen become weak. These lose their strength to support the spine which contributes to low back pain. On interacting with few working women while telling them about exercises for reducing low back pain, they had a common response that *"shaadi se pehle to hum saari exercises kar lete thay, but ab to hoti hi nai hai."– (Prior to getting married, we could do all these exercises so easily, but now it seems impossible).*

Here, the question arises, why is it difficult to do these exercises now when we were once able to do it easily. To know this, there is a need to test the strength of various muscles of the body that are important for maintaining a healthy back. This can be done by taking six simple tests shown below. These are known as the Kraus-Weber (K-W) tests.These are for everyone regardless of age, height or weight. These tests take into account different group of muscles including those of the back, hip, thigh and abdominal muscles.These together influence the condition of our back.

The pre-requisites of performing the test are:

- Take off your shoes.
- Make yourself comfortable.
- Breathe in and breathe out 2 times and try to relax your mind.

Test 1: To test the strength of hip muscles (Picture 1)

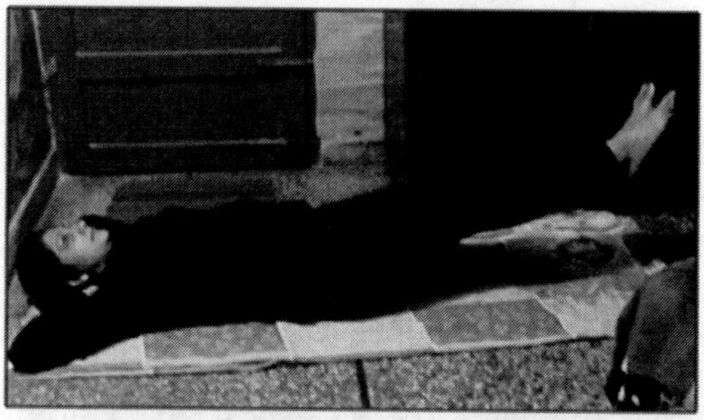

Pic. 1: Testing the strength of hip muscles.

1. Lie flat on your back
2. Put your hands with your fingers interlocked on the back of your neck.
3. Keep your legs straight and touching each other.
4. Now, while keeping your knees straight, try to lift your feet so that your heels are 10 inches above the floor as shown in picture 1.
5. You pass this test if you can hold this position for 10 seconds.

Test 2: To test if hip muscles and abdominal (stomach area and around) muscles combined are strong to handle your body weight (Picture 2)

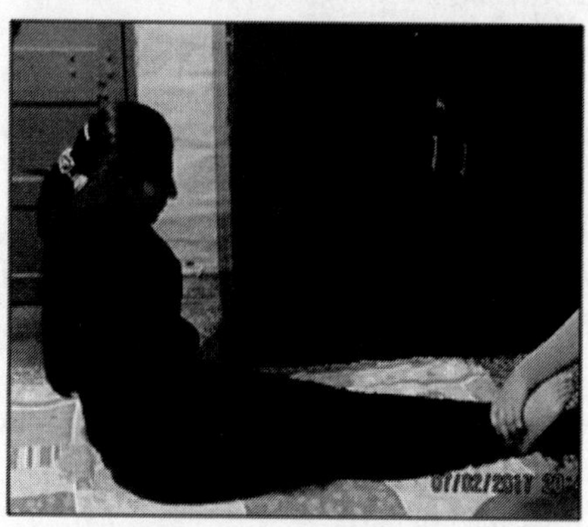

Pic.2: Testing the strength of hip and abdomen muscles.

1. Lie flat on your back
2. Put your hands with your fingers interlocked on the back of your neck.
3. Keep your legs straight and touching each other.
4. Ask someone to hold the ankles down your legs by holding (so that knees remain straight).
5. Now, try to roll up in sitting position (known as sit-up) without bending your knees.
6. You pass this test if you can do one sit-up.

Test 3: To test the strength of your abdominal (stomach area and around) muscles (Picture 3)

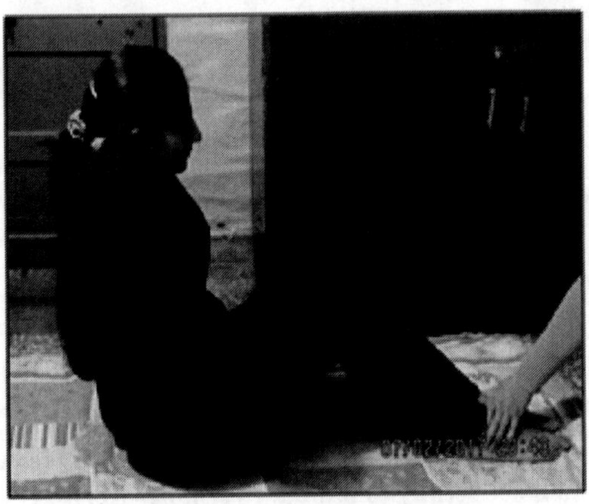

Pic. 3: Testing the strength of abdominal muscles.

1. Lie flat on your back
2. Put your hands (with your fingers interlocked) on the back of your neck.
3. Fold your knees. Make sure that someone holds your ankles.
4. Now, try to come to a sitting position as shown in the picture 3.
5. You pass this test if you can do one sit-up.

Test 4: To test if your back muscles are strong (Picture 4)

1. Lie over on your abdomen and put a pillow under it (i.e. under the stomach area and around).
2. Put your hands behind your neck.

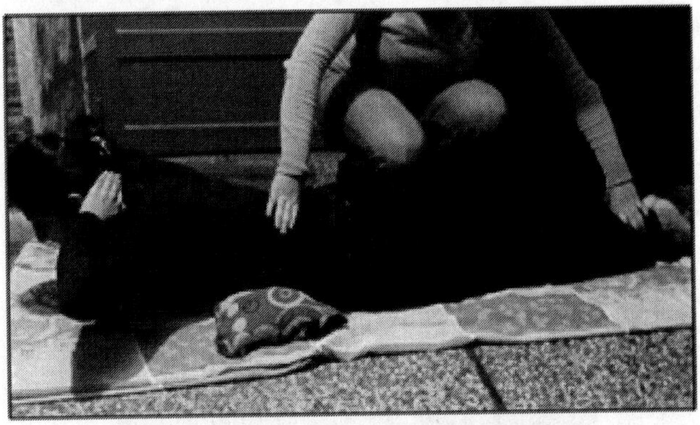

Pic. 4: Testing the strength of back muscles.

3. Ask someone to hold the lower half of your body by placing one hand on the lower back and the other on your ankles.
4. Now try to lift your trunk.
5. Your back muscles are strong if you can hold this position steady for 10 seconds.

Test 5: To test the strength of low back muscles (Fig. 16)

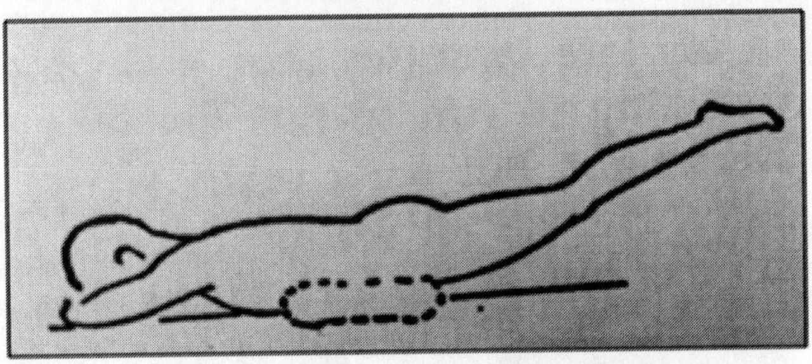

Fig. 16: Testing the strength of low back muscles

1. Lie on your abdomen and place a pillow under it.
2. Fold your arms under your head.
3. Now lift your legs 10 inches from the floor keeping your knees straight.
4. You pass this test if you can hold this position for ten seconds.

Test 6: To test flexibility of muscles of back, legs and back of thighs (Picture 5)

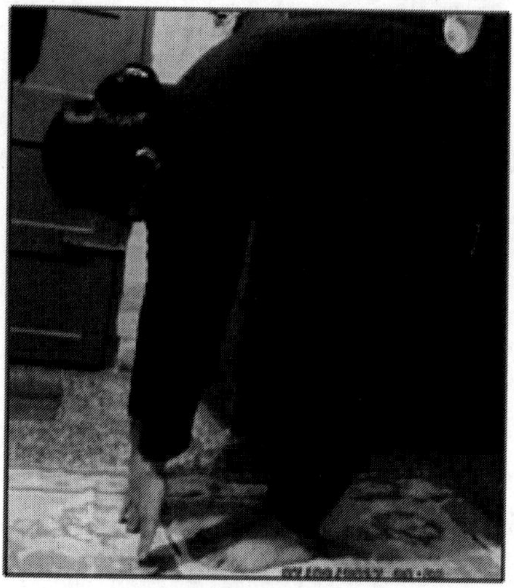

Pic. 5: Testing the flexibility of muscles of back, legs and back of thighs.

1. Stand up straight with feet together.
2. Now bend and try to touch the floor with your fingers by keeping the knees straight.
3. Keep your knees straight.
4. If you can hold this position, you pass this test. This shows flexibility of the muscles of your back, legs and back of the thigh.

These K-W tests are easy to perform and help to check our health. Passing all the six tests shows minimum level of muscular fitness i.e. there is enough strength and flexibility in the muscles to have a healthy back. However, if we fail or are unable to pass, even one of these six tests, it means that we are under- exercised and our muscles are stiff.

Clinical studies suggest that if you have failed one or more of the above mentioned tests and yet do not have back pain, you are likely to suffer from back pain in the future. So it is essential to exercise to have a healthy back and in-turn have healthy body. The details of exercises are discussed in following chapters.

Maintaining Correct posture

LBP is caused with the interplay of many factors. To treat and manage it, identifying the underlying cause is very important. If it is because of some underlying pathology, that needs to be treated. However, if it is because of factors such as lack of exercise/physical activity, wrong posture, wearing wrong footwear to using ergonomically incorrect furniture, etc., these need to be corrected.

LBP can be reduced and prevented by measures which can be divided into individual care and engineering methods. Individual care involves measures such as exercises and adopting a correct posture. Engineering methods include designing ergonomically correct workstation, kitchen, etc. In this chapter, we will discuss about the faulty postures we adopt while doing various activities and how can these be corrected. The suggested exercises and engineering measures for LBP are discussed in further chapters.

Individual care by adopting correct postures

Every day, we perform various activities like standing, sitting, driving and doing various household chores, etc. However, while doing these we unconsciously adopt wrong postures. Over time these become our habits. As it is said, bad habits die hard; it is not easy for us to correct our postures in a day or two. However, if we are aware about serious implications of our bad and wrong postures, we can correct them. The more we become conscious about harm of our bad postural habits; the more it is easy to change these.

A good correct posture improves our appearance and adds to a glowing personality. It also reduces pains and aches. Moreover, it helps in maintaining a healthy lower back. Various postures we adopt while performing some of the activities of the day are described below:

1. **Standing**: Most often, we casually stand in postures as shown in picture 6 & 7.

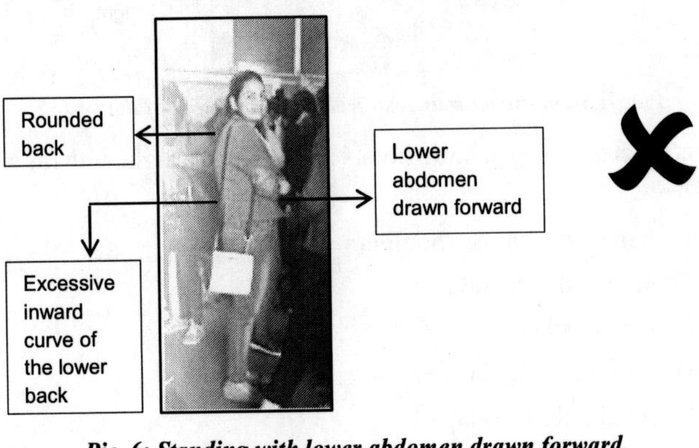

Pic. 6: Standing with lower abdomen drawn forward.

Standing for long period of time often causes severe pain that hurts the back, knees and the feet. The reasons for such discomfort are given below:

(a) Lower abdomen drawn forward: This may happen unconsciously as we stand. This posture is also often adopted, when our belly is hanging out, especially in overweight people. This puts pressure on the spine esp. lower part, causing it to curve more inwards/forward than usual. As a result the upper back becomes more rounded as shown in picture 6. Wearing tight jeans is also another factor which can cause the lower back to curve excessively inwards. Women often wear these to hide belly fat. This further causes the stomach muscles to become loose. This strains the muscles, joints, ligaments, etc. of the lower back. As a result, the surrounding nerves get irritated causing LBP.

(b) Uneven weight on one side of the body: As we stand, we have a habit of putting more weight on one side of the body as shown in picture 7. This puts pressure on one side of the spine sometimes causing LBP.

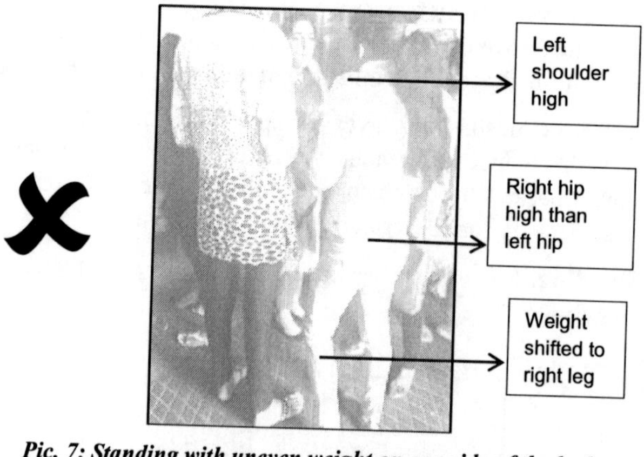

Pic. 7: Standing with uneven weight on one side of the body.

The correct standing posture involves standing straight with (as shown in picture 8):

(i) Ears in line with the shoulders.

(ii) Shoulders down and back.

(iii) Stomach tucked in.

(iv) Hips in line with the shoulders.

(v) Knees should be relaxed.

(vi) Feet need to be hip width apart.

With this posture, the weight of the body is evenly distributed on both sides (as shown in picture 8 & 9). In this position, the spine is least strained and chances of LBP are minimum.

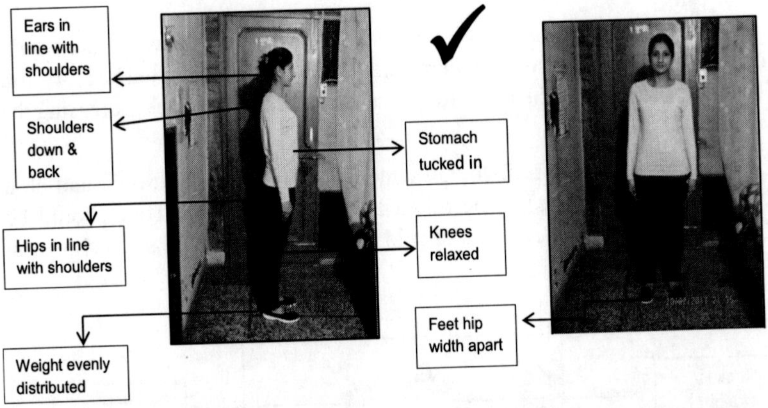

Pic. 8: Correct standing posture. ***Pic. 9: Correct standing posture.***

2. Texting while standing: Nowadays, the use of smartphones has definitely made communication easier. Phones are used not just for calling but also surfing the internet, texting, etc. However, the posture we adopt while using smartphones are often faulty. We often stand with neck bent down, shoulders rounded and putting weight on one leg as shown in Picture 10.

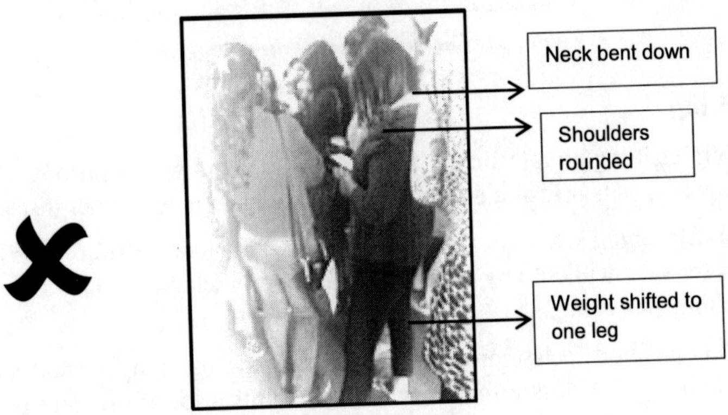

Pic.10: Usual texting posture.

This puts pressure on the neck/cervical spine. Sometimes, the cervical spine losses its natural curve (i.e. pushed forward). This irritates the surrounding nerves which causes neck pain. Sometimes, pain from the neck also runs down the arm. Often pain is accompanied with numbness in the arm and hand. This is referred to as cervical spondylosis.

Now due to bad posture, the cervical spine is pushed forward. As a result, in order to balance the body's alignment, the lower spine is also pushed forward. This puts pressure on the muscles, joints, etc. of the lower back increasing the chances of LBP.

The correct posture involves standing tall with neck straight and chin up. The shoulders need to be relaxed and squared. The phone should be raised to chin height. The feet should be kept hip width apart as shown in Picture 11.

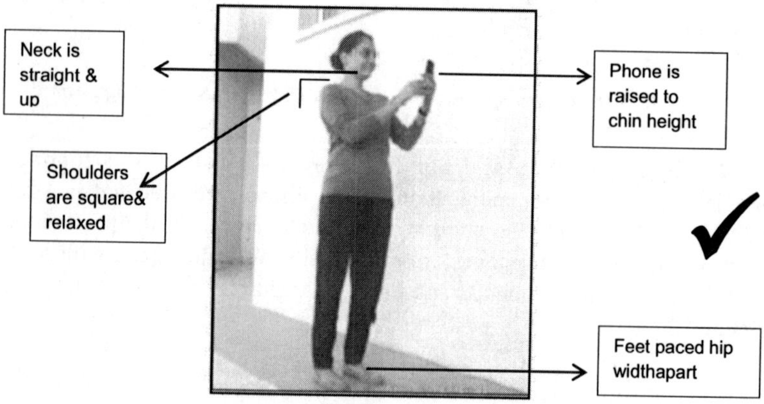

Pic. 11: Correct posture while texting.

3. Sitting

While sitting on a chair, we unconsciously adopt wrong postures. This unknowingly puts pressure on our lower back and compresses our discs.

(a) Slouching in a chair: Commonly, we sit on a chair with our lower back drawn forward without any support as shown in Picture 12. This is called 'slouching' in a chair.

This position feels more comfortable than sitting straight and upright because it requires less effort. However, this puts a lot of pressure on the lower back. In this posture, the lower abdomen is pushed forward, leaving the lower back to support the weight of the upper body. Moreover, the muscles of the abdomen and lower back that support the spine are weak due to lack of

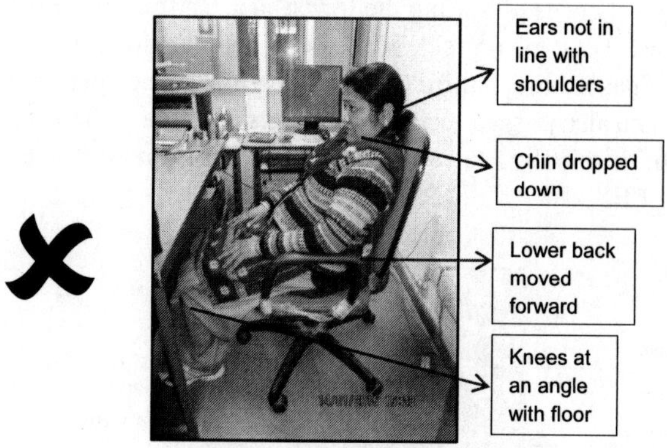

Pic. 12: Slouching in a chair.

exercise, etc. This puts pressure on the joints and ligaments of the lower back. As a result, the upper back becomes rounded and shoulders shift forward.

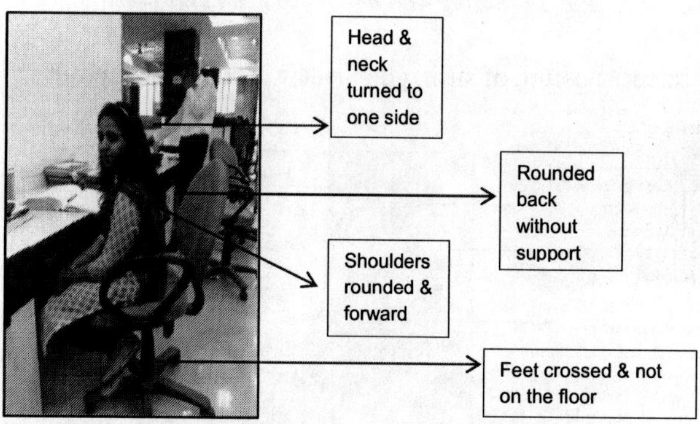

Pic. 13: Sitting on front part of chair.

(b) Sitting on the front portion of the chair: Another common sitting posture is, to sit on the front portion of the chair without any lower back support. The upper back and shoulders are also rounded as shown in picture 13. In this position the spine is C-shaped. Due to this the stomach muscles become loose and soft. This puts pressure on the lower spine muscles, joints, ligaments, etc. This irritates the surrounding nerves which cause LBP. Moreover, here, the feet and legs are crosssed and curled inside to rest on the base support of the chair. This puts pressure on the knees and feet also.

(c) Sitting with legs crossed: We are in a habit of sitting with legs crossed, keeping one knee above the other (picture 14). We unconsciously adopt this posture as it seems to be comfortable. However, sitting like this for long time increases the chances of hurting the lower back. In this position, the hips are at unequal level placing one side of the body higher than the other as shown in picture 14. Thus making it difficult to sit up straight. The lower spine is shifted to one side and also pushed forward. This puts pressure on the muscles, joints, ligaments of the hips and lower back. This overtime, increases the chances of developing LBP.

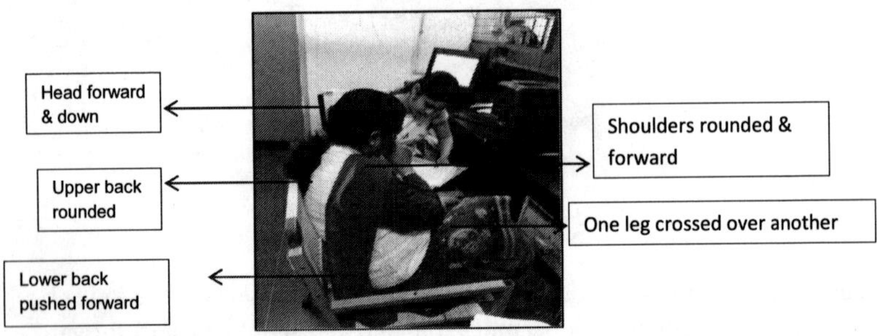

Pic. 14: Sitting with one leg crossed over other

The correct posture of sitting on a chair is shown in picture 15

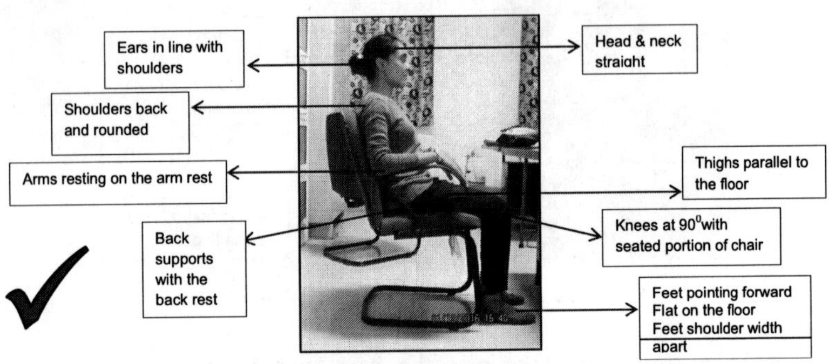

Pic. 15: Correct sitting posture on a chair

- The upper and lower back are supported with the backrest of the chair.
- The neck should be line with the shoulders.
- The shoulders in line with the hips.
- The arms should rest on the arm rest of the chair.
- Thighs need to be parallel to the floor.
- Knees should be at 90^0 with the seated portion of the chair.

- Feet flat on the floor and pointing forward.
- In short women, as the feet don't reach the floor, either the legs keep hanging or they shift to the front portion of the chair. Because of this, the lower back remains unsupported. To overcome this problem a footrest (known as *patara* in Hindi) or short stool can be used.

However, sometimes the lower back does not fit in to the lower curve of the back of the chair as shown in picture 16. Moreover, many times, the backrest of the chairs are hollow because of which the lower back cannot be supported (picture 17).

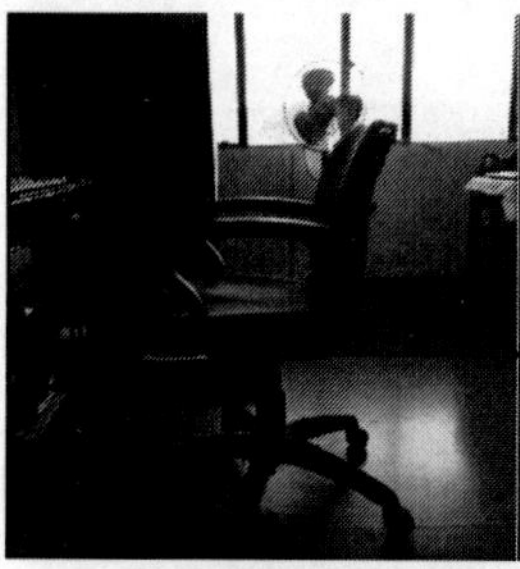

Pic. 16: Curve on the lower back of the chair.

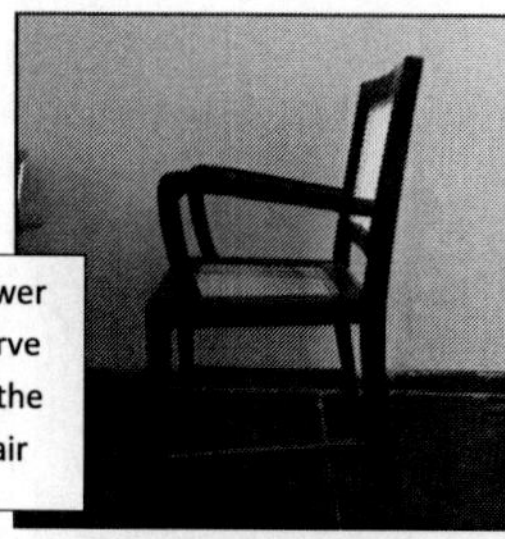

Pic. 17: Hollow back rest of the chair.

To overcome the above problems, keeping a cushion on the chair will support the lower back and decrease the pressure on it.

4. Working on the desk

We often adopt wrong postures while working on the desk. The head and neck are bent forward and down. The back is rounded and unsupported. Even the thighs and knees are wrongly placed. The common wrong postures while working on the desk are shown in pictures below. In most of these pictures, the upper back is rounded with shoulders dropping forward (picture 18; 19) or C-shaped as shown in picture 20 & 21. This posture is commonly known as hunching. This makes the stomach muscles loose putting pressure on the lower spine. This increases chances of developing LBP.

Moreover, as shown in the pictures, the neck and head are placed forward and down. Usually, the head and neck need support from the body to keep its movement effortless. However, rounded back, shoulders placed forward and chest drawn inwards do not give the head and neck adequate support. Due to this the neck muscles get strained and stressed as these try to support the head by themselves. This can cause neck pain.

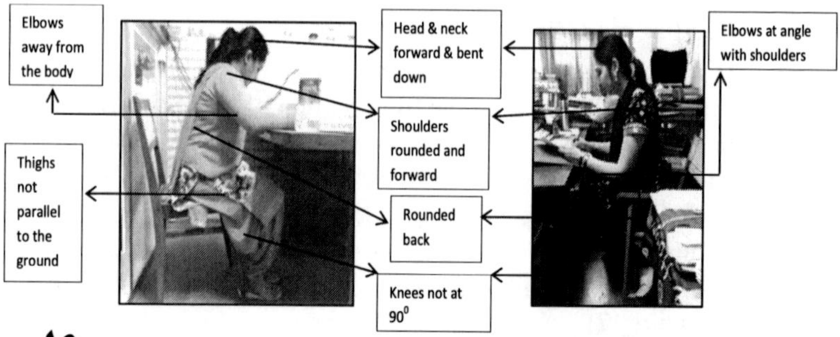

✗ *Pic. 18* *Pic. 19*

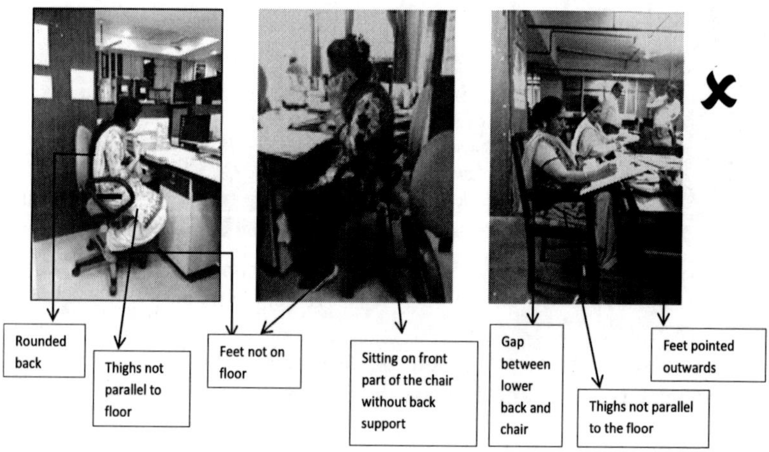

✗

Pic. 20 *Pic. 21* *Pic. 22*

Sometimes, as advised by our doctor we follow measures which can reduce LBP. These include, using a cushion while sitting on a chair to support our back; use a footrest for stability and comfort as shown in picture 22. Here, although the back is supported with a cushion, yet there is space between the cushion and lower back. Thus, this position is wrong. Moreover, the footrest is too high. Because of this, the knees are placed higher than the thighs. Thus, the thighs are not parallel to the floor and knees are also not at 90^0 to the seated portion of the chair. This puts pressure on the soft and weak knee muscles increasing chances of knee pain in the long run.

The correct posture for working on the desk is shown picture 23.

- The upper and lower back is supported with the backrest of the chair.
- The neck should be line with the shoulders.

- The chin is placed up and straight
- The shoulders in line with the hips.
- The arms should rest on the arm rest of the chair.
- Thighs need to be parallel to the floor.
- Knees should be at 90^0 to the seated portion of the chair.
- The feet point forward resting on the floor. In short people, the use of footrest is comforatble
- A table top or a hard board to work as table top can laso be used as shown in pic 22. This will avoid straining the neck.

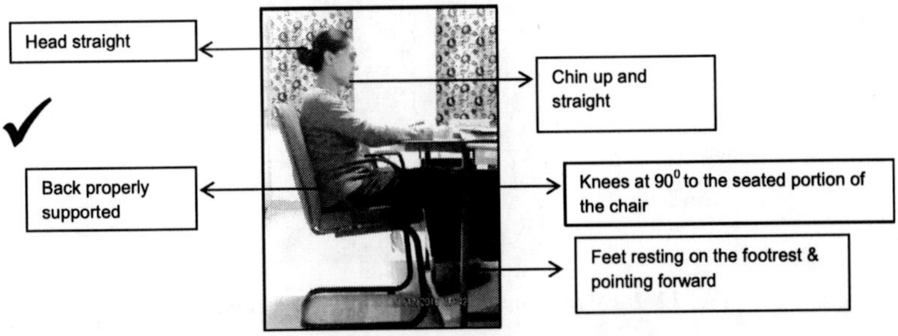

Pic. 23: Correct posture while working on desk.

4. Working on the desktop

We often either slouch or hunch our backs while working on the computer shown in picture 24 & 25. These wrong postures not only cause pain in the lower back but also cause pain in the neck and upper back. In picture 24, the desktop is placed too far from the body. In order to reach up to the desktop, the lower back and hips are shifted forward (slouch) causing LBP.

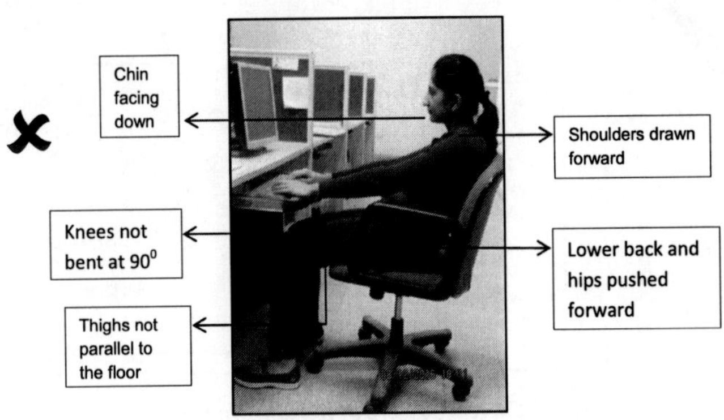

Pic. 24: Slouch while working on computer.

In picture 25, the body is placed too close to the laptop. The upper back is rounded and lower back is bent. Since, the laptop is placed far at the level of the shoulders the neck has to bend forward and down. This increases the chances of developing neck pain along with LBP.

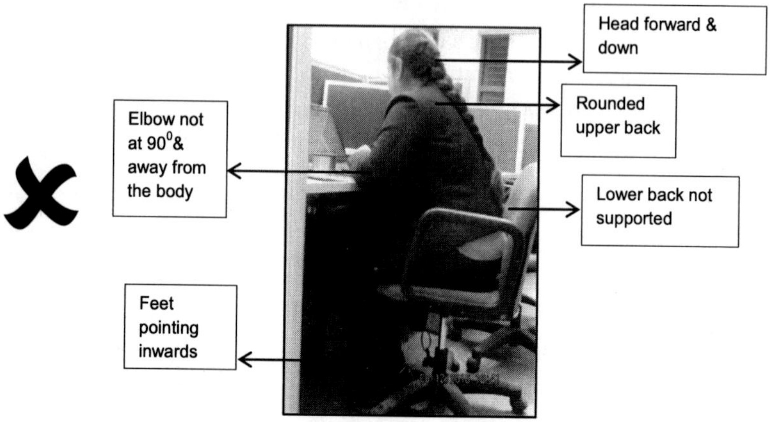

Pic. 25: Incorrect posture while working on computer.

While working on the computer the correct posture is (shown in Fig. 17):

- The monitor is roughly arm's length away.

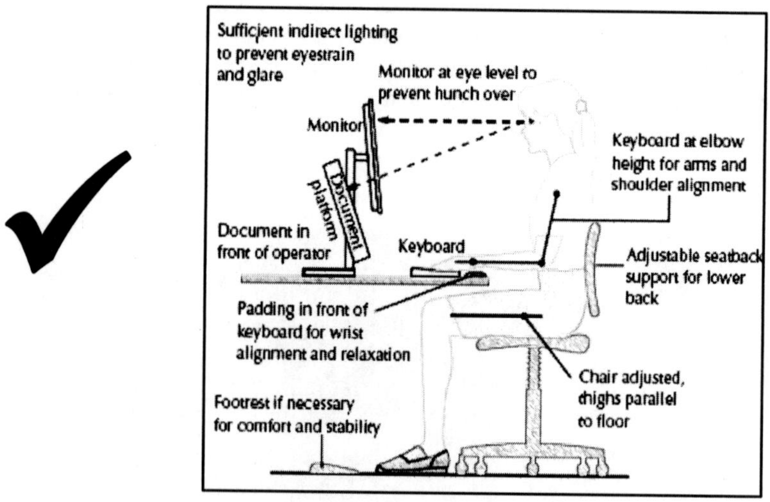

Fig. 17: Correct posture of working on computer.

- The monitor (upper edge of the screen) should be at or just below eye level to prevent hunch over. However, if this is not the case, the height of the monitor can be readujusted upto the eye level by placing a block or hard register below the monitor.
- The ears should be in line with the shoulders.
- The elbows must be close to the body and supported with armrests.
- The keyboard must be at elbow height.
- The lower back should be supported with the back rest of the chair.
- The thighs parallel to the floor
- Knees must be 90^0 to the thighs
- Feet pointing forward on the floor or footrest for comfort and stability.

6. Sitting on the sofa/couch

We often sit on the sofa in relaxed posture which most of the times is wrong and bad for the lower back. The common ways we sit on the sofa are shown below.

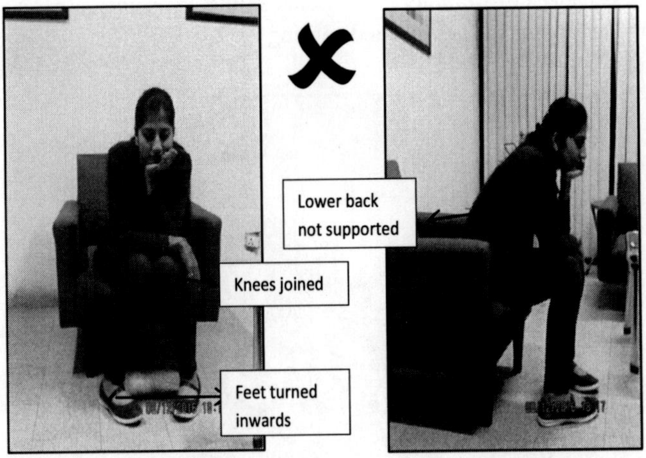

Pic. 26: Incorrect posture of sitting on sofa.

Pic. 27: Hunched posture on sofa.

In pic. 26 & 27, the lower back is not supported. Moreover, a hunched position also adds to the pressure on the lower back. This increases the chances of LBP. The knees are also bent and feet pointed inward which put pressure on the knees. This increases the chances of knee pain.

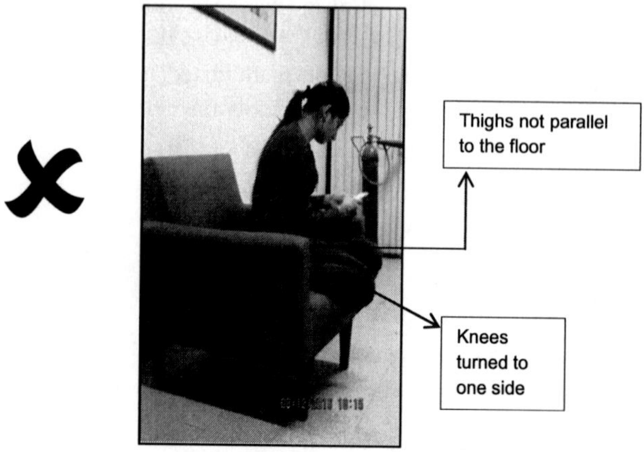

Pic. 28: Front view with knees turned to one side

In picture 28 & 29, the hips are at unequal level placing the right side of the lower back higher than the left. This causes the spine to shift to one side incresing chances of straining the muscles, joints, ligaments, etc. As a result the surrounding nerves get irritated causing LBP.

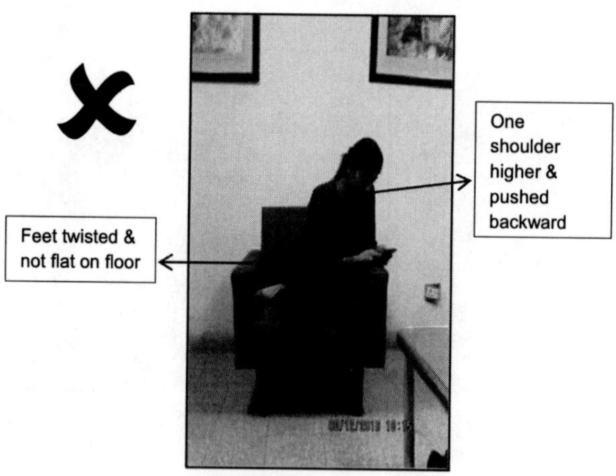

Pic. 29: Front view with knees turned to one side.

Moreover, the neck and head are placed down and forward putting pressure on the neck. This increases chances of neck pain. The knees are also turned to one side putting undue pressure on the knees.

Another common posture we adopt on the sofa is we slouch in order to sit comfortably as shown in picture 30 & 31. However, in this posture, the abdomen (i.e.stomach area) is pushed forward. The low back muscles have to bear the weight of the upper body increasing the chances of straining the lower back.

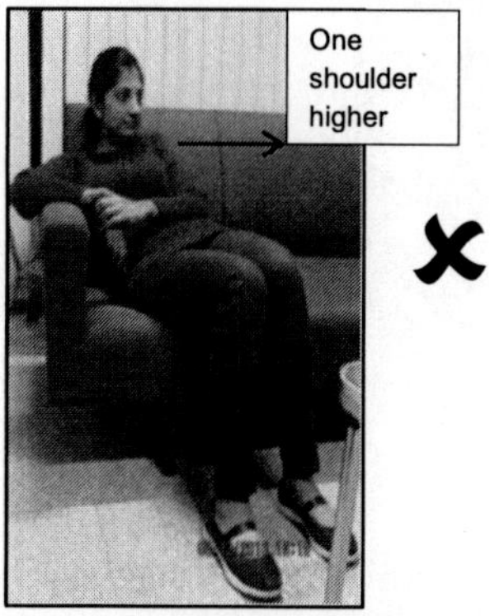

Pic. 30: Slouching on sofa-front view.

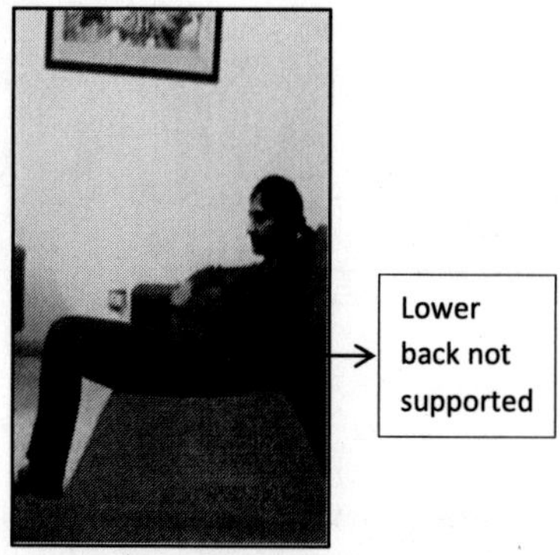

Pic. 31: Slouch on sofa-side view.

On the contrary, we should sit on the sofa as shown in picture 32 & 33.

- The upper and lower back needs to be supported (picture 32).
- The neck and head should be upright (picture 33).
- Ears should be in line with the shoulders.
- Shoulders should be in line with the hips.
- Knees should be at 90^0 to the seated portion of sofa (picture 7 ii).
- Feet need to be pointing forward and flat on the floor (picture 7 iii).

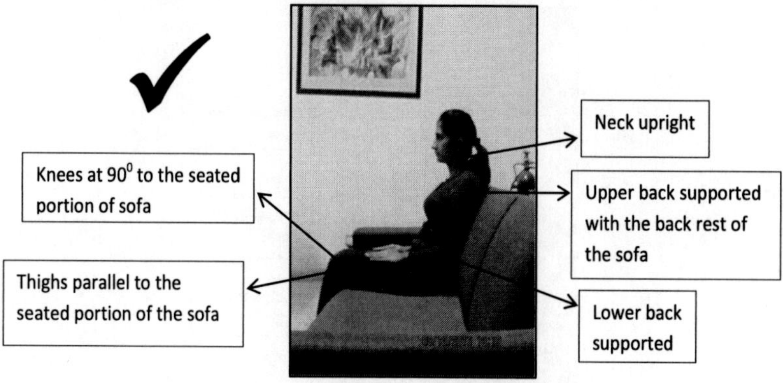

Pic. 32: Correct posture on sofa-side view.

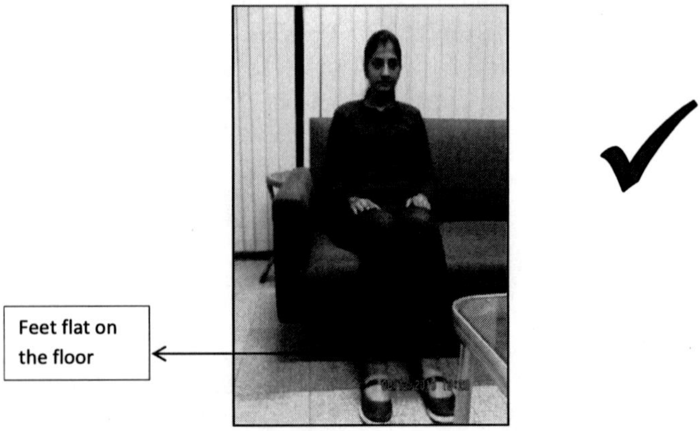

Pic. 33: Correct posture on sofa-front view.

However, we would still think that if sofas are made to sit easily then why should we sit in a posture that involves so much effort. In order to sit on the sofa with ease. We should sit with legs crossed i.e. *chowkari* in Hindi, with lower and upper back supported with the backrest of the sofa.

7. Lifting heavy things from the floor

We often carry or lift itmes that weigh 50-70% of our body weight. Ideally, it should weigh 40% of our body weight. Moreover, while doing this we unconciously adopt bad or faulty postures. Both these factors i.e. carrying heavy weight and faulty postures are not good for our lower back. This results in straining most commonly the lower back muscles, joints, tendons, ligaments, etc. causing LBP.

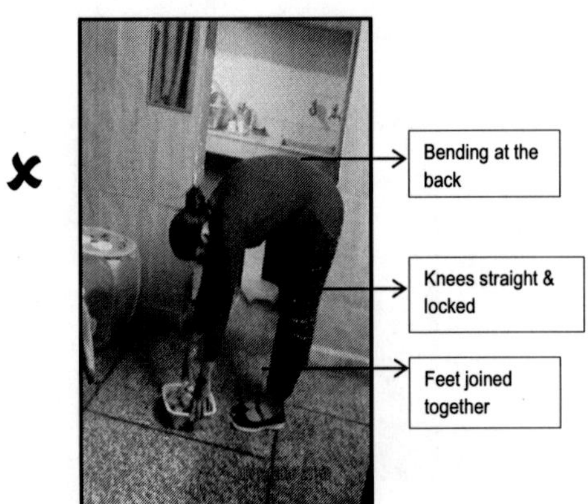

Pic. 34: Lifting with bending at the back.

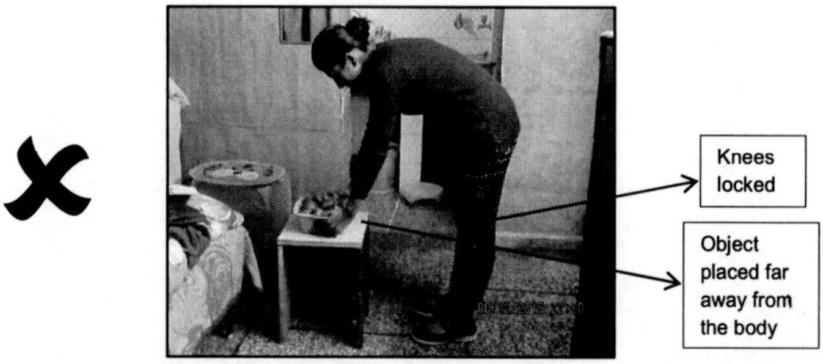

Pic. 35: Lifting with object far from the body.

The most common lifting postures we adopt in daily life are shown in picture 34 & 35.

In these postures, the object is placed away from the body. This causes the arms to outstretch in order to reach out to the object. This puts pressure on the lower spine while bending to lift the object. Moreover, the knees are kept straight with feet joined together. Also, the feet are not under the hips i.e. not in straight line. Due to this, the body might become unstable. So, to avoid a fall, the body tends to round from the back. This strains the lower back increasing chances of developing LBP.

The correct posture of lifting things is shown in pictures 36-38.

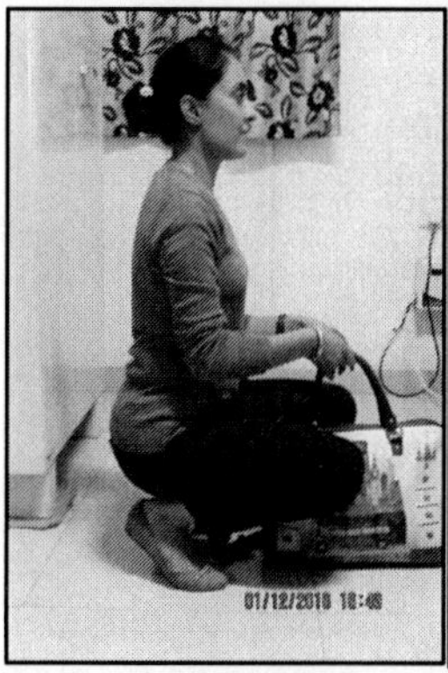

Pic. 36

- Sit on your toes with knees apart (squatting position) with the object between your knees.
- The back should be straight.
- Keep the head upright looking in front.

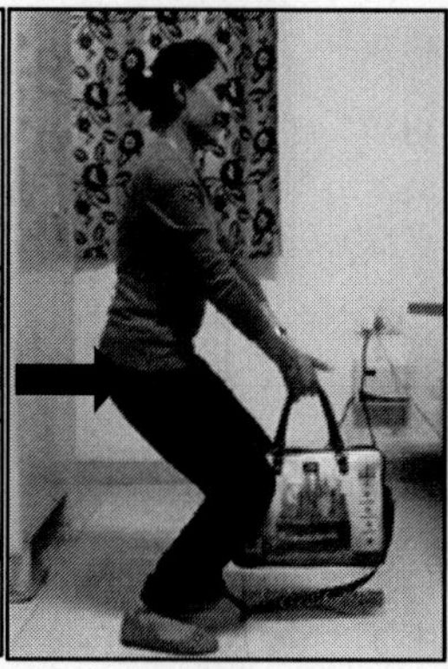

Pic. 37

Using your legs, stand up, bringing the object closer to your body.

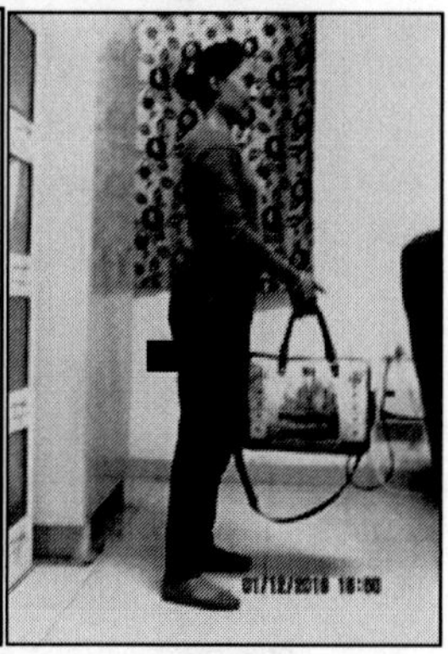

Pic. 38

Be sure to keep your back straight

There is another method of lifting things as shown in pic. 39 & 41.

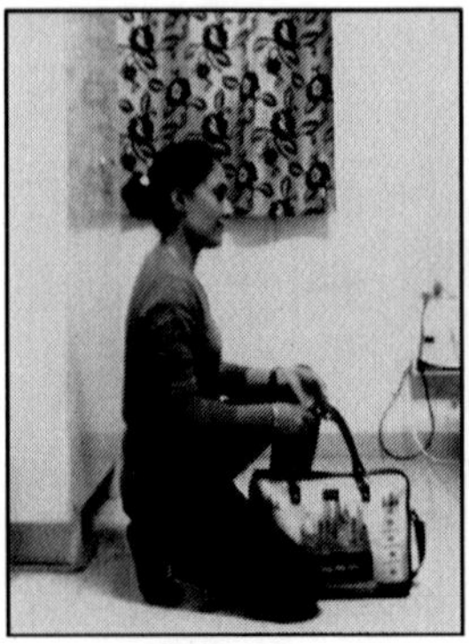

Pic. 39

- Keep one knee on the floor
- Keep your back straight
- Head and neck upright
- Look in front

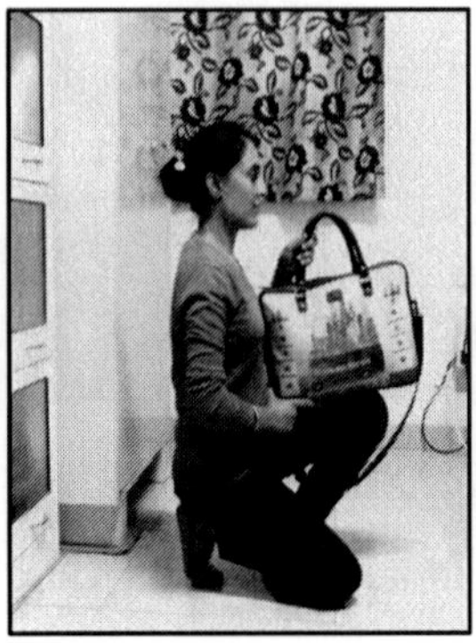

Pic. 40

- Using your arms, move the object up on the opposite thigh
- Keep your back straight
- Head and neck upright and looking in front

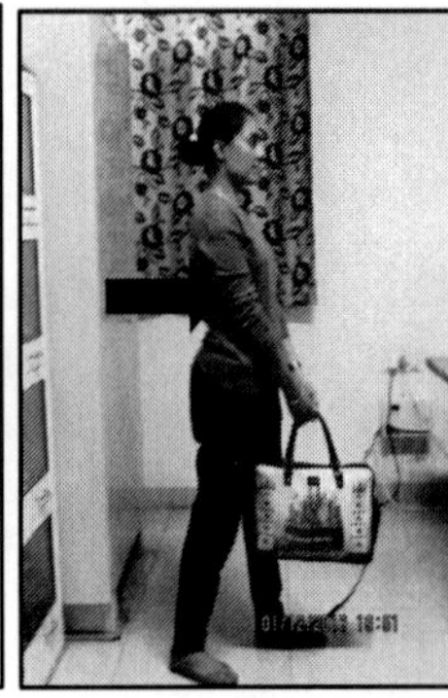

Pic. 41

Then, stand up keeping the back straight.

In both the methods discussed above, the knees and hips are used. This puts less pressure on the spine as it is kept straight. Thus, before lifting heavy objects we should keep few important things in mind:

- Assess the weight of the object before lifting it. Ask for help if the weight is more than 40% of your body weight.
- Keep the object close to body before lifting it.
- The feet should be shoulder width apart to provide balance to the body.
- Use the knees and hips and not the back when reaching out for the object.
- We should try and look straight and not down at the object. This is because when we lift the object our concentration is on the object itself. In this scenario, we chances of moving the neck up suddenly are high.This may cause a jerk in the neck which can cause neck pain.

8. Picking small things from the floor

While picking up small things from the floor, we hurriedly and unconsciously round our lower back. Such inappropriate bending increases the risk of jerk/strain or sprain in the back. Multiple factors acting together contribute to this condition. Some of them are:

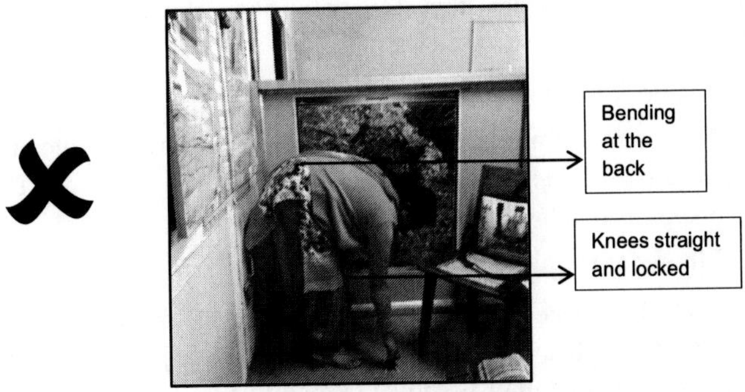

Pic. 42: Picking things with bend at back.

- The knees are straight. This causes to round our lower back as shown in picture 42.

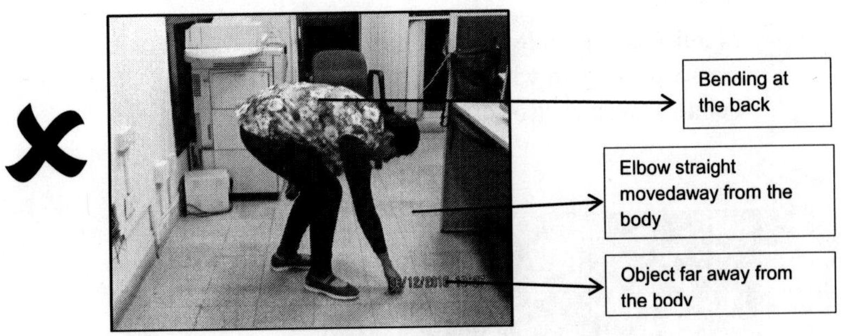

Pic. 43: Picking object kept far from body.

- Most often, the object is kept far from the body as shown in picture 43.

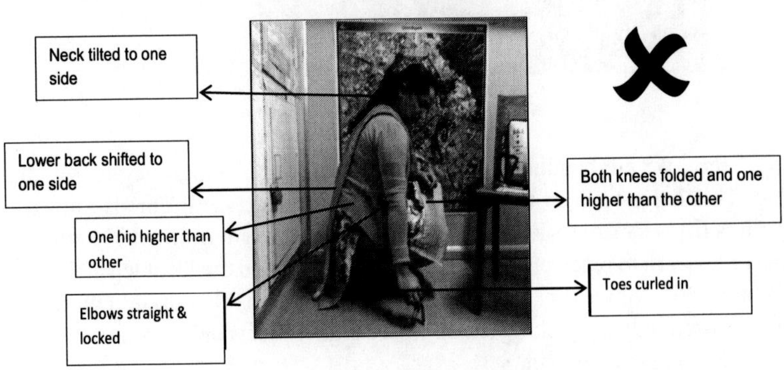

Pic. 44: Incorrect posture of picking things.

In picture 44 the object is kept close to the body. However, in this posture, as can be seen, there are some faults as follows:

- The neck is tilted to one side.
- The woman is sitting on the toes but both knees are at unequal level. Because of this, the lower spine is shifted to one side. This also positions one hip higher than the other.
- Elbows are straight and locked.

However, the correct way of picking small things from the floor should be same as for lifting heavy objects [refer pictures 47-53]. Another simple and correct way of picking things is shown in picture 53.

- Stand with feet hip or shoulder width apart.
- Support one hand on the shelf or some furniture.
- Now reach out for the object with the other hand by bending forward.
- Simultaneously slide or raise one leg out behind you. For example, if we are picking up with the right hand raise the left leg. This will be comfortable and also easier to maintain balance.

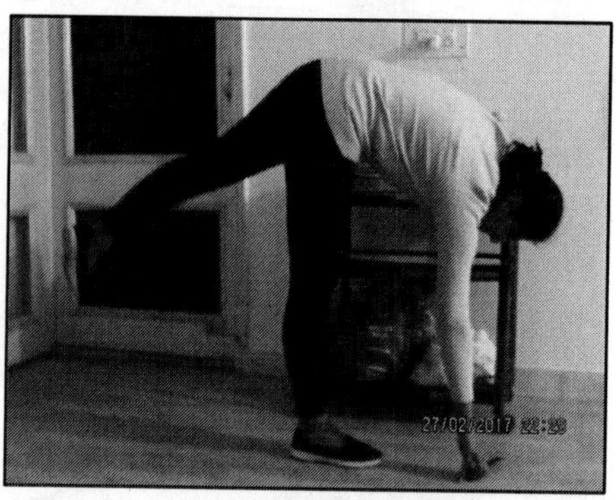

Pic. 45: Golfer's lift to pick up things.

Here, we are bending forward at the hip of the straight leg or standing leg. This helps to keep the spine straight and unstressed. This is known as golfers lift because it is similar to the lift used in the game of golf. Now, as we move forward to reach out for the object, we can bend the front leg at the knee [picture 46]. Moreover, we can also bend the leg that is raised behind. This can be used only for picking small/ lightweight objects or when we cannot get close enough to an object.

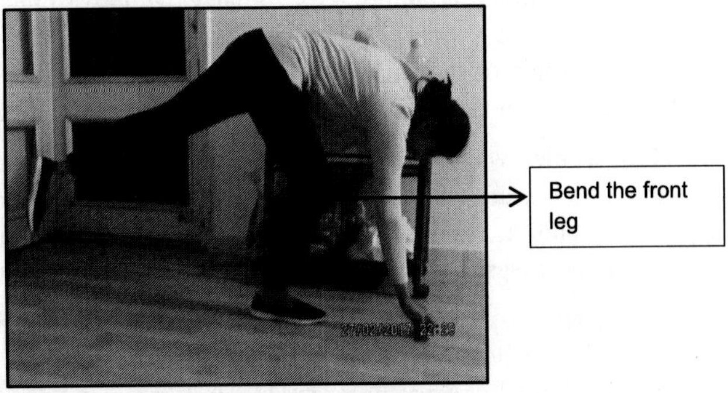

Pic. 46: Variation of golfer's lift by bending the forward leg.

One mistake which can happen, while adopting this posture is, we might first bend our body forward to reach out for the object and then raise the leg out. However, bending forward and raising the leg out must happen simultaneously.

9. Performing household chores

Women are in a habit of finishing their household chores as quickly as possible. However, while doing this, they often unconsciously adopt wrong postures because of which they commonly strain their backs. Thus, correcting postures while performing various household activities is important. Postures adopted while doing a few household activities are discussed here.

I. Cooking/Washing Utensils: Working in modern kitchens involves standing for long hours. We often stand with our lower back bent. Also the upper back is rounded. While cooking, often the shelf of the kitchen is not suitable to the height of the woman. This leads the woman to wrongly bend

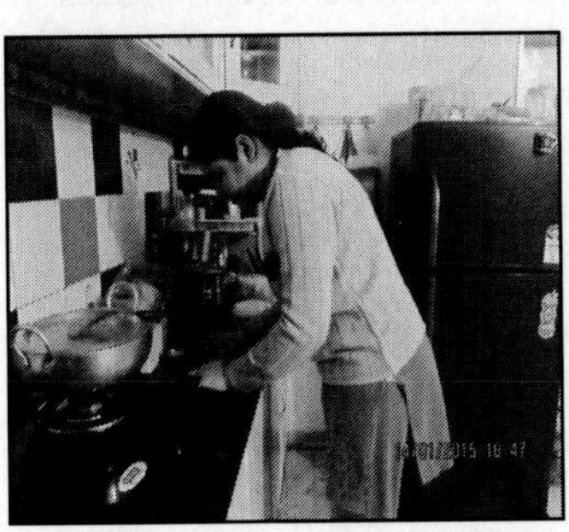

Pic. 47: Bending the back.

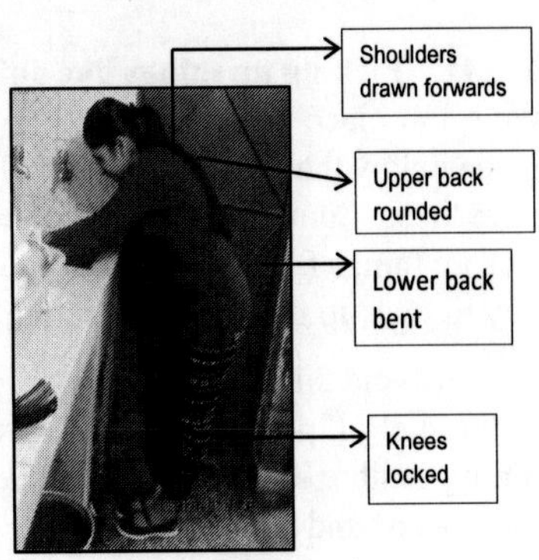

Pic. 48: Bending the back.

their backs as shown in picture 47. Similarly, while washing utensils at the sink, the lower back is bent inappropriately [picture 48]. This occurs mainly because the height of the sink is not according to the height of the woman. Mostly, the distance of the tap is paced far from the edge of the sink.

Thus, women while washing utensils, outstretch their hands. As a result the shoulders are drawn forward, upper back becomes rounded and lower back is also bont as shown in pictures 47 & 48. This wrong position of the lower back increases the chances of stress/injury causing LBP.

The correct posture involves, bend at the hips keeping the lower back straight. This can be done by standing close to the sink and using a small footrest commonly known as *patara* in Hindi. With its use, the bend will be at the hips and not the lower back. The ears should be in line with the shoulders and elbows resting at the edge of the sink [picture 49 & 50].

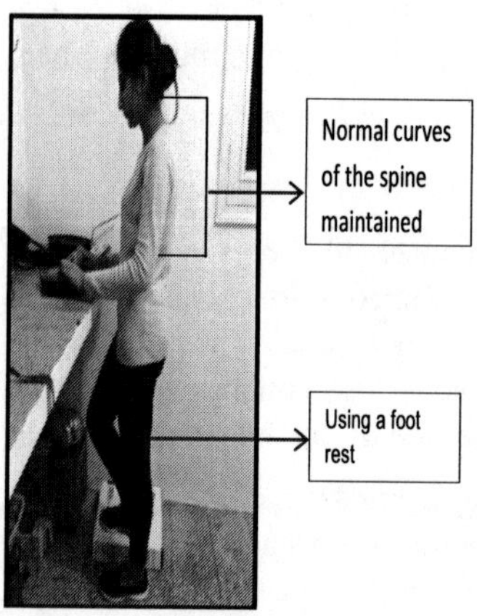

Pic. 49: Correct posture while cooking.

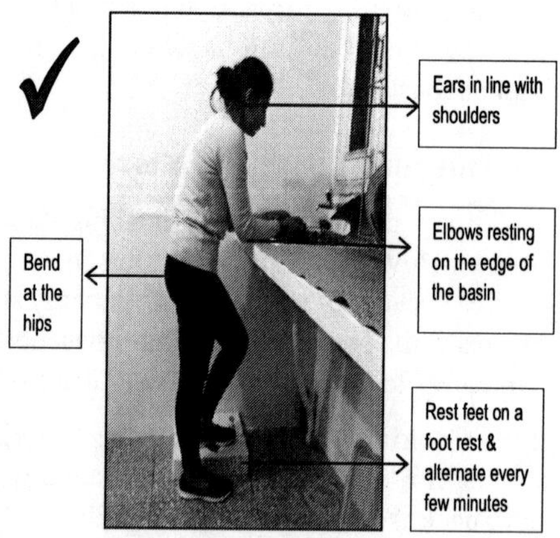

Pic. 50: Correct posture while washing utensils.

II. Picking up things like onions/potatoes from the vegetable basket: We often place onions/potatoes in a vegetable basket in the kitchen in the space below the shelves. We usually bend our backs to pick onions/potatoes from these. Sometimes, our back hurts while bending so we ask someone to pick up things from the basket. This is because we bend our backs in a wrong way to pick up things as shown in picture 51.

To avoid this pain in low back, we should try placing the vegetable basket on the shelf, if possible, so that we don't bend our lower back. However, if it is not possible, we should stand close to the basket and sit on our toes with knees apart and pick things from the basket as shown in picture 52.

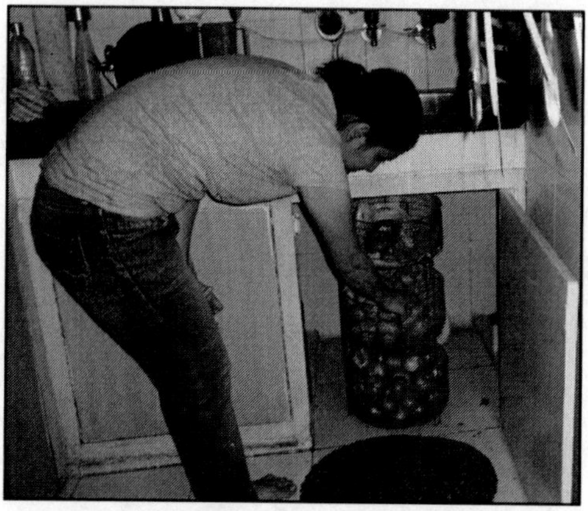

Pic. 51: Wrong posture while taking things from vegetable basket

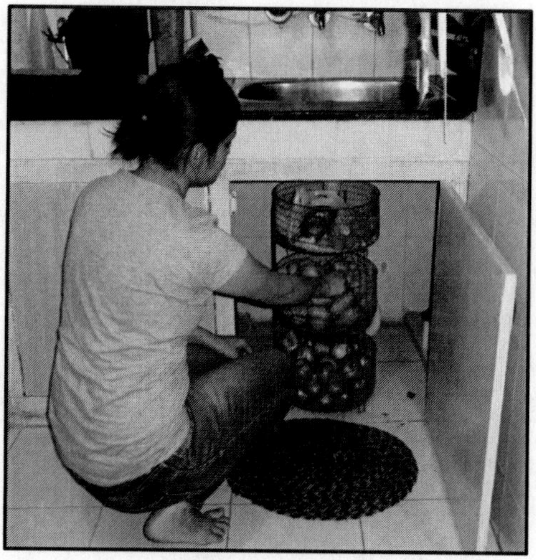

Pic. 52: Correct posture while taking things from the basket.

III. Sweeping the floor using a broom (*jhaadu* in Hindi) and mop (*pochha* in Hindi): We commonly in the desire to clean the floor, using a broom quickly, bend and round our lower back as in picture 53. This puts strain on the lower back muscles, joints, etc. causing discomfort or pain in the lower back.

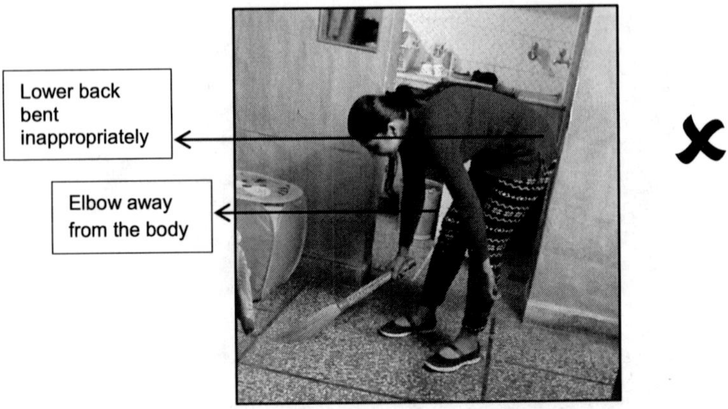

Pic. 53: Incorrect posture while sweeping the floor.

Instead, the floor should be swept, by sitting on the toes with knees apart (squatting position). The knees should be kept at the same level as shown in picture 54. In this posture, the chances of hurting the back muscles are minimum as the back is kept straight.

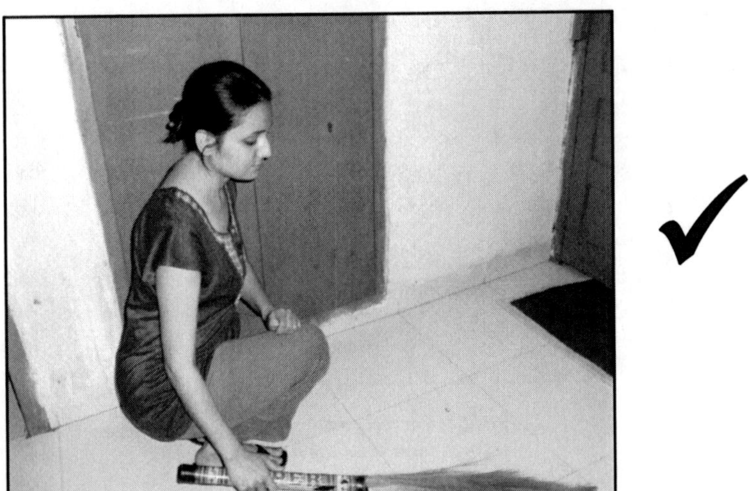

Pic. 54: Correct posture of sweeping the floor.

Moreover, we should keep in mind, some important tips while sweeping the floor:

- Keep the broom or mop close to the body.

- Try sweeping small sections so as not to reach out too far, with the broom/mop. Keep moving or shifting the feet as we sweep, so as to avoid straining the lower back muscles.

The above discussed points are important; otherwise we might twist or bend the lower back inappropriately. This increases the chances of developing LBP.

IV. Taking out things from the refrigerator: When taking out things from the refrigerator, we unconsciously bend our lower back as shown in picture 55. Moreover, many times after taking out the things from the refrigerator when we straighten up, we feel discomfort and pain in our lower back. It is also difficult to straighten our back. This is because the underutilized back muscles are strained by the sudden bending. This happens usually the most used part of the refrigerator is lower to the waist portion of the body.

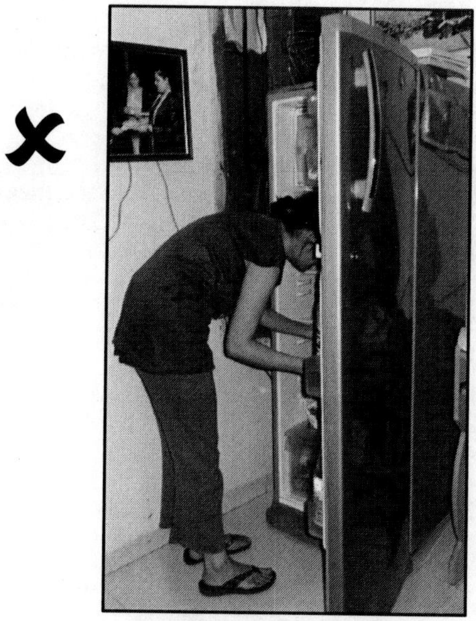

Pic. 55: Usual posture of taking things from refrigerator.

To avoid this strain, we should try to sit on the toes with knees shoulder width apart. Another technique is to use a stool. After opening the door of the refrigerator, we should sit on the stool in front it and reach out for things needed as shown in picture 56. To practice this, the stool should be kept near the refrigerator itself (making healthier choice an easier choice).

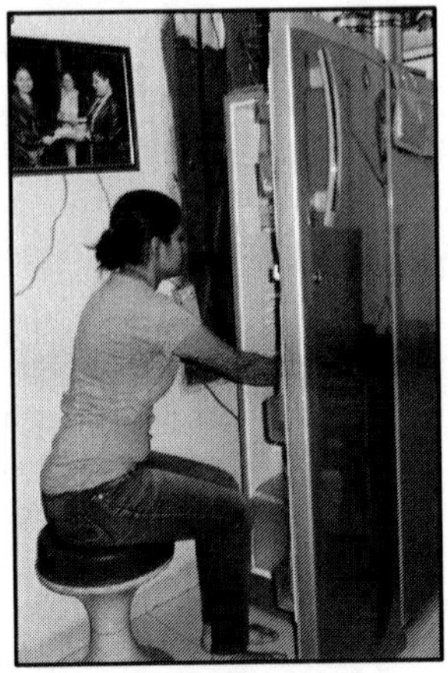

Pic. 56: Using a stool for taking out things from the refrigerator.

V. Ironing clothes: Every morning in a hurry, we iron clothes on the bed as shown in picture 57. We rarely use the ironing table.

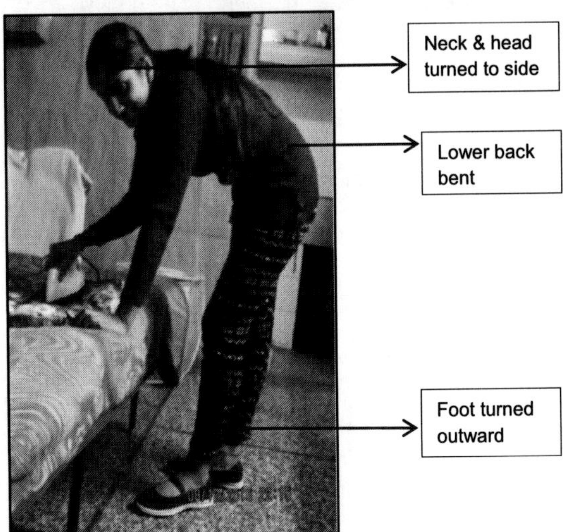

Pic. 57: Faulty posture of ironing clothes.

However, clothes should be ironed preferably an ironing table. However, any hard surface which is up-to the height of the waist or above should be used. Moreover, the feet should rest on small footrest i.e. *patara* or foot stool and alternate every few minutes. This will cause bending at the hips and not the lower back Fig. 18.

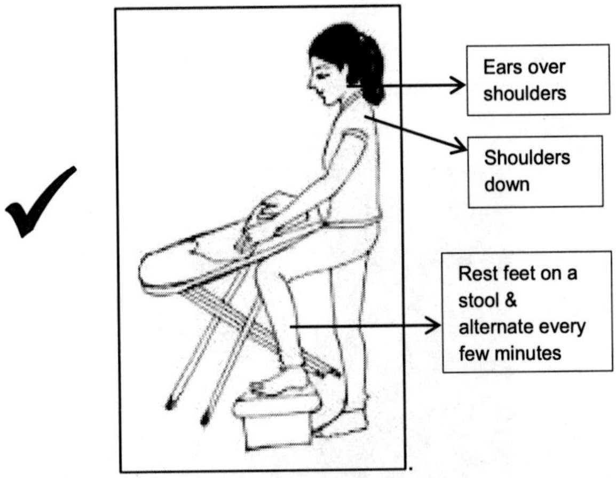

Fig. 18: Correct posture of ironing clothes.

VI. Lifting a bucket of water: It is very common to hear about a lower back strain while lifting a bucket of water or flower pot. We usually lift a bucket by bending at the forward and sideways. Moreover, the bucket is

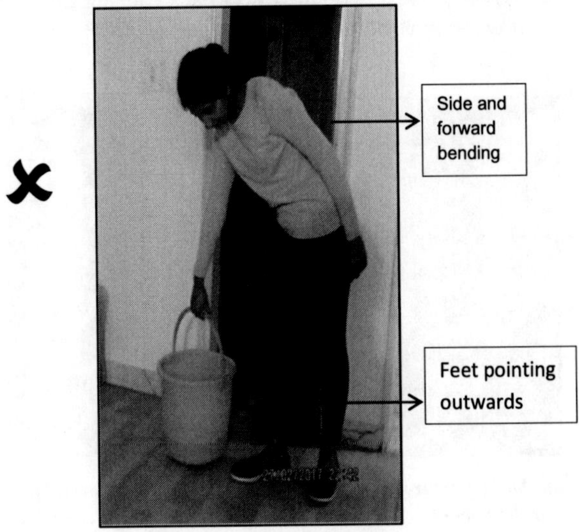

Pic. 58: Faulty posture of lifting bucket- front view.

often too far from the body. So, as we lift the bucket, the chances of having a sudden jerk in the lower back are maximum. This condition is very painful. For example as shown in picture 58, the woman is bending on the right side and forward to pick up the bucket.

Moreover, as we lift the bucket, we bend our bodies again but to the opposite side as shown in picture 59.

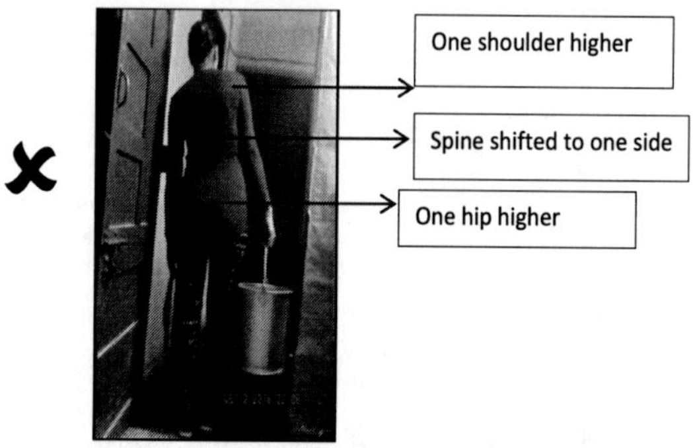

Pic. 59: Faulty posture after lifting the bucket.

Here after lifting the bucket, the woman bends on the left side with right shoulder higher than the left. Moreover, sometimes, we carry this heavy bucket of water up and down the stairs. Carrying heavy bucket in wrong postures, almost every day, puts pressure on the lower back causing LBP. Thus, lifting heavy bucket of water in wrong posture often causes LBP.

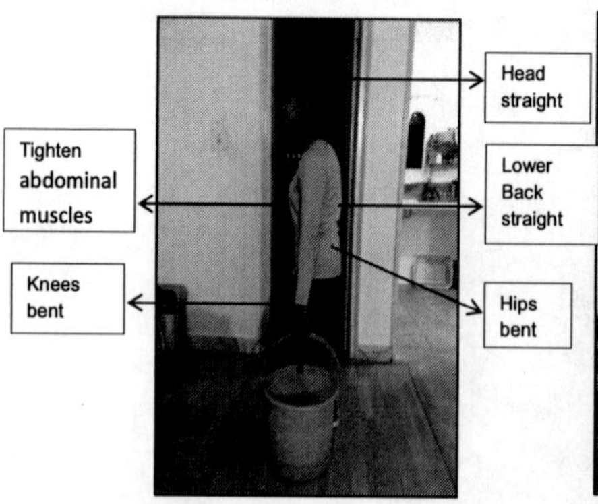

Pic. 60: Squat posture to lift the bucket.

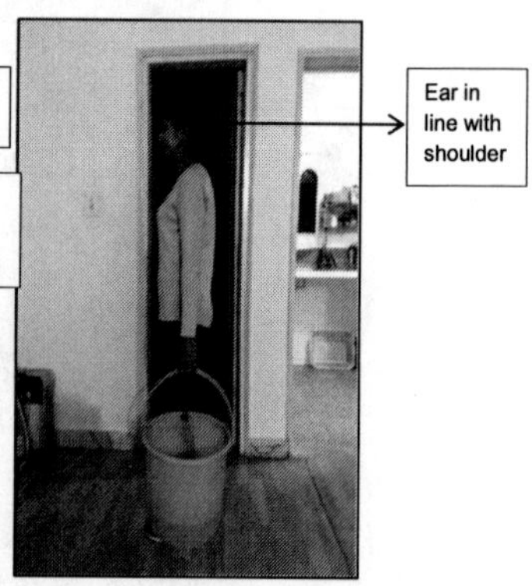

Pic. 61: Correct posture to carry bucket-side view.

However, if we lift the bucket adopting a correct posture, the chances of straining the lower back are reduced. The correct method of lifting the bucket is shown in pictures 60 & 62.

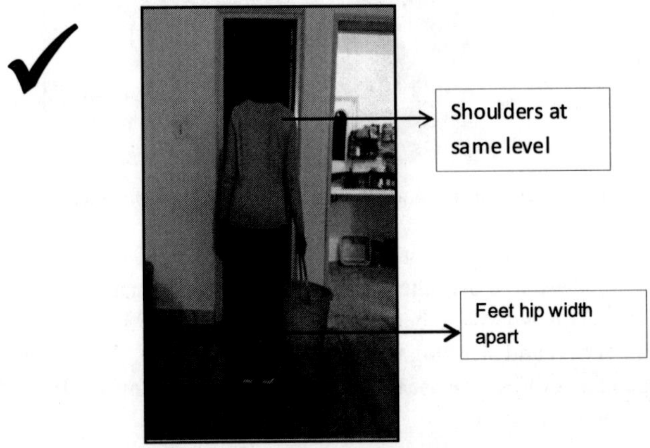

Pic. 62: Correct posture to carry the bucket- back view.

- Stand close to the bucket. Make sure the bucket is at your side.
- Feet should be kept hip width apart [picture 62]
- Tighten the abdominal muscles
- Bend your knees and hips to get into squat (as if sitting on a chair) posture. Back is kept straight [Picture 60]
- Head is upright and forward.
- Keep the bucket close to your body, lift the bucket and straighten your knees into a standing position [picture 61].
- The pressure should be on the heels as you straighten and not on the toe.

Moreover, we should not lift bucket full of water. The bucket must always be half full so that it is easy to carry. This will help in maintaining a straight upright standing posture after we have lifted the bucket [picture 61 & 62.

VII. Washing clothes using semi-automatic washing machine: While moving clothes from the main tub to the dryer of a semi-automatic washing machine, woman often bend their backs in an unhealthy way. Sometimes, they round their backs [picture 63]. This puts pressure on the lower back causing LBP.

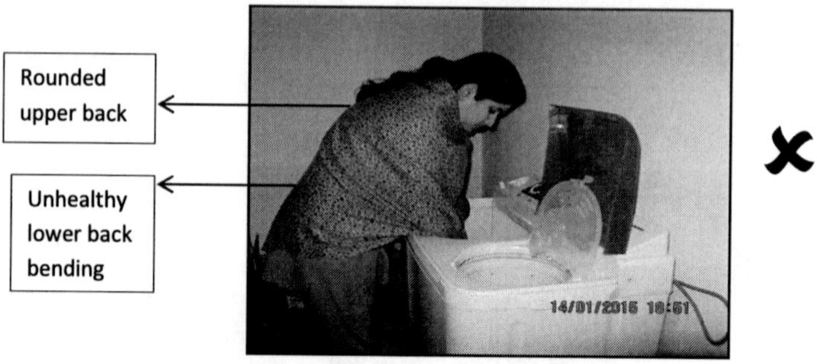

Pic. 63: Faulty posture using semi-automatic washing machine.

A simple solution to correct our posture is keeping one foot on the footrest/ footstool or *patara* and the other on the floor. Keep alternating the feet every few minutes. This will avoid bending of the lower back. Moreover, the lower back will not hurt and standing will be more comfortable. This is because, by standing on the footrest, we use the hip muscles for standing and bend the hips instead of the lower back.

Another, wrong posture we adopt is while unloading or picking clothes at the bottom of the dryer. Here, also we commonly bend our lower back. The correct posture to unload clothes from the dryer is using the golfers lift (refer to section on picking small things).

VIII. Dusting/Wiping: (i) Furniture below our waist level: We usually do this by standing and bending our lower back in order to reach out to the furniture as shown in picture 64. This is because we are unconsciously in a habit to adopt this posture. Moreover, we also think it would be time saving. However, bending at the lower back, in an improper way, puts pressure on its joints, ligaments, etc. increasing chance of LBP.

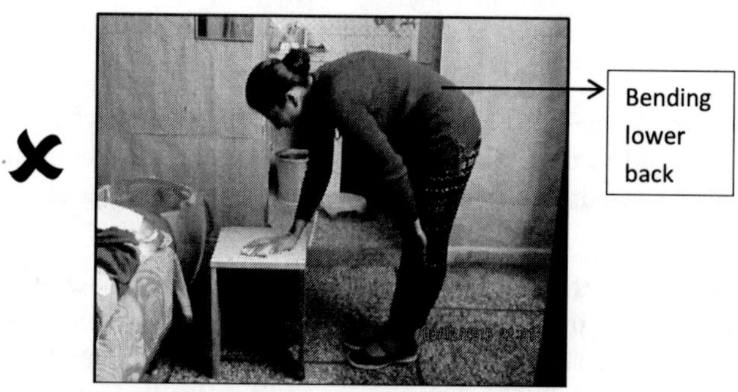

Pic. 64: Incorrect posture while dusting.

However, instead we should position ourselves as close to the working surface. This can be done by kneeling down on the knees [picture 65]. In this posture we are using our legs and hips and not the lower back. So, chances of straining the lower back are less.

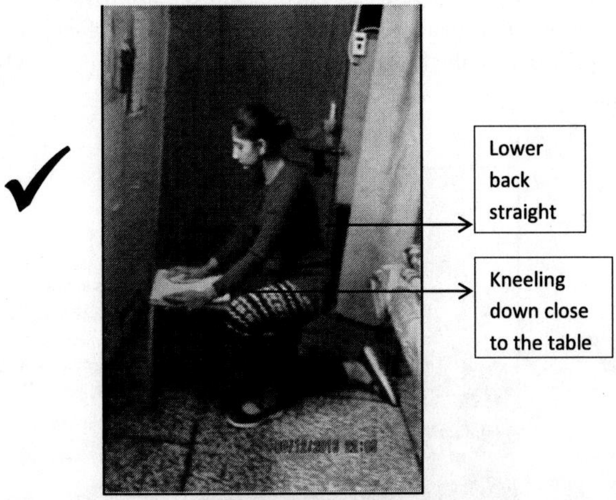

Pic. 65: Correct posture while dusting.

(ii) For things above our head: We usually overstretch ourselves, stand on our toes and outstretch our arms. While doing this, we also push our chest (also upper back) forward and upwards. In order to avoid a fall, the body

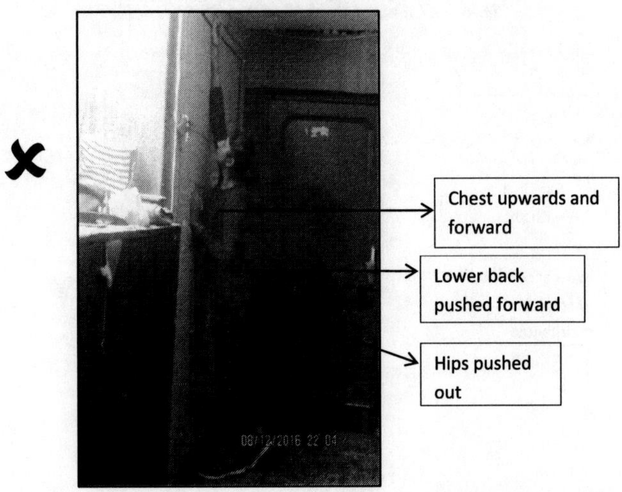

Pic. 66: Incorrect posture while dusting things kept above our head.

adjusts itself by pushing the lower abdomen forward. As a result, lower back is also pushed forward and hips out. This puts pressure on the upper as well as lower back. Moreover, in order to look up to the surface, the neck is also over stretched as shown in picture 66. Here, the legs are also straight and locked.

Thus, while wiping overhead surfaces, we should raise ourselves on a stool to reduce overhead reach. We should wipe surfaces within reach [picture 67]. This way the normal curves of the spine while standing will be maintained.

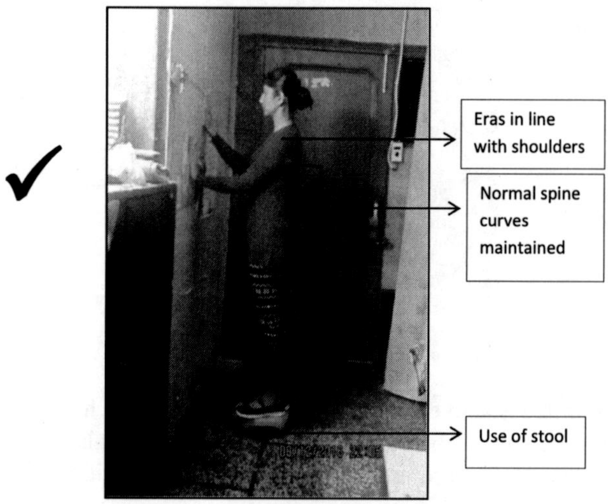

Pic. 67: Use stool to reduce overhead reach.

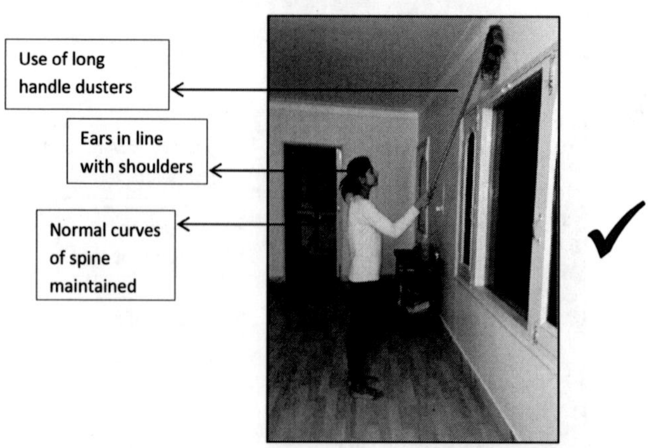

Pic. 68: Use long handle dusters for hard to reach areas.

For hard to reach areas dusters with long handle must be used [picture 68].

IX. Moving objects like pushing almirah: While doing this, we stand facing the almirah with hands on it with outstretched arms. We usually stand too far from the almirah. Now as we push, the upper back is shifted forward. The lower back is curved more inwards. In order to maintain body balance, the hips are pushed out. This puts most pressure on the lower back causing LBP. This is shown in picture 69.

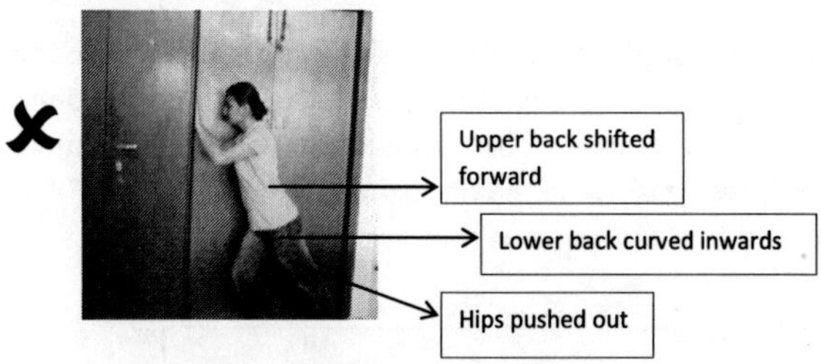

Pic. 69: Faulty way of pushing almirah.

It is suggested that adopting a correct posture, while moving heavy things such as an almirah, will reduce chances of having LBP. The correct posture [Fig. 19 involves:

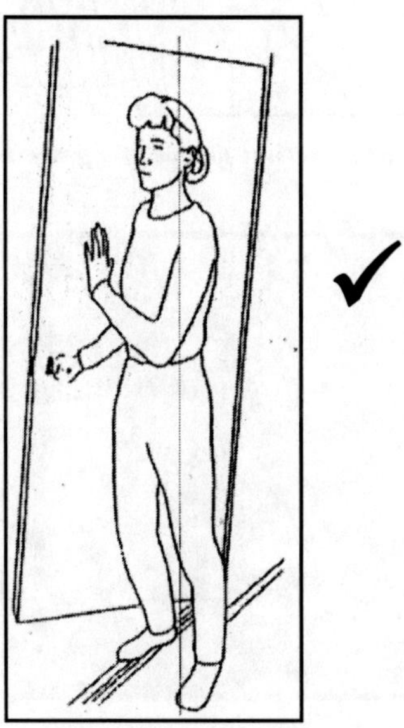

Fig. 19: Correct way of pushing almirah.

- Stand close with the almirah on the side
- Keep one elbow such that it touches the almirah.
- Use total body weight and legs to push the almirah

10. Out of the house to shop for:

I. Groceries in the supermarket: In the supermarkets we use carts for carrying groceries. However, while reaching out for the groceries in the cart we bend our lower back in a wrong way. This puts pressure on the muscles, joints, ligaments of lower back irritating the surrounding nerves causing LBP.

However, for adopting the correct posture, we should use the golfers lift (refer to section on picking small things). This is done by keep the other hand on the edge of the cart basket. Now, as we reach out for the things in the cart, with one hand, we must raise the opposite leg behind [Fig. 20. This way we use our hips and legs putting less pressure on the lower back.

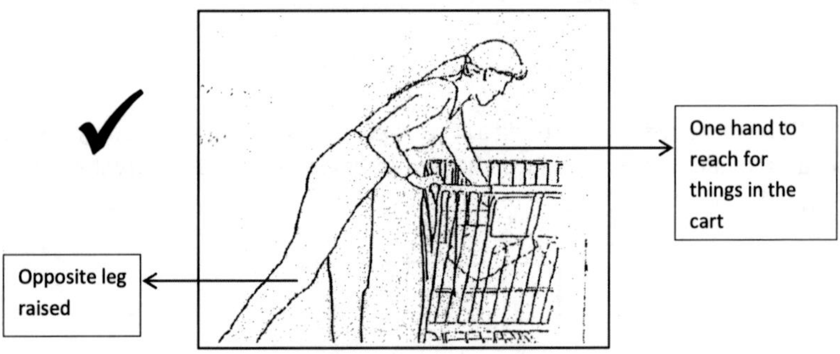
One hand to reach for things in the cart
Opposite leg raised

Fig. 20: Correct way to reach for groceries in the cart.

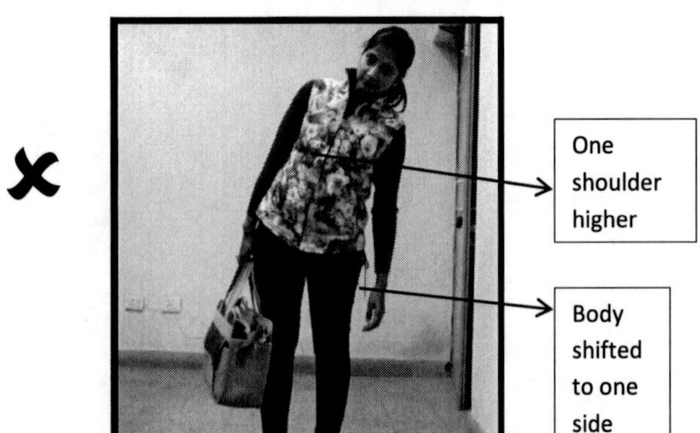

Pic. 70: Incorrect posture of carrying bag.

II. Carrying fruits & vegetables from *sabzi mandi* (fruit and vegetable market): While and after shopping from the fruit and vegetable market we often carry one heavy shoulder or hand grip bag. This causes the body to shift to one side as shown in picture 70-71.

In this posture, one shoulder is higher than the other. As a result to hip are also not at the same level. Doing this once will not harm your body. But adopting this posture, every now and then for months and years can cause shifting of the spine from its normal position, disc bulge, etc. This way the spine is strained and we may complain of LBP.

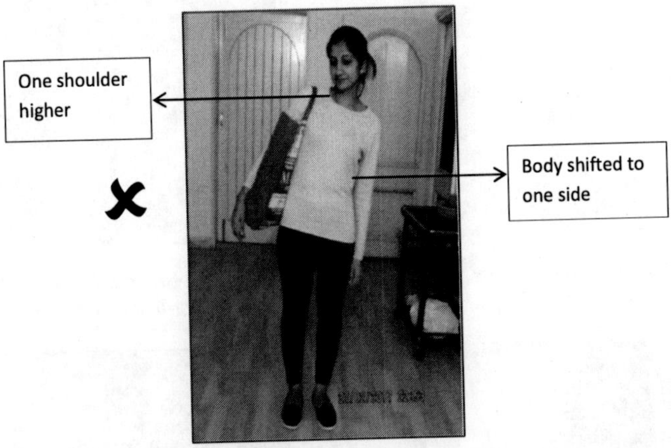

Pic 71: Incorrect posture of carrying bag.

In order to avoid straining of the spine, we should carry two bags. Preferably, one a shoulder bag hanging on one shoulder and the other a handgrip bag held on the other side shown in picture 72.

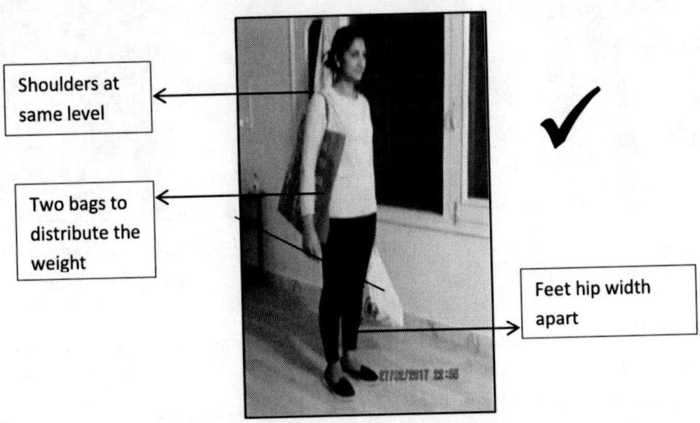

Pic. 72 : Correct posture of carrying bag.

III. To the mall carrying heavy handbags: We carry handbags as shown in the Pic. 73-76.

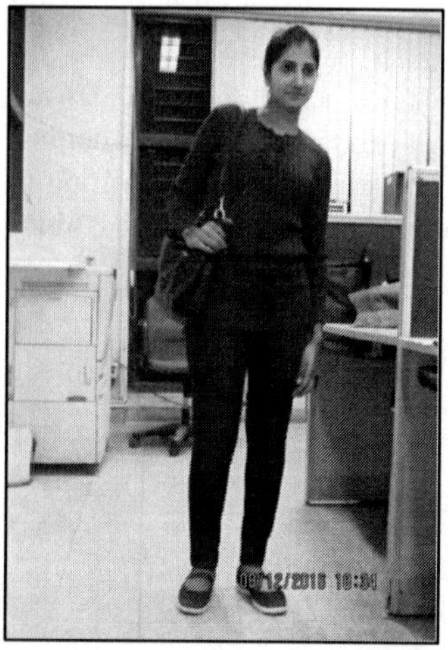

Pic. 73: Incorrect way to carry handbag

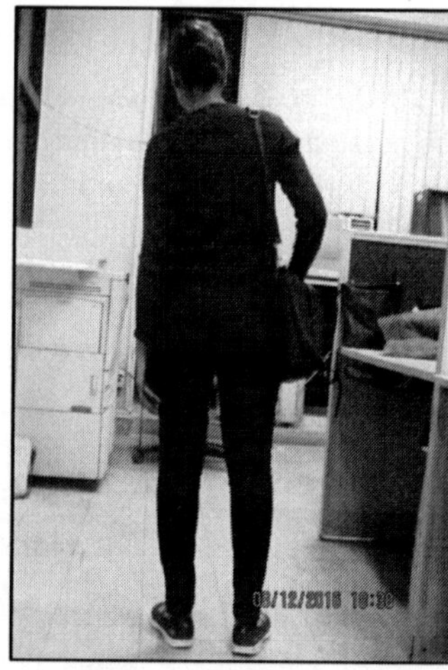

Pic. 74: Incorrect way to carry handbag-back view-front view

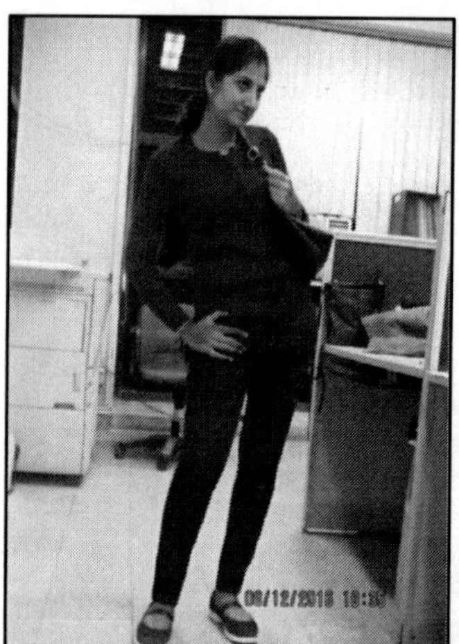

Pic. 75: Incorrect way to carry handbag.

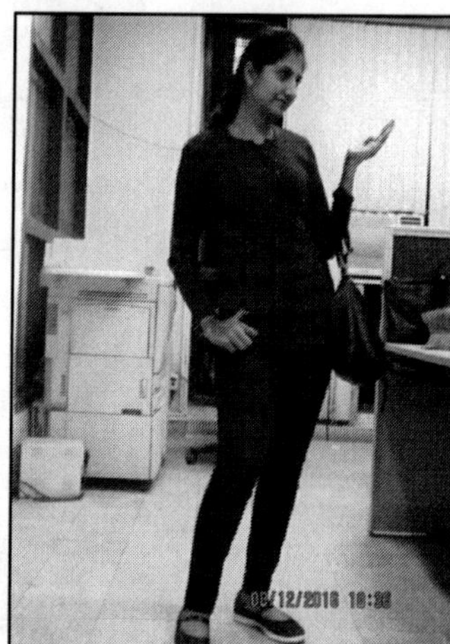

Pic. 76: Incorrect way to carry handbag

In all these postures, one shoulder is higher than the other and one hip is also higher than the other. This causes the lower back to shift to one side causing straining of the muscles, joints, ligaments, etc. causing LBP. Due to this the body is strained as shown in Fig. 21:

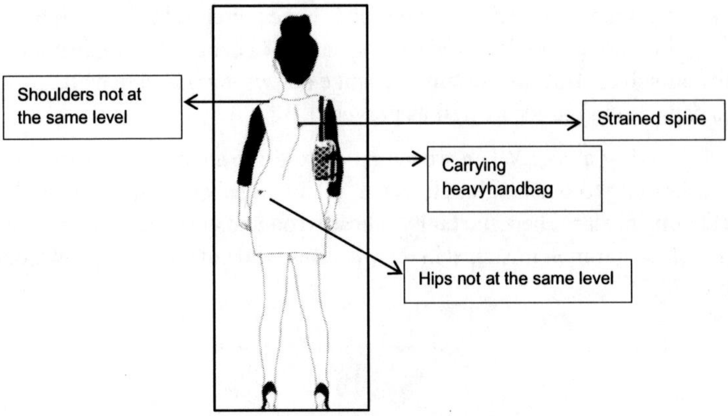

Fig. 21: Shifting of spine to one side when carrying heavy handbag on one shoulder.

In order to avoid this problem, we must:

- Try to distribute the weight by carrying two bags (Pic. 77).

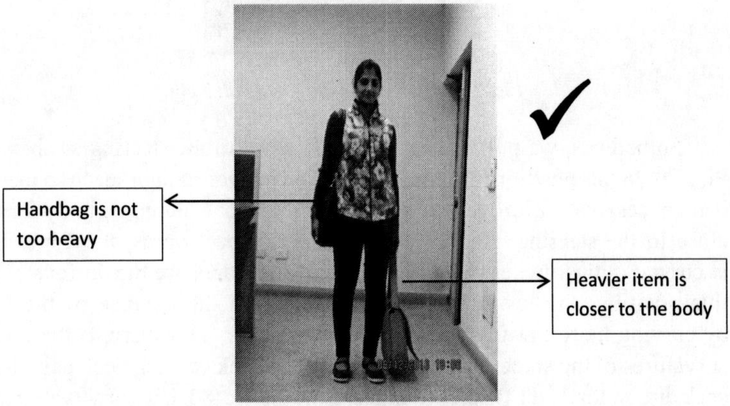

Pic. 77: Correct way to carry handbags

- When carrying one bag, keep alternating sides to carry the bag. This will give the muscles on either side some rest.
- Try to use short strap bags so that the handbag is as close to the body as possible. But make sure it is not too heavy so as to disrupt your posture.

11. Driving

Faulty postures along with long hours of driving, unexpected speed breakers, bumpy /rough and uneven roads have increased the problem of low back pain among people. However, we cannot change the condition of the roads ourselves. But we can surely change our wrong postures while driving. This can help to reduce as well as prevent LBP.

I. Driving a car: When we get ready to drive a car, we position the car seat according to our height. However, many times we do it wrong and thus our driving postures become faulty. These wrong postures often are a cause of LBP. A few common mistakes in our postures while driving are shown below in pic. 78.

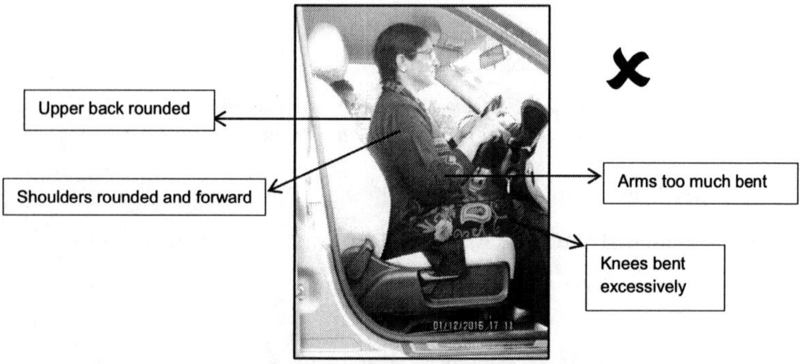

Pic. 78: Incorrect posture while driving.

Sometimes, we pull our car seats too close to the steering as shown in Pic. 80. In this position, the arms and legs do not get enough space so they are bentt excessively. Morover, we are in a habit to move our upper body forward close to the steering. Here, the neck is drawn backwards; the upper back is curved outwards i.e. more rounded and shoulders are drawn forward. In this position, the lower back tries to maintain the balance of the body by curving more inwards than normal. Moreover, This disrupts the normal curvatures of the spine straining the complete back causing neck pain, upper back discomfort and LBP. For example in the the Pic. 80, if we observe carefully the position of the neck, upper back and lower back, we realise that the curves of the spine from the neck to the lower back, are not as they should be normally (refer to text on anatomy).

Another, common posture we adopt while driving is shown in picture 79. Here, the head and neck are drawn forward, chest is drawn inwards rounding the upper back. The elbows are kept too far away from the body. In this position, the neck muscles are strained and chances of neck pain increase. Sometimes, this pain extends to the shoulders and arms. This may also be due to the faulty positioning of the shoulders or arms.

Moreover, our lower backs do not fit into the curve of the backrest of the car seat. That is there is a gap between the lower back and the lower portion of the backrest of the car seat. Because of this, the hips are pushed forward. Since, the lower back is without support, strain on the muscles, joints, ligaments of the lower back is maximum causing LBP.

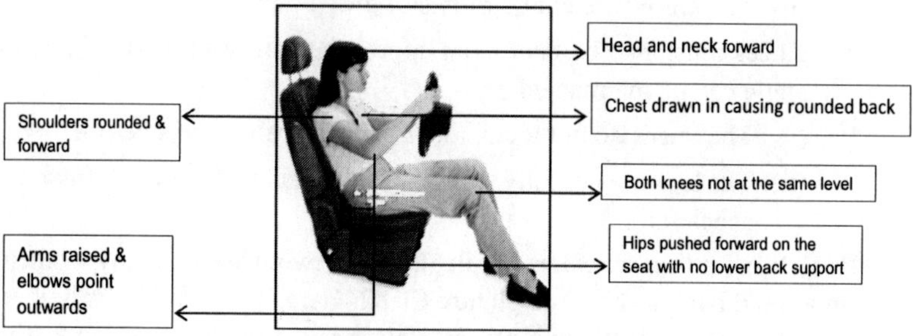

Pic. 79: Incorrect posture while driving.

While driving a car, the following things must be kept in mind. These are shown in picture 802:

- Head needs to kept upright and straight.
- Ears should be in line with the shoulders.
- Chest must be raised.
- Shoulders need to be in line with the hips.

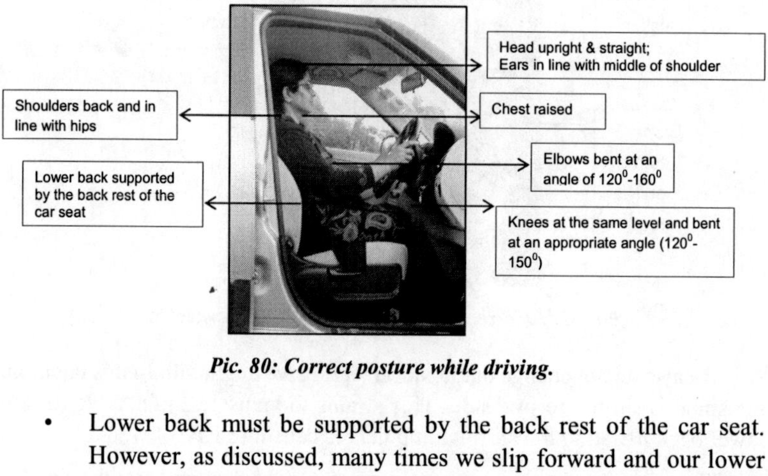

Pic. 80: Correct posture while driving.

- Lower back must be supported by the back rest of the car seat. However, as discussed, many times we slip forward and our lower backs do not fit into the curve present in the lower portion of the back rest of the car seat. To overcome this problem keep a firm cushion so that the lower back remains supported.

- Elbows must be bent an appropriate angle (120^{0}-160^{0}) and held close to the body. This angle can be maintained if:
  (i) The hands (while on the steering) are not too close to the chest.
  (ii) The elbow are not be fully straight.
- Knees must also be bent at an appropriate angle (120^{0}-150^{0}). This angle can be maintained if:
  (i) The knees do not touch the dashboard below the steering.
  (ii) The legs are not fully straight while pushing the brake, clutch or accelerator.

II. Driving a two-wheeler: While driving a two wheeler, many women sit with a tilted back a shown in picture 81-82. Here, one shoulder is higher than the other. As a result one hip is also higher than the other. This mostly happens when we try to stop the vehicle on the red light by putting one foot on the road and unconsciously we keep sitting in the same position when we restart the vehicle.

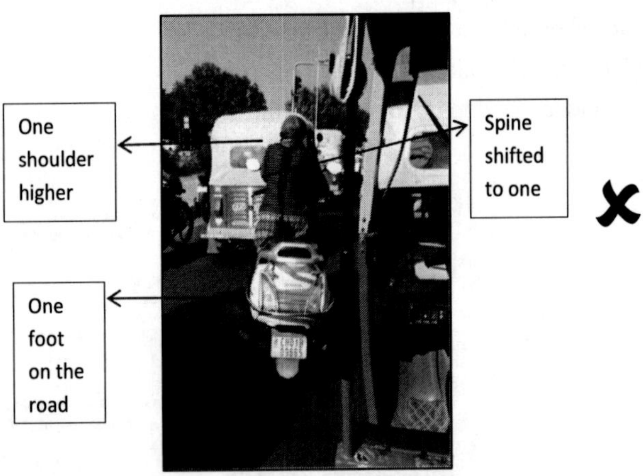

Pic. 81: Incorrect posture while driving two-wheeler.

We also do not change our position fearing we might fall. In this position, the spine is shifted to one side. This strains the muscles, joints, etc. of the lower back irritating the surrounding nerves causing LBP.

The correct posture while driving a two-wheeler we should keep the following things in mind as shown in picture 82:

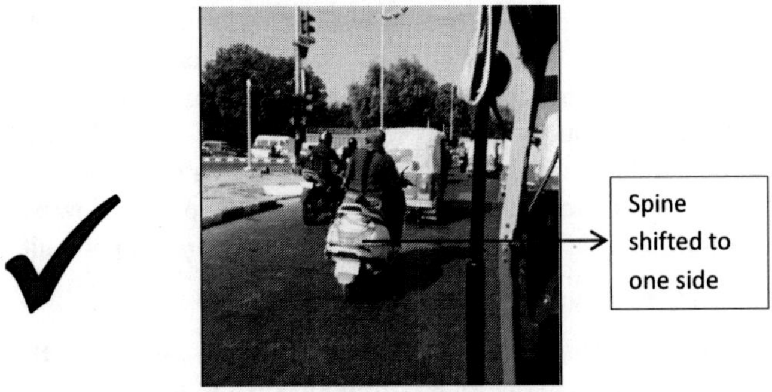

Pic. 82: Incorrect posture while driving two-wheeler.

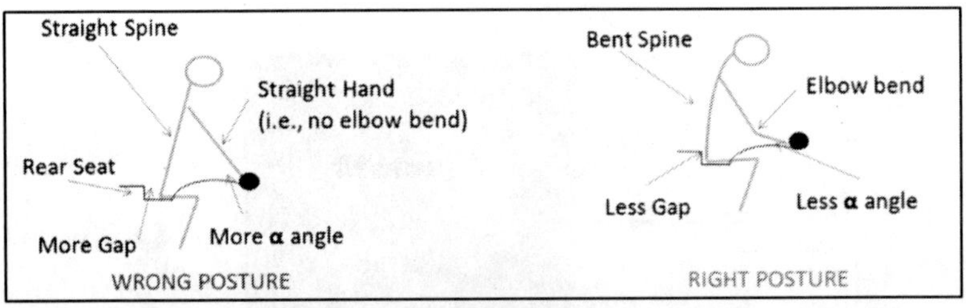

Fig. 22: Correct posture while driving two-wheeler.

- We should have a slightly curved back. If we keep a straight and a stiff back, the chances of jerk or impact on the lower back is high esp. when we ride on an uneven surface. So the back should be slightly curved. Moreover, in case of straight back with shoulders pushed backwards, the angle between the shoulders, elbow and hand will increase that will cause more stress on the lower back while driving.
- The elbows must be bent and relaxed.
- Shoulders need to be relaxed and not stiff
- Stop the vehicle using brakes. However, even if we have to use our feet to stop the vehicle, we should do it with both feet. This helps to maintain balance over the two-wheeler as well as not strain our lower back.
- Long continued driving can also cause low back pain. Therefore, it is necessary to take breaks when driving for long hours.

12. Sleeping postures

Sleep is important for a healthy body and mind. It is a natural way to relieve all our tiredness. We spend nearly five to eight hours of a day sleeping i.e. one third of a day and almost one-third of our life span. Think about sleeping in our favorite position in the hope to get up all fresh and ready for the day's work. In fact, sometimes that is the only time of the day when we get to lie down and straighten our backs. However, we need to check if our favourite position is the right one for our backs. Certain sleeping postures, put pressure on the spine. They increase the chances of us waking up with a low back pain, neck pain and stiffness. So, sleeping in the right posture is important.

Some of the faulty sleeping postures are as follows:

I. Sleeping on the belly with one leg higher than the other: In this position the head turns to one side. This puts pressure on the neck. Also the lower back (incl. tailbone) curves more than the normal [picture 83]. This puts pressure on the lower back.

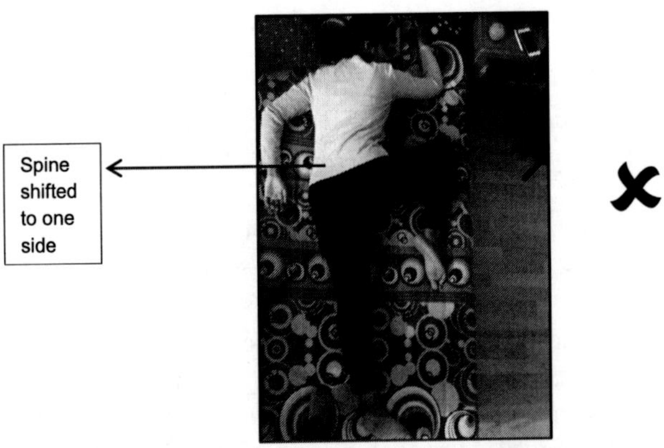

Pic. 83: Sleeping on the belly with one leg higher.

II. Sleeping on the stomach: In this position, the hips become tight as they do not get support. This causes the lower back to curve inwards [picture 84]. This puts pressure on the lower back causing LBP.

III. Sleeping on the side with a deeply rounded back: This is also known as foetal position as this is similar to the baby when it is still in the mother's womb. Here the legs are too bent. As a result, the lower back is also bent. Thus, the spine adopts a C- position (picture 85).

This C- puts pressure on the muscles, joints, ligaments and other structures of the lower back irritating the surrounding nerves. This causes LBP. Moreover, sometimes the shoulders are also drawn inwards causing pressure on the upper back and neck. Remember that pain we get in the neck and surrounding area after getting up in the morning as if beaten up by someone. This sore pain is mostly because of sleeping in this position.

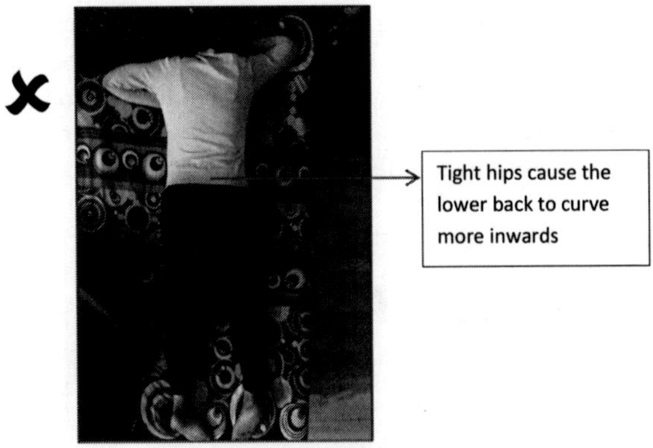

Pic. 84: Sleeping on the stomach.

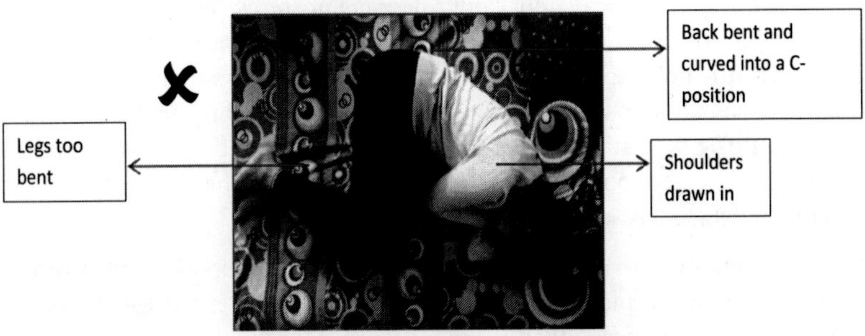
Back bent and curved into a C-position
Legs too bent
Shoulders drawn in

Pic. 85: Sleeping on side with rounded back.

IV. Sleeping on the side with straight legs [picture 86: In this position, the legs are straight. This causes the lower back to curve outwards causing pressure on the surrounding muscles, joints which causes LBP.

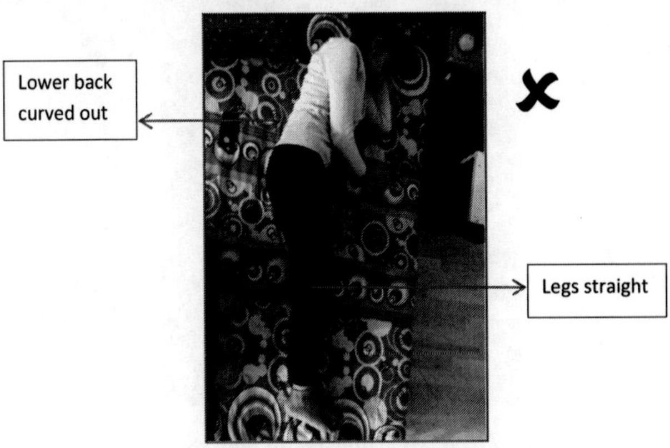

Pic. 86: Sleeping on side with straight legs

V. Sleeping on the back [Fig. 23]: Some people have a habit of sleeping on the back. In this position, the lower back does not touch the bed. There is always a gap between the lower back and bed such that a hand can fit in. In this position, the muscles of the lower spine do not get relaxed and remain tensed. This is the reason most often we get up with a sore back.

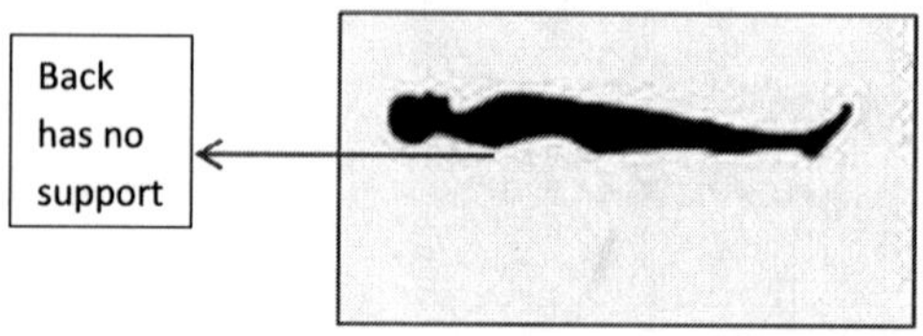

Fig. 23: Sleeping on the back

It is difficult to correct our faulty sleeping postures. We have got so used to these that we do not get sound sleep until we sleep in that particular posture. However, it is not impossible to do so. Moreover, with simple modification we can correct our postures. As we try to change our habits, in the beginning it will be difficult to adjust to the new postures. But with time as we would get use to them correct postures will become our habits. The suggested correct sleeping postures are as follows:

VI. Sleeping on the side: While sleeping on the side, add a pillow between the knees [picture 87]. This will relax the lower back muscles and also keep the spine normally aligned.

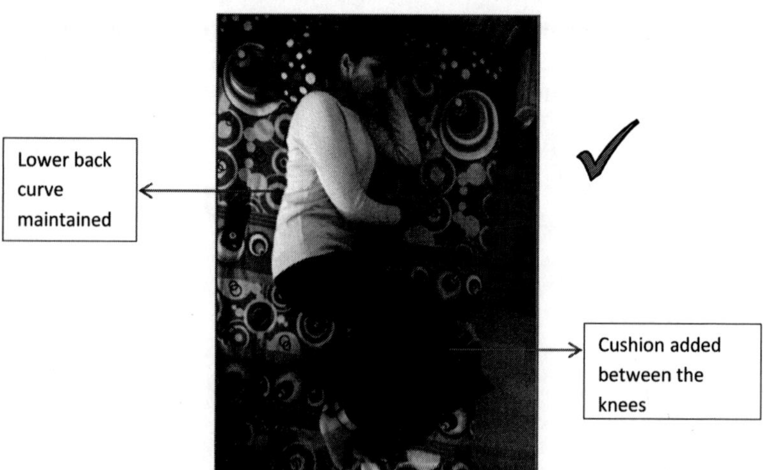

Pic. 87: Sleeping on the side with cushion between the knees.

VII. Sleeping on the back: When sleeping on the back, keep a pillow below the knees [picture 88. This will relax the hip muscles and allow the lower back to maintain its normal curve. Moreover, add a thin towel or pillow below the neck. But it should be kept such that it does not raise and push the head beck. The head must be kept in line with the neck.

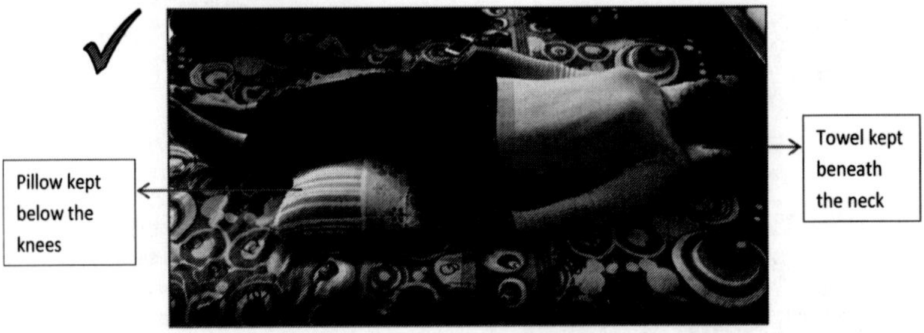

Pic. 88: Sleeping on the back with pillow below the knees.

13. Getting out of bed

As sleeping postures are important so is the posture to get out of bed. We often get out of bed as shown in picture 89. This puts a lot of strain on the lower back. In this position, the lower back is twisted and bent which can often cause a jerk causing LBP.

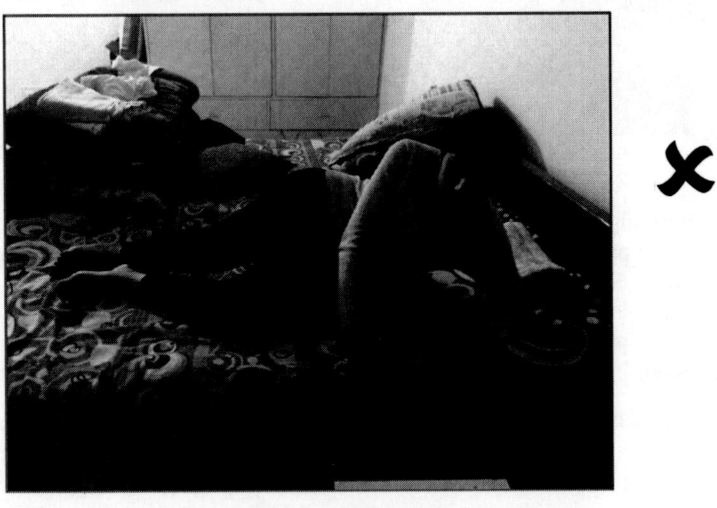

Pic. 89: Incorrect way of getting out of bed.

The correct method to get out of bed is as follows:

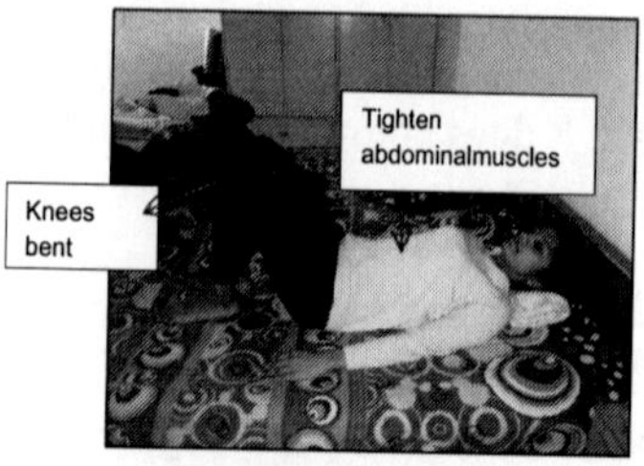

Pic. 90: Bend the knees

- Lie on your back
- Breathe in and gently draw in the abdomen by pulling the belly button towards the bed
- Slide one leg up at a time to bend the knees as shown in picture 90.

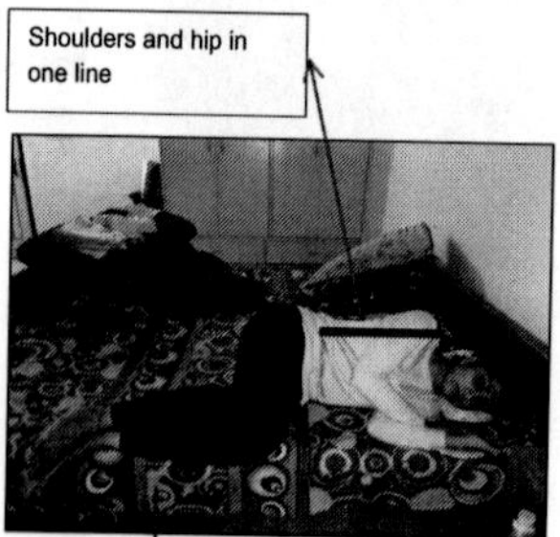

Pic. 91: Turn to one side.

- Turn to your side (Preferably your non-involved or less involved side)
- Keep your shoulders and hips in line with each other (known as log rolling to reduce stress because of twisting and bending of the spine)
- Bend your knees so that your feet and lower legs are almost over the edge of the bed as shown in Picture 91.

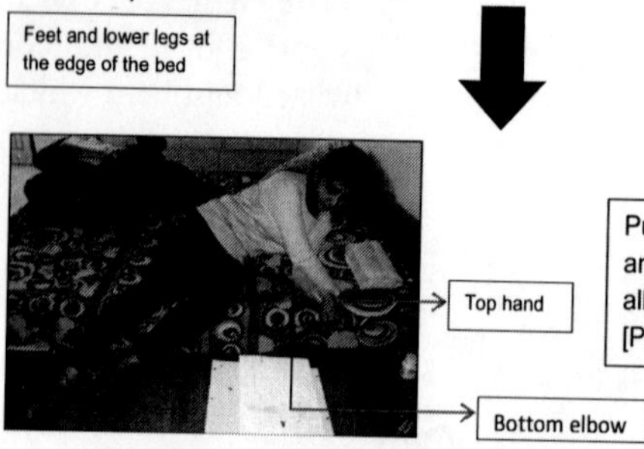

Pic. 92: Getting out of bed.

Push into the bed with your top hand and bottom elbow while simultaneously allowing your feet to drop to the floor [Picture 92].

Adopting these changes in posture in our routine life is suggestive to reduce and prevent LBP. However, nothing is 100% effective for everyone. What works for one person may not work for another. Thus, using the approach of "whatever works" can be helpful in management of LBP.

Exercises

As discussed before, loose muscles aggravate LBP. Therefore, toning up and adding strength to the affected muscles can help in its treatment and management. Regular exercises of the back, abdomen, hip and leg muscles strengthens the underlying weak muscles and help in management of LBP. Some exercises that can help in reducing LBP are discussed in this chapter.

The exercises are divided into 3 groups viz. start-up exercises; strengthening exercises and pain relieving exercises. Start-up and strengthening exercises can be done by those who do not suffer from LBP. These help in preventing LBP as this strengthens the muscles of the back and abdomen.

DISCLAIMER!!!! These exercises may seem easy to perform but should only be done under the guidance of qualified expert physiotherapist or trained yoga professional.

I. START-UP EXERCISES

(a) Ankle Pumps (Picture 93-94):

1. Lie on the back with straight legs.
2. Alternately move ankles up and down
3. Repeat it 10 times on each ankle.

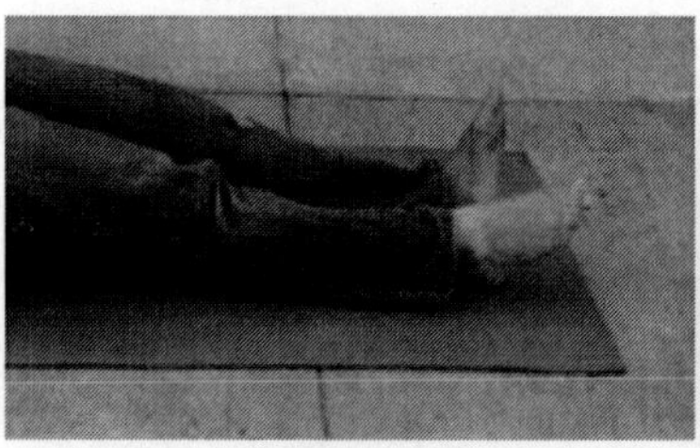

Pic. 93

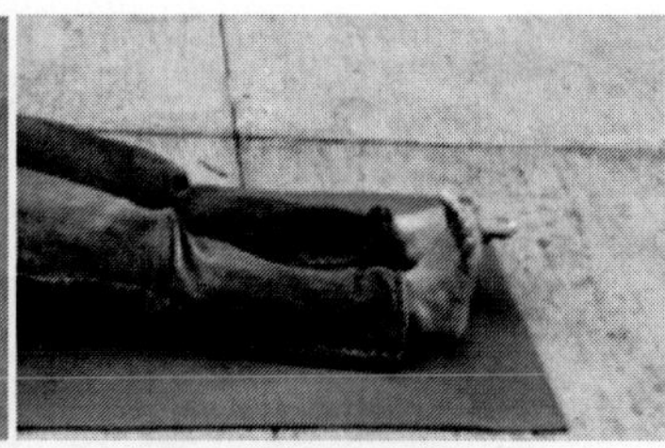

Pic. 94

(b) Heel slides (Picture 95-96):

1. Lie on the back with knees bent, shoulders relaxed and abdominal muscles drawn in.
2. Breathe in and as you breathe out, slide the heel down away from your body.
3. Breathe in and bring it back.
4. Keep the lower back firm and steady when you move your leg.
5. Repeat 5 times on each leg.

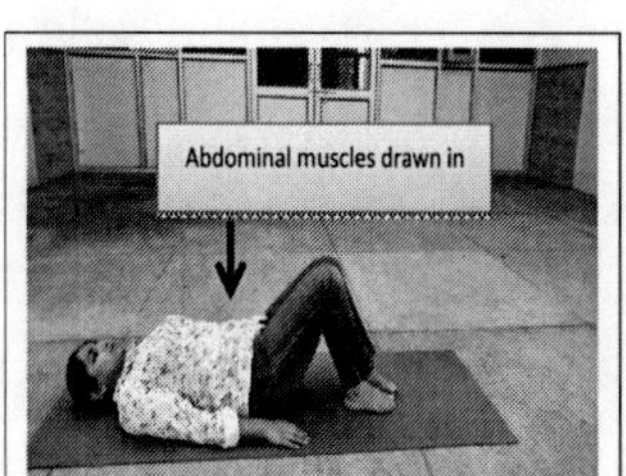

Pic. 95

Heel Slides

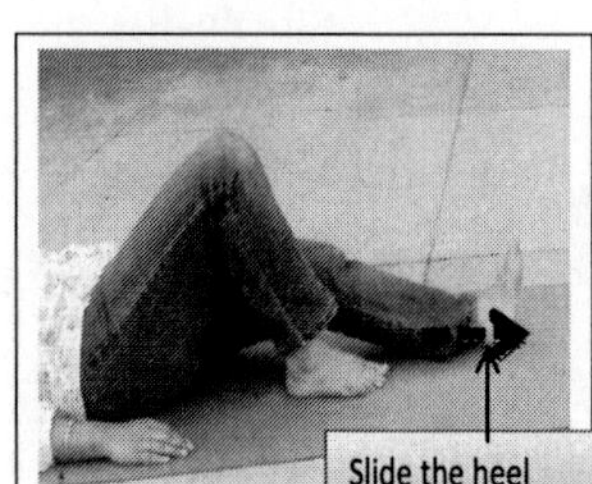

Pic. 96

(c) Abdominal Contraction (Fig. 24-25):

1. Lie on your back with knees bent.
2. Find the bony prominence on both sides of the lower abdomen (known as the anterior superior iliac spine).
3. Now move your hand 2-inches towards the middle of the body from this bony prominence (this point will be in line with the navel).
4. Draw your lower abdomen towards the spine.

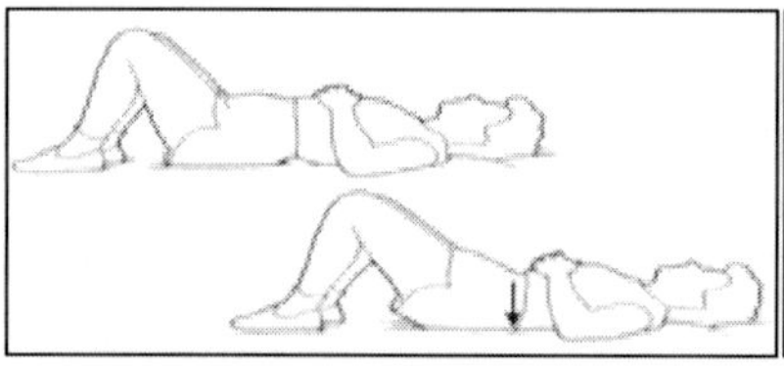

Fig. 24: Move lower abdomen towards spine.

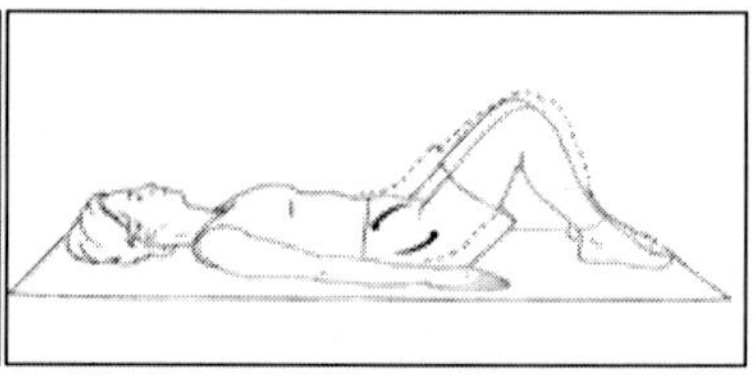

Fig. 25: Move the spine up.

5. Try to move your spine upwards (slightly contracting the hip muscles) (Picture 90)
6. Breathe in and out with the abdominal muscles contracted.
7. Hold the position for 5 seconds and relax
8. Repeat 5 times.

   Caution: Do not hold your breath at any time while doing this exercise.

(d) Straight leg raise (Picture 97-98):

This exercise strengthens the front and back muscles of the thighs and tones up the abdominal muscles

1. Lie on your back with one knee bent and one leg straight (Picture 8e).
2. Tighten the abdominal muscles i.e. move the abdomen towards the spine.
3. Slowly lift the straight leg upto 6-12 inches from the floor (Picture 8f).

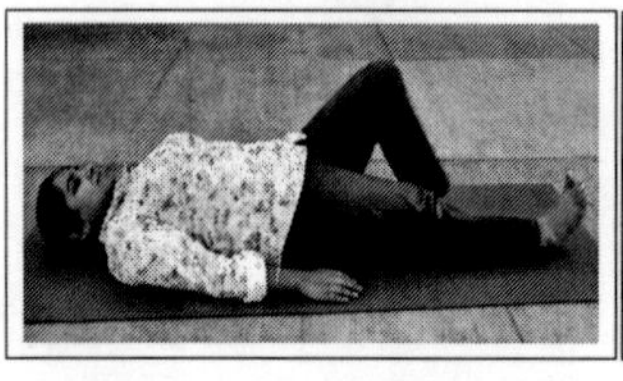

Pic. 97

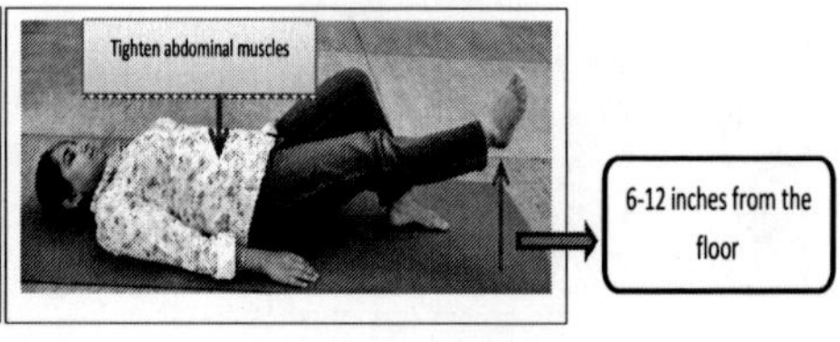

Pic. 98

4. Hold the position for 5 seconds and lower the leg slowly.
5. Repeat 5 times on each leg.

II. PAIN RELIEVEING EXERCISES

(a) Cobra pose (*Bhujang asana*): It has 4 levels. Out of these three levels are discussed here whereas the fourth level is discussed later under strengthening exercises.

This exercise builds up the back and neck muscles and stretches the abdominal muscles

Level 1 (Picture 99-100):-

1. Lie flat on the stomach with hands besides the chest, feet together, chin touching the ground and elbows on the side of the rib-cage.
2. Breathe in and slowly raise the chin, neck and head to look straight in front.
3. Avoid tightening your back and allow it to curve. The concentration should be on the low back.
4. Hold the posture for 10 seconds. A stretch is felt on the back of neck and low back
5. Exhale/breathe out and come back to the lying-down position.
6. Repeat it 5 times.

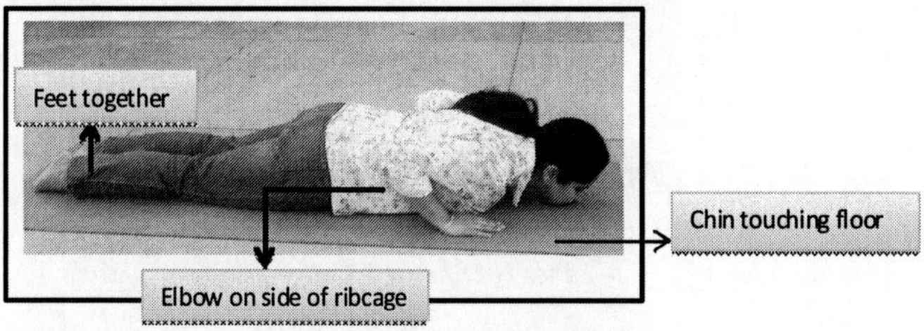

Pic. 99: Lying position for cobra pose.

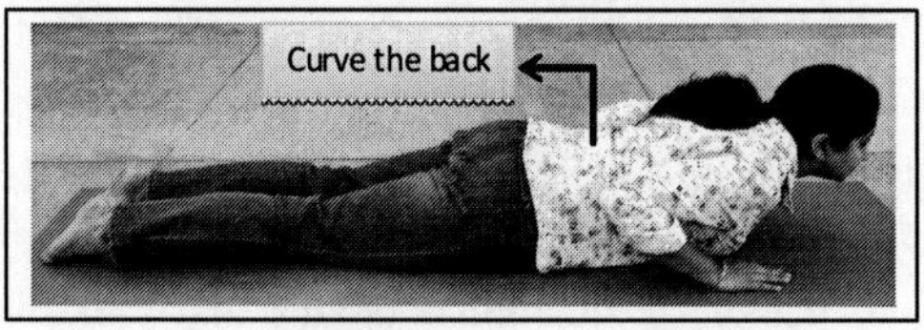

Pic. 100: Level 1 Cobra pose.

Level 2 (Picture 101):-

1. Breathe in and raise the chin, chest and abdomen up-till the naval with the head to look in front.
2. The elbows point backward and inwards.

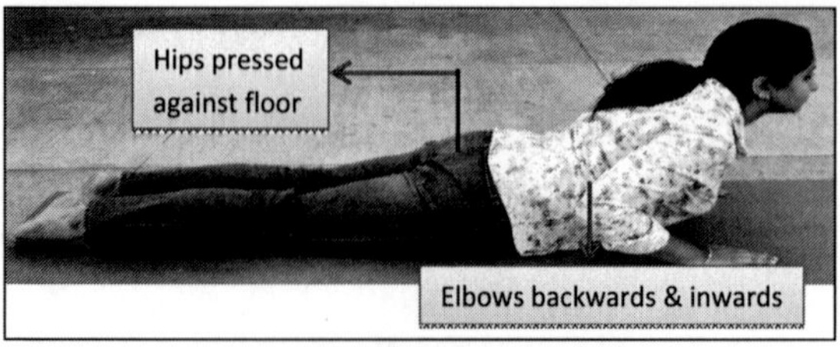

Pic. 101: Level 2 Cobra pose.

3. The hips are pressed against the floor and back is curved.
4. A slight stretch is felt on the back of neck and low back

Level 3 (Picture 102):-

1. Breathe in to raise the chin, chest, abdomen and head to look towards the ceiling of the room.
2. The shoulders and elbows are in a straight line with elbows bent at 90^0 to the floor.
3. Hands flat on the ground in front of the body.
4. A stretch is felt on the low back as well as back of neck

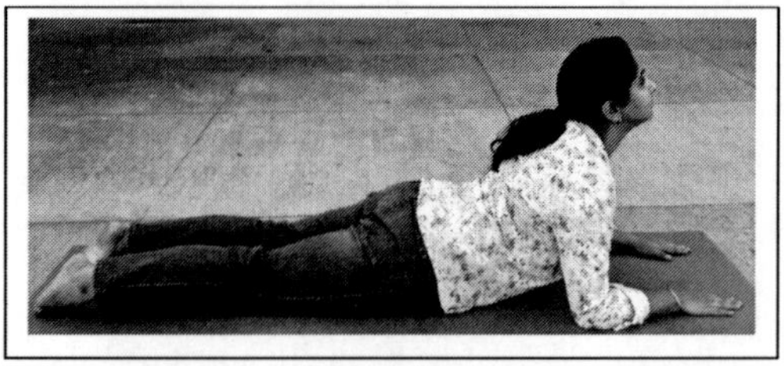

Pic. 102: Level 3 Cobra pose.

Precautions: The exercise should be done gradually and very slow as a stiff spine can lead to LBP. Moreover, raise the body only to a point when you feel a slight stretch. Do not over strain.

(b) Knee to chest (*pawan mukta asana*)- (Picture 103-104):

This exercise improves upper abdominal and lower abdominal muscle tone, massages abdominal organs and the spine. Also stretches the hip muscles.

1. Lie on your back with both knees bent and feet flat on the floor.
2. Lift one knee and while breathing in, bring it (knee) up towards your chest. Do not lift the head or neck).

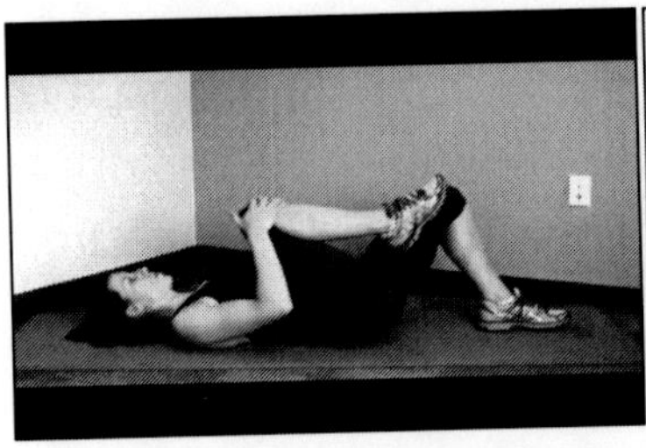

Pic. 103: Single leg- knee to chest.

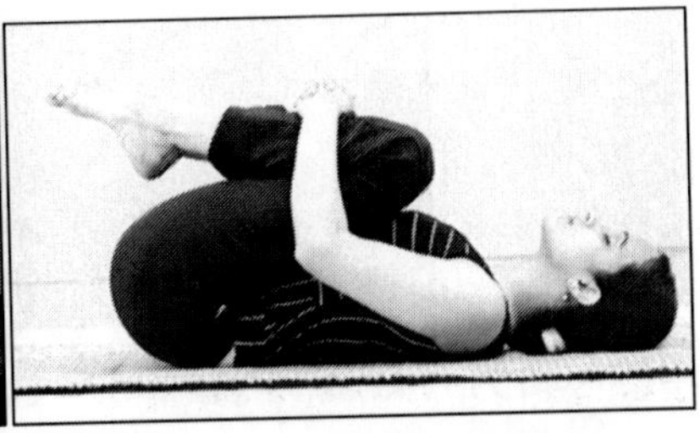

Pic. 104: Both legs- knee to chest.

3. Hold for 10 seconds.
4. Breathe out and return to the staring posture.
5. Repeat with other leg.
6. Then, from the knees-bent position with feet flat on the floor, breathe in and bring both knees up towards your chest. Hold for 10 seconds.
7. Repeat the exercise 5 times.

Note: As you progress with the exercise, start with keeping your legs straight than with bent knees (Picture 105)

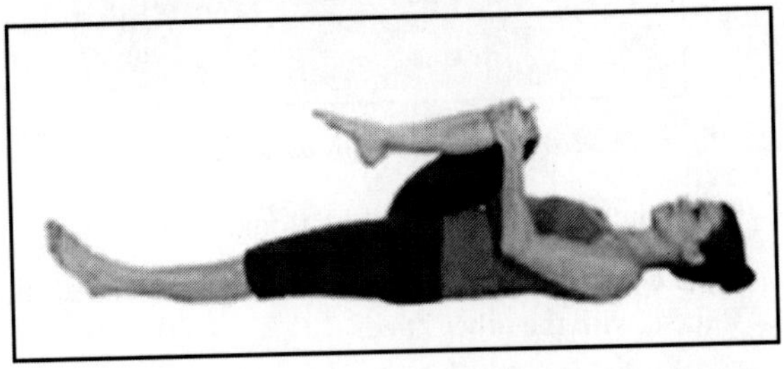

Pic. 105: Single Knee to chest- by keeping one leg straight

Contraindications:

- Must be avoided in case of recent abdominal surgery
- Anyone suffering from piles, hernia should not practice this exercise

(c) Lower back rotation (*Markat asana*):

This exercise tones the abdominal muscles. It strengthens the muscles of the back, neck, hips and legs.

(i) Single knee (Picture 106-107):-

1. Lie flat on the back with arms extended out to the sides.

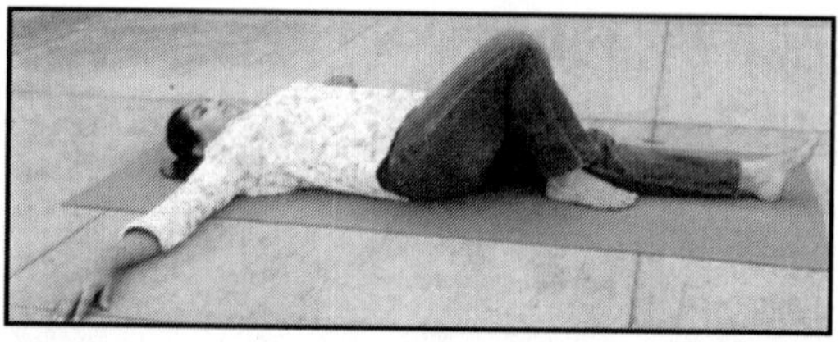

Pic. 106: Single knee lower back rotation- starting position

2. Bend the right knee and keep the left leg straight (Picture 6p).
3. Slowly cross over the right (bent) knee over the left leg, trying to let it touch the floor (on the opposite side) (Picture 6q). A stretch is felt from the right arm extending to the lower back to the right (bent) knee.
4. Turn the head to the right.

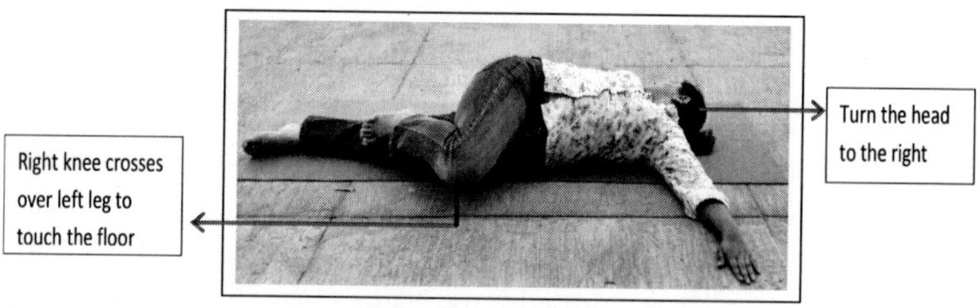

Pic. 107: Single knee low back rotation.

5. Keep the shoulders flat on the floor.
6. Hold the posture for 10 seconds and return to the starting position. Repeat with the other knee.
7. Repeat 5 times for each side.

(ii) Double Knee (Picture 108-109):-

1. Bend both the knees with feet flat on the floor (Picture 6r).

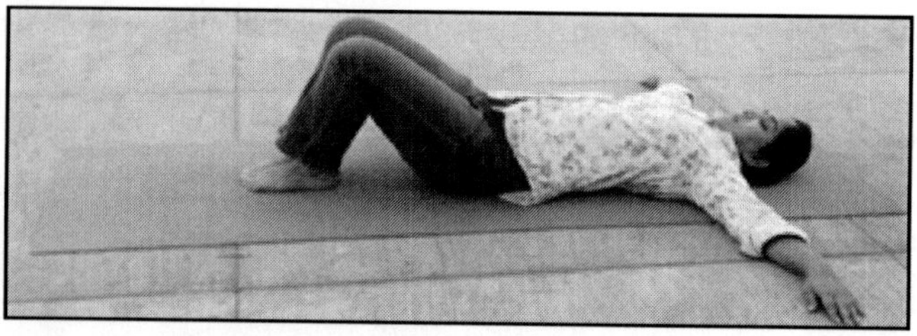

Pic. 108: Double knee low back rotation.

2. Slowly lower both the knees (together) to one side, trying to touch them to the floor.
3. Turn the head in the opposite direction.

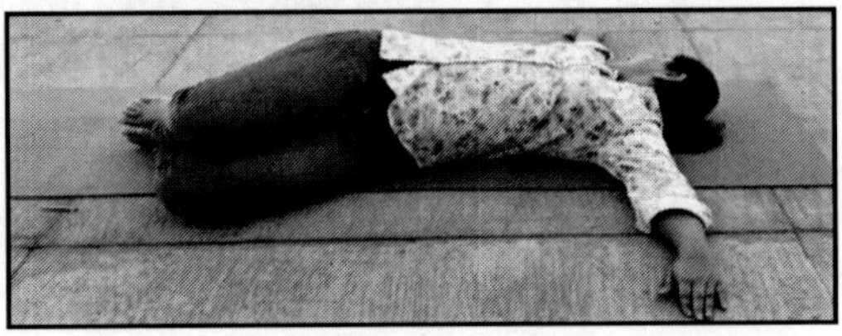

Pic. 109: Double knee low back rotation.

4. Keep the shoulder flat on the floor.
5. Hold for 10 seconds and get back to the starting position.
6. Repeat 5 times for each side.

Contradictions: People suffering from hernia should not practice this exercise.

(d) Cat-camel pose (Picture 110-111):

This exercise massages the abdominal muscles. It also strengthens the muscles of the low back, wrist and shoulders

1. Begin on your all fours- hands and knees.
2. Breathe out and draw your chin towards the chest by arching/ curving your back i.e. curve is directed upwards

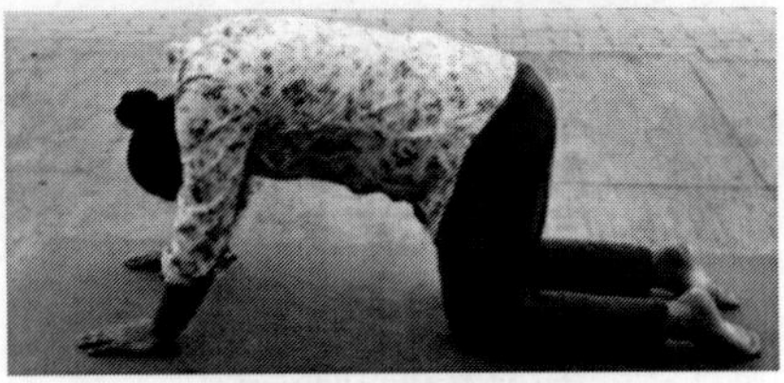

Pic. 110: Camel pose.

3. Hold this posture for 10 seconds.
4. Slowly bring your head up by curving your back in the opposite direction i.e. downwards. Breathe out while doing this step.

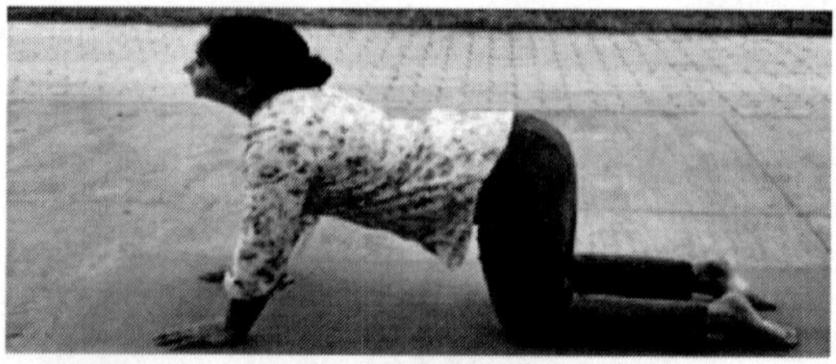

Pic. 111: Cat pose.

5. Hold for 10 seconds. In this posture, a stretch is felt in the lower back.
6. Alternate between these two postures 10 times.

Contraindications:People suffering from neck problems should do this exercise carefully.

III. Strengthening Exercises

(a) Abdominal strengthening diagonal curl: This exercise strengthens the abdominal muscles which support and protect your back muscles from strain.

1. Lie on your back with knees bent, feet flat on the floor, and hands across the chest (Picture 112-113).
2. Breathe in.

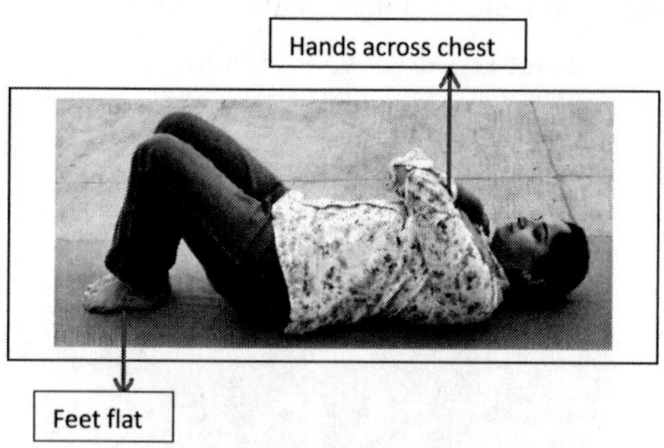

Pic 112: Diagonal curl.

3. Breathe out as you partially sit-up with your right elbow pointing towards the left hip with the left upper arm touching the ground. Then repeat it on the other side. Stretch is felt in the upper abdomen.

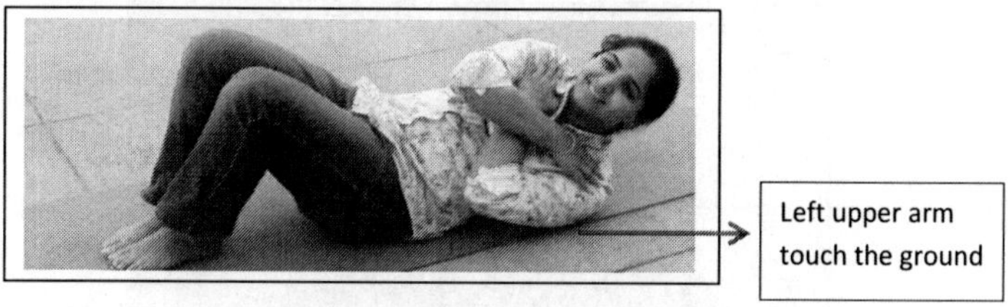

Pic. 113: Abdominal diagonal curl.

4. Do it 10 times on each side.

Caution: Keep your neck straight (imagine a fruit between your chin and chest)

(b) Bridging/Bridge pose (Setubandh asana) (Picture 114-115):

This exercise strengthens the muscles of low back, neck, hips and legs. It also massages the abdominal organs and thus strengthens the abdominal muscles

1. Lie flat on the floor on your back with knees bent, palms facing the ground (or try holding the ankles with your hands).
2. Keeping your feet flat on the floor, exhale and slowly raise your hips upwards as far as you can without discomfort. Try to bring the knees in line with the hips. While doing this exercise stretch is felt on the sides as well as central area of the lower back.
3. Inhale as you slowly lower to the starting posture.
4. Repeat it 5-10 times.

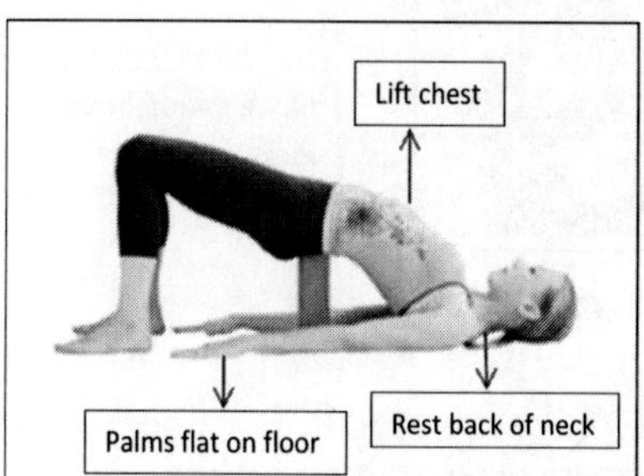

Pic. 114: Bridge pose with palms flat on the floor.

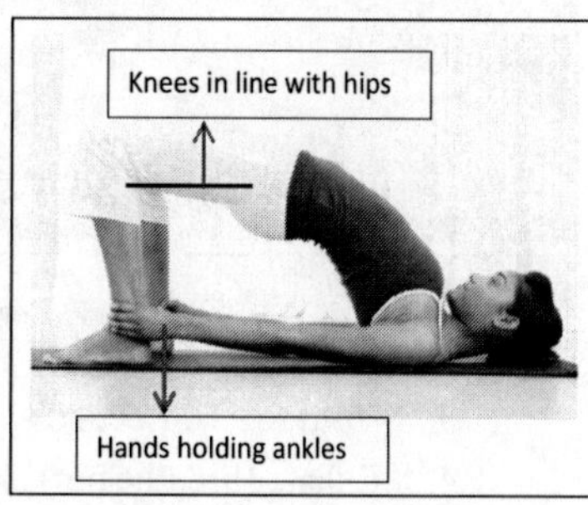

Pic. 115: Bridge pose hand holding the ankles.

(c) Hamstring stretch (Picture 116):

1. Lie on your back with legs bent.
2. Hold one thigh behind the knee
3. Slowly straighten knee until a stretch is felt in the back of thigh.

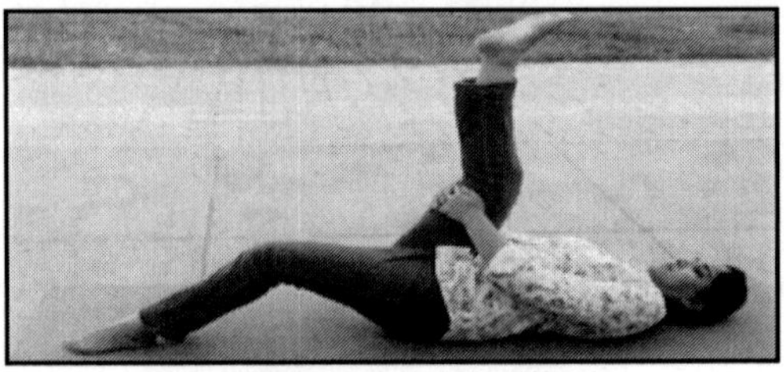

Pic. 116: Hamstring Stretch

4. Hold for 10 seconds and relax.
5. Repeat 5 times on each leg

Contraindications:People suffering from neck injury, shoulder injury, knee pain should avoid doing this exercise

(d) Advanced press up (level 4 of Cobra pose/ bhujang asana) :

1. Lie on your stomach with hands besides the chest, feet together, chin touching the ground and elbows touching the rib-cage. (Picture 5a).
2. Breathe in and slowly raise the chin, chest, abdomen (till little below the naval) off the ground. Look up towards the ceiling. Ensure that the arms and elbows are straight and locked (Picture 117).

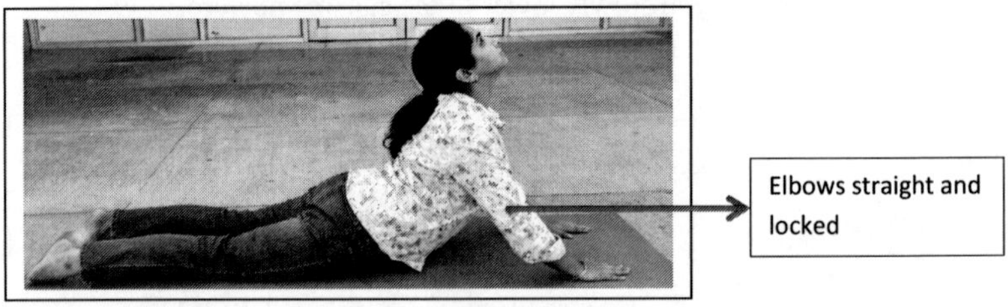

Pic. 117: Level 4- Cobra pose.

3. Hold for 3-5 seconds.
4. Exhale (breathe out) and return to the starting posture.
5. Repeat 5 times with 30 seconds rest between each repetition.

IV. Exercises at Office

Sitting in awkward postures in desk jobs or working on computer for long hours often leads to LBP. To avoid this it is suggested to:

- Get up every 20 minutes from the desk.

- Do stretching exercises which help reduce pressure on the intervertebral discs, muscles, joints and ligaments of the spine.
- They should be performed regularly (every 1-2 hours) during the day.

1. Bending [Picture 118-119]:
    - Sit comfortably in your chair, with the back evenly in contact with the chair.
    - Keep your feet flat on the floor and around 2 inches apart
    - Now slowly slide your hands down in front of your legs until you reach the floor.
    - Try to bend further down with each breath.
    - You will feel slight stretch in low back and on back of legs.
    - Hold the posture for 30 seconds. Repeat 3 times

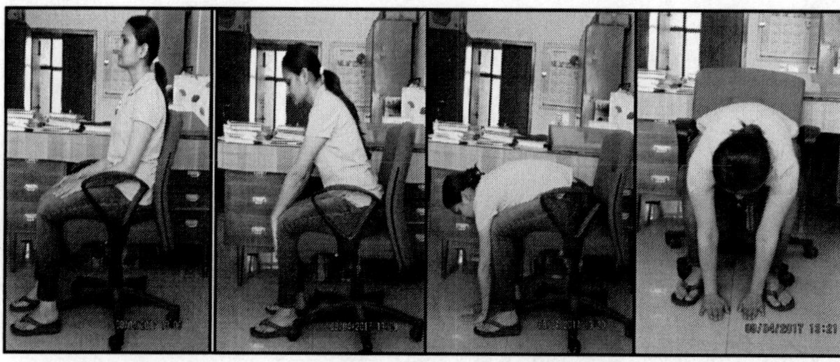

Pic. 118 ***Pic. 119: Bending***

2. Seated twist [Picture 120]:
    - Sit in your chair around 2 inches away from the back rest of the chair.
    - Keep your feet flat on the floor and knees in line with each other
    - Inhale and place your right hand on your left knee and left hand behind your back.
    - As you exhale, tighten the lower abdomen
    - Twist to the left by focusing on the upper back,
    - You will feel a stretch in the back and side of the neck, upper back, low back and shoulders.
    - Return to the starting position.
    - Repeat with the other side.

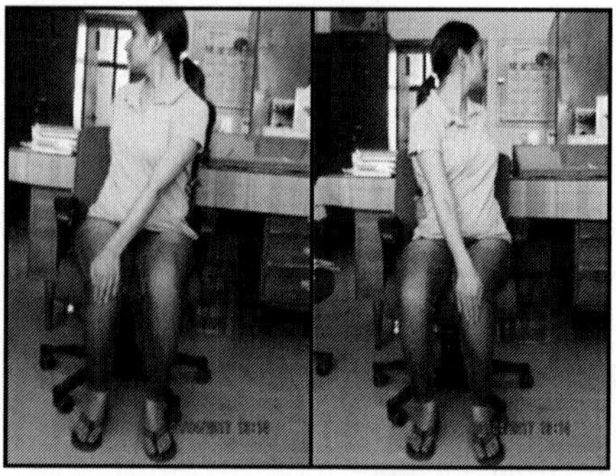

Pic. 120: Seated twist.

3. Back Arching [Picture 121]
    - Stand up
    - Support your lower back with hands as shown in the picture
    - Gently arch back from the waist as shown in picture
    - Hold for 5-10 seconds and then straighten up
    - Repeat 3-5 times.

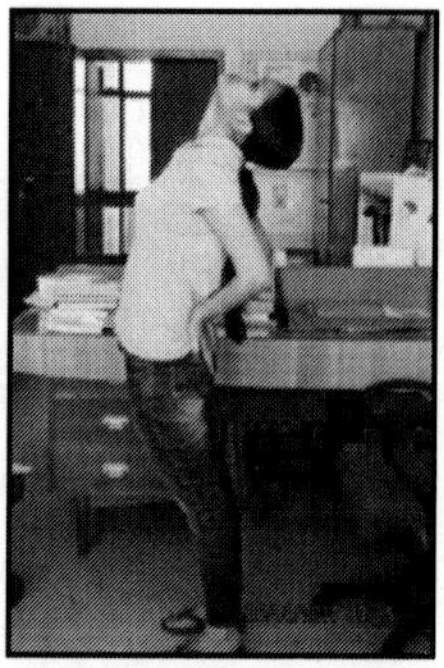

Pic. 121: Back arching.

4. Upper and lower back stretch [Picture 122]
    - Interlace your fingers and turn palms upwards above head
    - Straighten your arms and try to reach out for the ceiling
    - Hold for 10 seconds

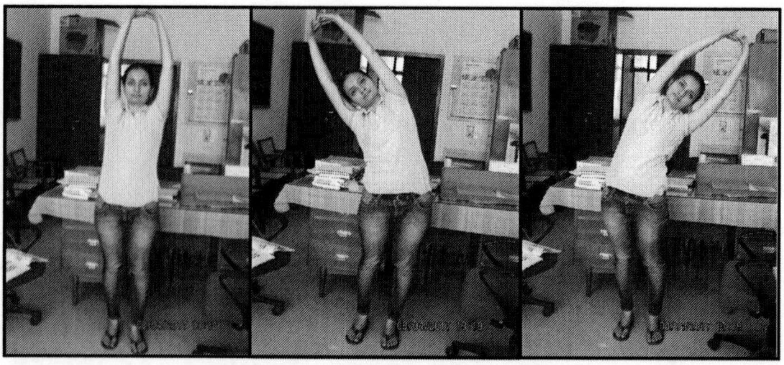

Pic. 122: Upper & lower back stretch.

- Slowly, bend slightly on one side. A stretch is felt on the opposite side of waist extending up the arm.
- Come back to the starting position and then bend to the other side.
- Hold for 10 seconds. Repeat movements several times

The exercises discussed in this chapter are suggested in management of low back pain. But these should be performed only under the guidance of a doctor or physiotherapist/yoga expert, etc.

Moreover, there are other exercises also available which act on various groups of muscles and are beneficial for low back pain. However, patients should choose exercises that 'suit them best' only after consultation with experts as different presentations/phases of low back pain require different kind of management.

Engineering Measures to be adopted at workplace and at home

In modern society, we spend a lot of our time sitting in chairs/sofas. Much of our job involves table work. Hence, our furniture should be ergonomically sound. Otherwise it may lead to low back pain (LBP). For example, in offices, we are forced to use the chairs and tables which are not comfortable. The chairs do not support the lower back. Also, they are either too high or too low with respect to the table. Thus, the user either bends forward or pushes the hips forward in order to reach the table (as discussed in section on postures). Similarly, in our homes, furniture once brought or the one that came as dowry some 20 years back is used for years. Mostly, these are not comfortable and cause pain esp. in the lower back and neck. For example, the seats of fancy big sofas available in the market are quite in its horizontal portion. Because of this, our feet usually hang down. We are not able to put these flat on the floor. In order to reach the floor, we adopt wrong postures (as discussed earlier in the chapter on posture). This hurts the lower back, knee, ankle, etc. Moreover, the ergonomic aspect of the design of the kitchen often decides the incidence and prevalence of LBP. For example, the height of the shelf; the height of the sink; distance of the tap from the edge is also important in order to maintain a correct posture while working in the kitchen. Thus, engineering measures play an important role in maintaining healthy back and preventing as well as reducing LBP. Some measures ensuring design of an ergonomic office workstation and kitchen are discussed in this section.

I. Design of office workstation: The office furniture is often purchased in bulk. The chairs, writing tables, computer tables, etc. are usually not according to the need of the user. Moreover, in many cases tables and chairs are purchased separately. These often mismatch. Thus, while working, the individuals are forced to adopt wrong postures that cause pain mostly in the neck and lower back. Furniture used in offices should be according to the need of the user. Some important points that need to be kept in mind while designing office workstations are discussed here.

The workplace should be according to the users' need. There are two main factors that should be kept in mind while designing office workstations. These are as follows:

- It should be suitable for all people as per their height, weight and body build. For example, if shorter people can reach objects at higher shelves, there is a possibility that everyone else can do the job. On the other hand, when bulky people can fit in a defined area, all the other people can also be accommodated.
- The working area needs to be comfortable for the user. This will prevent the user from inappropriate bending and adopting postures that cause neck and back pain. Also, it will help to increase work productivity.

Components of workstation: The office workstation comprises mainly of the following things:

(i) Chair: The office chair needs to be comfortable and suitable for the user. Usually offices have chairs with fixed height which are not suitable for people of all statures (height). Thus, adjustable chairs should be preferred. The Bureau of Indian Standards (BIS) has suggested dimensions for office chairs (table 1).

The various components of office chair are as follows:

(a) Seat height ('H'): The chair should be adjustable on a five-point star base. A range of 390-480 mm from the floor should suit most users (picture 7a). The height of the chair should be such that the thighs are parallel to the seated portion of the chair. The lower legs should be vertical i.e. legs below the knees are 900 to the thighs. The feet need to be flat on the floor or on the footrest. The seat height should also allow a 900 angle at the elbows for writing or typing. Moreover the elbows need to be at the level or just below the working surface.

(b) Seat depth ('B'): The chair should be deep enough to allow the lower back to come in contact with the lumbar i.e. lower backrest of the chair. Moreover, the front of the chair should be rounded so that it does not put pressure on the back of the knees/thighs/legs. According to BIS, the chair should be 390-450mm deep depicted as 'B' (Fig. 26).

Table 1: Recommended dimensions of office chair.

Seat			***Dimension in mm***
'A' Seat height:	Chair with fixed height seat		435 ± 5
	Chair with adjustable height seat		390 to 480
'B'Effective seat depth:	Chair with fixed back		390 *Min,* 430 *Max*
	Chair with adjustable back		390 *Min,* 450 *Max*
'C' Seat width Slope of the seat in relation of horizontal from front to back			450 Min 0° —6° backward
ARMRESTS (if provided)	**'G'** Height of armrests above point *Z* of the seat		200 ± *5*
	'Gi' Inside distance between armrests		440 *Min*
	'Gt' Set back of armrests in relation to the front of the seat		100 *Min*
	'Ga' Length of the armrests		200 *Min*
	'Gt' Width of the armrests		50 *Min*
BACKREST	**'W'** Centre of the backrest above *Z*	Chair with fixed backrest	250 ± 10
		Chair with adjustable backrest	200 to 250
	V Vertical height of area of essential lumber support (having *X* at its centre		200 *Min*
	F Width of area of essential lumber support		360 *Min,* 420 *Max*
	V Horizontal curvature of lumber support, radius		400 *Min,* 450 *Max*

(c) Seat width ('C'): The width ('C') of the seat should be slanting from front to back. The slope should be 0°-6° backwards (Fig. 27).

(d) Backrest: The backrest should provide firm support especially to the lower back region. It should be adjustable both in angle (i.e. forward – backward) and height while sitting. While

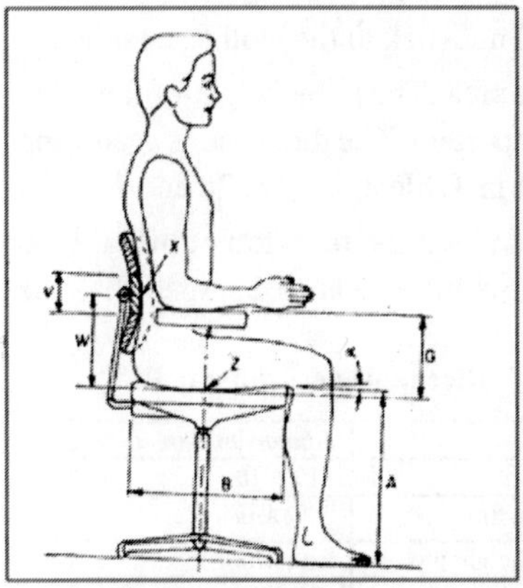

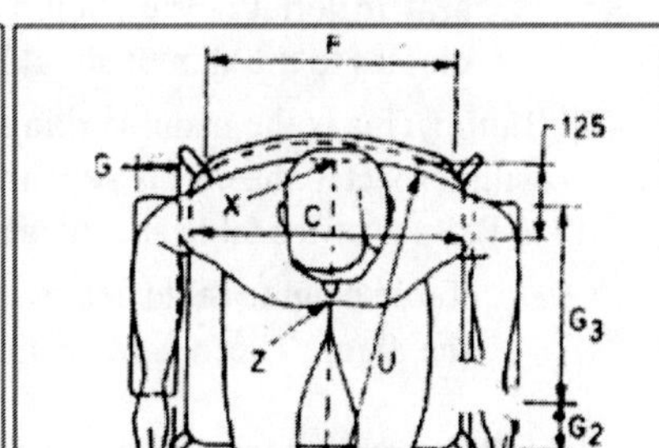

Source: Dimensions of tables and chairs for office purpose- Bureau of Indian Standards.

Fig. 26: Dimesions of adjustable revolving chair.

Fig. 27: Dimensions of chair-overhead view.

working,the angle between the spine and thighs should be at least 900. As per BIS, the height ('W') of the adjustable backrest should be 200-250mm whereas for fixed backrest it should be 250+/- 10mm. The width ('F') of the lumbar support of the backrest needs to be 360-420mm (Fig. 26-27). The top edge of the backrest should be raised up to the shoulder level or it should be below the thoracic vertebrae 8 i.e. T8 of the vertebral column.

(e) Armrest: These are optional depending on the user preference and task to be performed. They should not restrict the user from getting close to the work surface. The user, preferably, should not rest forearms on the armrest while using the keyboard. This is because mostly the keyboard is not placed at the level of the armrest of the chair. So, the wrists may bend up or down which can cause pain in the wrist sometimes going up the arms. However, BIS have suggested dimensions for armrest given in Table 1; Fig. 26-27.

(f) Footrest: Sometimes, the user is comfortable to work on the desk or computer with lower back well supported. Also, the keyboard as well as monitor is located at the correct place with respect to the user. However, the feet do not rest on the floor or are pointed inwards or outwards as discussed in the section on posture. In this case a footrest should be used.

(g) Seat material: The chair seat and back should be padded. The seat material/fabric should allow air circulation through the clothes to the skin. It should not stick to the clothes or skin.

(ii) Table: This is the main working area. Thus, the height of the table with respect to the user is very important. The dimensions according to BIS for office table are shown in Table 2; picture 28 and 29.

- Table height: Table height is measured form top of the table to the floor. The height of the table needs to be such that the

Table 2: Recommended dimensions of office table according to BIS.

Table		*Dimension inmm*
'H' Height of top surface: Fixed height top		710 ± 10
'R' Clearance below desk top:	Fixed height top	640, *Min*
	Adjustable height top	610, *Min*
'T' Clearance across the kneehole		580, *Min*
'S' Leg room, front to back (upperside)		450, *Min*
'Si' Leg room, front to back (lowerside)		600, *Min*

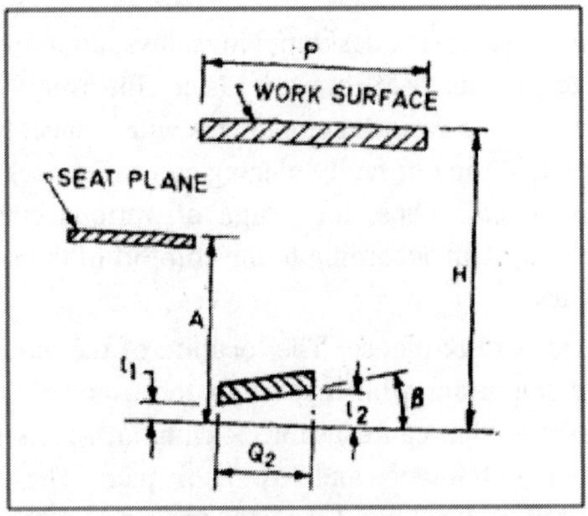

Source: Dimensions of tables and chairs for office purpose- Bureau of Indian Standards.

Fig. 28: Height of the table.

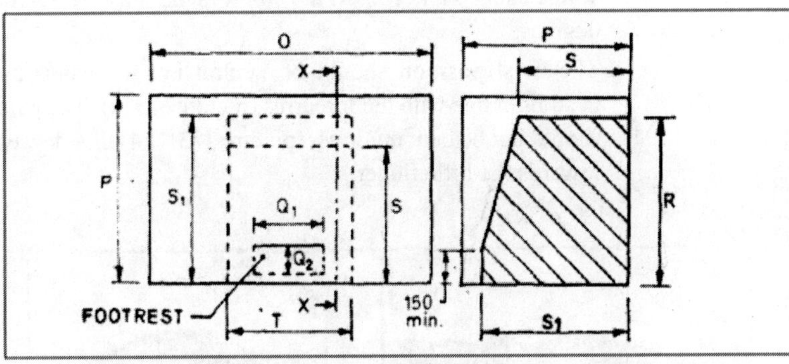

Source: Dimensions of tables and chairs for office purpose- Bureau of Indian Standards.

Fig. 29: Dimensions of a table as per BIS.

working area, i.e., the table top should be at the level or just below the level of the elbow of the user.

- Leg room: There should be enough space under the table such that the user is able to stretch legs also. There should not be any drawers in the space where legs need to fit.
- The table top should be big enough to allow space not just for paperwork, files, books but also for computer related equipment.
- Moreover, in order to avoid forward bending while writing on the desk, a writing board should be used. This board covers the space between the table and the user.

(iii) Computer system i.e. desktop: Nowadays, digitalization with use of computers has made office work easier. However, the correct position and place of the various components with respect to the user is very important. Wrong or faulty placing can cause neck pain, back pain, knee pain, etc. Thus, the usage of various components of the computer system according to the comfort of the user are discussed as follows:

(a) Keyboard & mouse: The location of the mouse and keyboard are important with respect to the user so as to avoid faulty postures that can cause neck pain, arm pain, numbness in the hand and fingers and low back pain. The important points regarding location of the keyboard and mouse are as follows:

- The keyboard and mouse location must allow the elbow and upper arms to be kept close to the body.
- While using the keyboard the elbow angle must be 90-100 degrees.
- The wrist position should be neutral i.e. the hands are in straight line with the forearms (picture 8xxiii). The wrist should not be bent up/down (picture 123-124) or sideways towards the little finger.

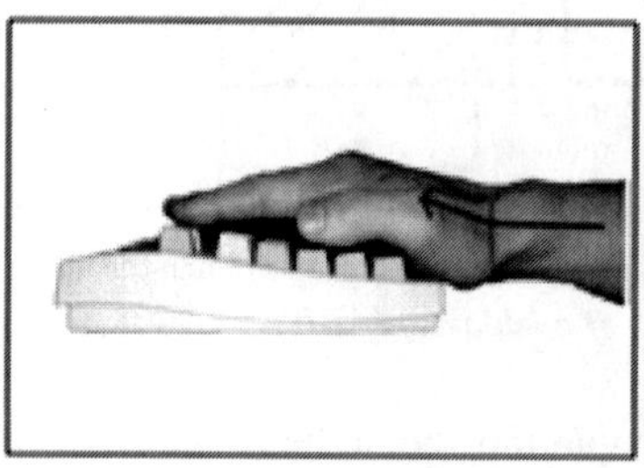

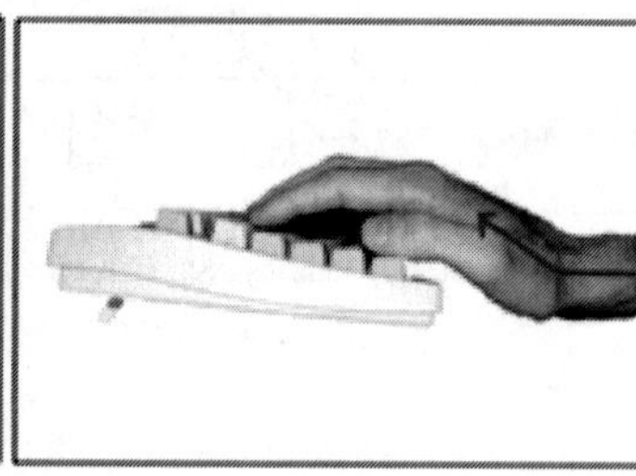

Pic. 123: Correctposition of the wrist. Pic. 124: Incorrectposition of the wrist.

- The wrist rest should be used to support the wrist during in between breaks. Placing the wrist on the wrist rest while typing can cause pressure and bend in the wrist commonly called as carpel tunnel syndrome.

(b) Monitor: The following points need to be kept in mind with respect to location of the monitor:

- The screen must be kept directly in front of the user so as to avoid any twisting of the head or neck

- The top line of the screen should be at or slightly (0-30 degrees) below eye level. It should be located at least an arm's-length away
- The monitor should be located such that user can read the screen clearly without bending the head/neck or trunk forward or backwards.
- There should not be any glare on the screen, because if present; the user will adopt awkward posture to read the screen.
- Document holder: It should be used instead of keeping the document on the table. The document holder must be kept close to the monitor and at an arm's length away from the users face. This helps to avoid strain in the neck, upper back and lower back.

Other considerations: there are some other important things which need to be kept in mind while designing and working on a workstation.

- The chair and table should complement each other. For example, the armrest of the chair should be at the level or just above the level of the top of the table.
- The desk should be set up so as to keep frequently used items within a forearm's length and less frequently used items within a stretched out arm's length.
- Follow the 20-20-20 rule: Every 20 minutes focus on an object 20 meters away for 20 seconds.
- Take regular breaks: Get up from your seat every 20-30 minutes and stretch your body.
- Keep hydrated: Drink plenty of water. To keep a check on this follow a simple rule. Keep a 1L bottle full of water on your desk. Try finishing it once before lunch i.e. between 9 a.m. 1 p.m. and once post lunch i.e. between 2-5 pm.
- Avoid eating lunch at your desk.
- Try doing stretching exercises at your desk.

II. Kitchen design: Indian women spend a major part of the day cleaning dishes or cooking in the kitchen. Nowadays, people buy already constructed houses which have well build modular kitchens. These are beautiful to look at. But most of the times these are not comfortable to work in. Many times, the woman of the house often complaint of LBP. During the preliminary days of my research I met women who complaint of LBP just while working in the kitchen. One of them said, "rasoi ich wadde hi kamar dukhan lag jandi ha" which means "low back pain begins as soon as I enter the kitchen". This is mainly because the food preparation area and cooking area are far apart. For example, rolling out (belna in Hindi) chapattis on one shelf of the kitchen whereas the cooking gas is placed on the opposite shelf. This involves moving (turning) here and there in the kitchen every minute. This can be tiring and may also cause LBP.

Moreover, another factor that contributes to LBP is the height of kitchen shelf or the sink is not according to the height of the woman. They adopt wrong postures and inappropriately bend their back while working in the kitchen. Thus, designing of the kitchen should be done according to the woman who has to work in it. Some of the important points regarding kitchen shelf and sink are discussed here.

(i) *General design of the kitchen-the work triangle:* The flow of activity in the kitchen follows a triangle. It starts with the food washing area which is generally the sink. Here, food from the storage or refrigerator is washed and cleaned. The next stage is food preparation area where cutting, mixing or rolling out chapattis, etc. is done. The third stage is the cooking area where the gas stove or cooking range is kept. Here the food is cooked and should be close to the food preparation area (picture 8xxv). All these three areas need to be arranged in a triangular pattern to conserve energy. The most efficient design is L-shaped. This is where two adjacent walls for a natural triangle (picture 125-126).

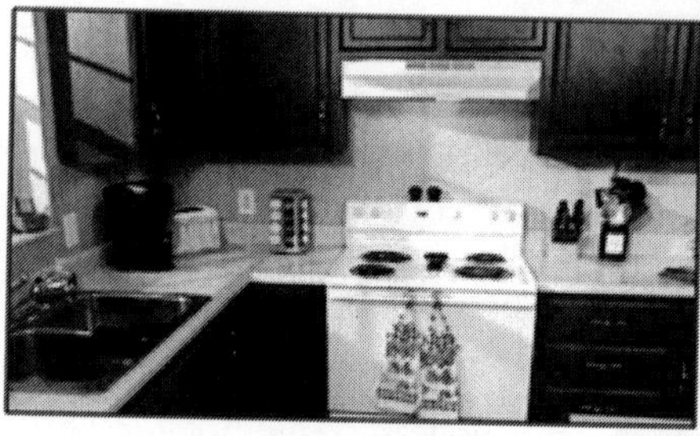

Pic. 125: Kitchen design.

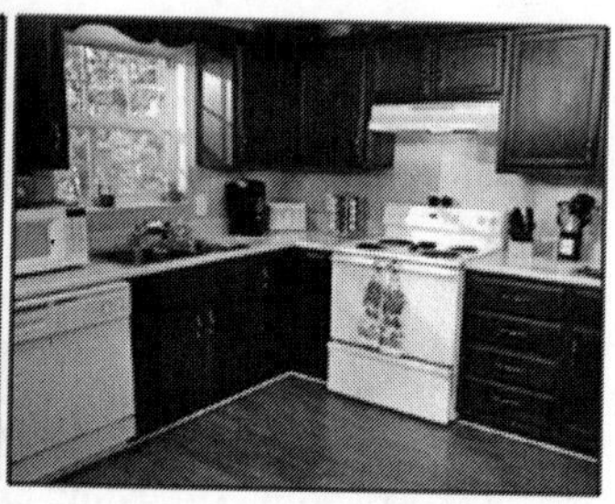

Pic. 126: Work triangle in the kitchen.

The work stations should be separated with the least amount of steps, but with the proper amount of work space. That means the distance between any two appliances should be no less than 3 feet and no more than 7 feet. This can avoid unnecessary moving and also reduce the standing and working time in the kitchen. Thus, reducing chances of developing low back pain.

(ii) *Kitchen shelf:* With respect to Indian kitchens, all the shelves are of the same height. However, different jobs in the kitchen require different kind of hand movement and bending. Thus, height of the shelves should be according to the task to be performed. For designing the kitchen shelf, its height should be measured with respect to the woman's elbow bent at 90 degree angle and not her body height. For example:

- For Chopping/slicing/dicing: It requires up and down movement of the forearm. This can be done easily without bending our backs when the shelf height is three-four inches below the elbow when it is bent at 90° angle as shown in Fig. 30.
- While cooking over the gas stove: We make different motion like stirring or mixing with a tablespoon having a long handle. In this situation, if the gas stove is 5-6 inches below the bent elbow, cooking will be comfortable and the woman will not have to bend her lower back (Fig. 30). This will also avoid spilling of oil to the height of the woman's face.

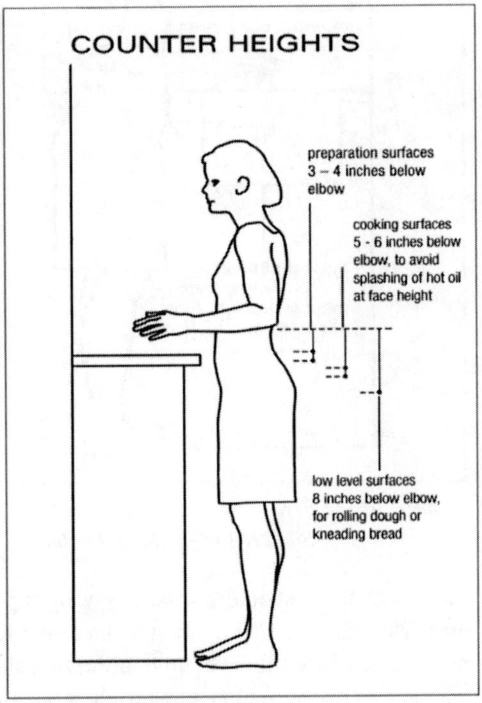

Source: Johnny grey.

Fig. 30: Height of the kitchen shelf.

Apart from height, the shelf should be light coloured. This will help in pointing any dirt or dust on the shelf easily without unnecessary bending. The chances of missing dirt/filth/dust are more in dark or black coloured shelves.

(iii) Washing utensils:The actual working surface for washing utensils is bottom of the sink. Therefore, the bottom of the sink should be 8-11 inches below the bent elbow as shown in Fig. 31. Whereas the shelf height on either side of the sink needs to be 2 inches below the bent elbow.

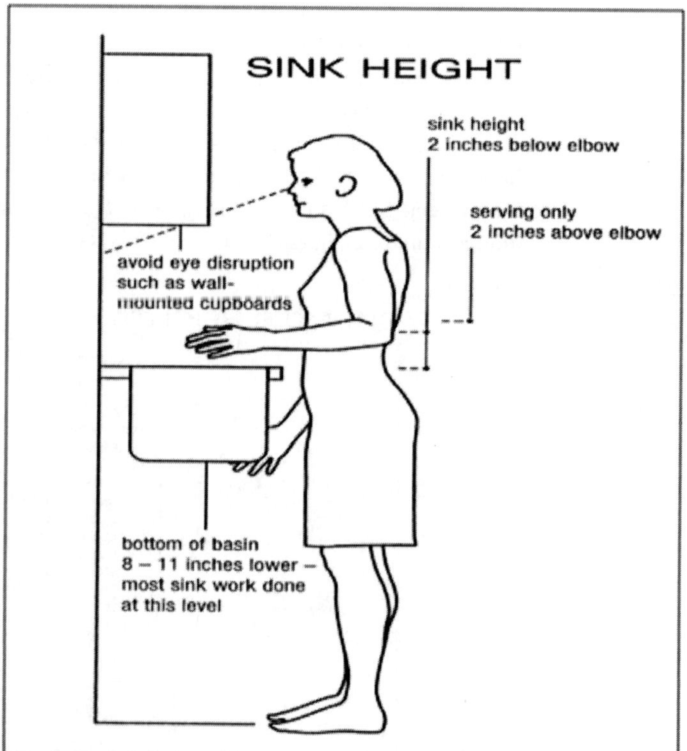

Source: Johnny grey

Fig. 31: The height of the sink.

Moreover, there should not be any wall cupboards over the sink area. This may obstruct lighting in the sink. Moreover, the user may not be able to see till the bottom of the sink clearly.

Another important thing which needs discussion is how to manage the shelves height if a newly married girl comes into the house and has to work in the kitchen. For this, it is suggested that if the height difference between the two ladies of the house is more than 12 inches, then the kitchen shelves need to be designed according to person who spends more time in the kitchen. Moreover, in India, there is a tradition of renovating the house before a wedding. Also, new electrical appliances are purchased. That is the time, re-designing the kitchen and buying new electrical appliances, if needed, should be considered.

(iv) Water storage area: Nowadays, due to shortage of clean drinking water in many cities, a tradition of using big plastic jars of distilled water is catching up. These jars are delivered by various agencies and dropped at our doorstep. Although clean drinking water reaches us.But these have added to the incorrect ergonomics in our kitchens. These jars are very huge and heavy as shown in picture 127.

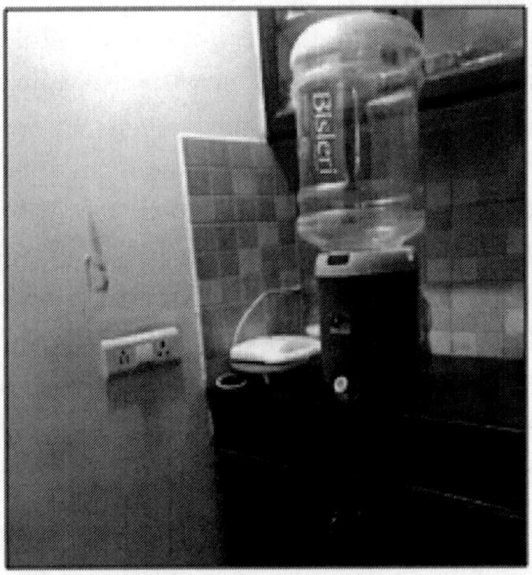

Pic. 127: Big jars of distilled water.

Picking them up alone and taking them to the kitchen takes a toll on the lower back. This can strain the back and cause LBP. Moreover, the cap of this jar has to be opened up over the utensil in which water is to be stored. A woman alone cannot hold this heavy jar on the utensil and open it up. But unfortunately, as expected of women, they will do it and over exert themselves!!! Moreover, they will adopt wrong postures, twist and turn their lower backs in order to reach the top of the jar. This increases the chances of straining the back and may cause LBP.

(v) Electrical appliances: Various electrical appliances like refrigerator, oven, microwave, etc. are used in the kitchen. All these should be ergonomically sound i.e. according to the comfort of the user otherwise its constant usage can contribute to low back pain, neck pain, etc. For example, in top freezer refrigerators, there is a lot of bending and stooping because the most used portion of the refrigerator is lower than the waist portion of the body. This can cause low back pain.

Ergonomically, the main refrigerator should be at the level that is between the waist and shoulders. This will prevent unnecessary bending of the lower back. Thus, refrigerators with bottom freezer units are better. In these, the main refrigerator is on the top which is usually at a level above the waist. However, these refrigerators are costlier than top freezer refrigerators. Moreover, size of the refrigerator is also a factor that needs attention. Some large/big refrigerators have deep shelves that require more bending to reach out for things kept on it. Therefore, depth of the shelves must be according to the user so that unnecessary bending can be avoided.

(vi) Lighting: Women working in the kitchen may not be able to clearly see very small things. This will force them to bend their neck and back in a wrong way. This may strain their low back and neck.

Thus, there should be proper lighting in the kitchen. This will allow the woman to work easily and comfortably without bending their back or neck unnecessarily.

Thus, workstations whether at office or house should be according to the users' need. These office and the kitchen workstations should be designed such that the user is comfortable and is also able to maintain correct posture while working over them. This way the user will not bend their back inappropriately. This will help in preventing and reducing LBP.

Other common treatments and remedies

Apart from exercises and correction of posture, there are other common remedies for LBP. There are many other treatments which we resort to in times of LBP. These range from applying the modern gels and tubes to traditional remedies in the form of churanas and also some self -home based treatments. Some of these are discussed in this chapter.

1. Hot Fomentation: It has a great pain relieving effect. It decreases muscle tension which is helpful in relaxing the affected muscles of the lower back.

Methods of applying hot fomentation

(a) Hot water bottle/bag: These are generally made of rubber or plastic. Hot water is poured in it to apply heat on the painful area in the lower back. This relieves congestion in the lower back. It maintains heat for around 20-30 minutes.

Steps of applying hot water bottle:

(i) Fill up a hot water bottle (the bottle should be ISI marked)

(ii) Expel the air carefully before putting the cap tightly; check for water leakage.

(iii) Check the temperature & wrap the hot bottle in a towel before application. This is done to protect the skin from burning.

(iv) Apply the bottle to lower back for 15-20 minutes.

(b) Moist hot towel: This is the easiest method of applying heat in case of low back pain. Dip the towel in hot water. Squeeze it to drain out extra water so that it is just damp and keep it on the lower back. This maintains heat for only 5-10 minutes.

(c) Electric heating pads: These pads provide heat as long as plugged in. However, we should avoid falling asleep while the pad is on. To remove the pad after 20 minutes set an alarm clock. Remove the pad when the alarm rings.

(d) Heated gel packs/microwave packs: These gel filled packs are available in different shapes that are appropriate for low-back and neck. These can be microwaved or heated in water and tend to stay warm for 30 minutes.

(e) Heat wraps: These are wrapped around the lower back and waist to provide heat. These are generally worn under the clothing to provide convenient and several hours of low level of heat application.

(f) Hot baths, sauna and steam baths: All of these relax the body which may reduce muscle spasm and pain.

Precautions: There are some precautions that need to be taken when applying heat. These are as follows:

(i) If there is increased swelling or warmth in the painful area, heat can deteriorate the pain by increasing blood flow to the skin. In such cases cold packs need to be used after consultation from experts.

(ii) A towel must be used between the skin and the heat source to prevent overheating or burns.

(iii) Heat should never be taken by lying on the back. It is best to apply heat by lying on the side or on the stomach. This is because, if the heat source is applied by lying on the back, there are chances that spinal curvature may increase.

2. Cold application: This method is generally used for acute inflammation or swelling. Use of cold application shuts down the blood supply close to the surface of the skin and helps to decrease swelling and inflammation. It also relieves pain as it numbs the nerve endings. Cold application should generally be used in the first 48 hours after an injury when the skin is not broken. It is also helpful when pain becomes worse after exertion.

Methods of cold application:

(a) Ice towel: Wet a towel with cold water. Then squeeze it until it is just damp. Fold the towel and put it in a plastic bag. Let it freeze for 15 minutes in the freezer. Remove the towel from the bag and place it on the painful area of the low back.

(b) Ice pack: These are available in different sizes in stores. Once brought these need to be kept in the freezer until used. These remain cold for about 20-25 minutes. If keeping the ice pack is uncomfortable at first, we can cover the icepack with a warm towel. This will give us few minutes to get use to the cold temperature.

(c) Local ice massage: For smaller areas of pain this method is most effective. Hold the ice in a cloth and rub it on the affected area in small circular pattern until the area feels numb (sunn hona in Hindi) and warm. This takes about 3-5 minutes. Once this sensation is achieved, remove ice and warm the area with a towel.

Precautions:Certain precautions need to be taken before cold is applied for relieving low back pain.

(i) Some people tense up their muscles when cold pack is applied on the painful area. If the muscles are not relaxed there are chances that the pain may increase.

(ii) If the area being treated becomes warm, remove the cold as continuing longer may cause frostbite ('sheetadansh' in Hindi- it is an injury caused by excessive exposure to extreme cold starting with initial redness and tingling ('jhunjhunahat' in Hindi) to gangrene).

3. Massage: This method is widely used by women to relive LBP nowadays. Massage generally improves circulation and can help in muscle relaxation. However, women take help of untrained household maids for getting massage. This can make the pain even worse. This should be avoided.

Another variant of massage available nowadays are the hand held vibrators. These are available easily in the market. These also act by increasing circulation which relaxes the muscles. One important thing that we need to keep in mind is the amount of vibration required to relive LBP. So, if these are used, it should be done under the supervision of physiotherapy experts.

4. Physiotherapy: All the methods discussed above are techniques used in physiotherapy. The difference is that these are done in a clinical setting under the supervision of experts. Thus, it is suggested to resort to physiotherapy when the acute phase of LBP (i.e. after 4-5 days) is over. There are other physiotherapy methods such as traction, spinal manipulation, kinesio-tape, etc. available for relieving LBP.

5. Ayurvedic Medicine: This is the most traditional form of medicine prevalent in our country. According to Ayurveda, all diseases arise from imbalance of doshas i.e. tri-energies vata, pitta and kapha. These doshas govern the equilibrium of the body. Thus, imbalance in any of these is responsible for developing a disorder. According to Ayurveda literature, imbalance/disturbance mainly in Vata dosh is responsible for LBP. It is referred to as Kati shoola in Ayurveda. Kati can be referred to as waist or hip area and shoola as pain.

As for management of LBP, there are two types of treatments available in Ayurveda viz. shodhan and shaman. Shodhana refers to curative treatment and involves procedures like Panchkarma; Snehan, Svedan, Kati Vasti, etc. whereas Shaman is considered equivalent to palliative treatment given in the form of drugs, churanas, herbal supplements & tablets.

Shodhana: These are many treatment procedures available for shodhana. Only a few are discussed here as follows:

(i) Abhyanga: This involves massage with medicated oils this is generally followed by swedana i.e. steaming. Swedana is given only in accordance with the decision of a qualified Ayurveda physician after proper diagnosis of the condition of the patient.

(ii) Swedana: This involves inducing sweating by providing steam or hot fomentation. There are many types of swedana according to Ayurveda text. Which kind of swedana is to be given depend on the condition of the patient as is diagnosed by a qualified Ayurevda physician.

(iii) Snehana: This is oleation (giving a person any kind of fat) therapy and is a part of procedure done before panchkarma. This involves external and internal oleation. In internal oleation, patient is asked to drink cartain amount of medicated ghee/oil for few days. In external olaetion, Ayurvedic massage is done with medicated oils.

Kati vasti is a part of snehana (external oleation) therapy. According to Ayurevda literature, Kati Vasti is very effective in LBP.The waist area of the body is called Kati. Holding warm medicated Ayurvedic oil on the affected areas is called Vasti. Kati Vasti involves retention of warm thick medicated oil over the lower back for some time. Here, the patient is asked to lie on the stomach. Then medicated oil is applied around the lumbo-sacral region. Then, a basin made of black gram dough is built around the lumbo-sacral area. Thereafter, little warm medicinal oil around 200-300ml is slowly poured into it. The temperature of oil is maintained by continuously adding more oil. This is done for 30-40 minutes. After this the affected area is gently massaged, followed by a steaming for 10-15 minutes for better absorption of the medicine.

(iv) Panchakarma: This involves detoxifying the body of impurities and toxins through 5 main procedures viz. vamana (therapeutic vomiting), verachana (therapeutic purgation), vasti (medicated enemas), nasya (nose cleaning) and raktamokshana (blood letting).

Shaman involves giving ayurveda medicine and formuations for treatment of low back pain. To name a few are Rasna Kwath (Pluchea lanceolata); lasuna (Alium sativam); Erandamula (Ricinus communis); Dasamula Kwatha; Maharasnadi Kwatha; Mahayograja Guggulu; Trayodasanga Guggulu; Naryana Taila. However, these should only be taken under the prespriction of a qualified and trained Ayurveda physician.

Ayurveda also involves the concept of ahara (referred to as diet correction) and vihara (activity correction) to reduce LBP.

In Ahara, it has laid downdefinite rules about do's and don'ts of eating according to the dosha involved. According to Ayurveda literature, in LBP, wheat and rice except special variety of rice like samvaka/kodrava; black gram pulse can be taken. However, pulses like peas (matara); Chickpea (chana); pigeon pea (arahara) should be avoided. As for fruits and vegetables,garlic; drum stick; paravala; brinjal; pomegranate; mango; phalasa; jujube plum (badara, bera); grapes can be taken. However; Jambo (jambu); bitter gourd (karella); lotus stem;cauliflower; lady finger should be avoided. Other food items which can be taken includesesame; milk; sour vinegar; coconut water; clarified butter; oil but beetle nut and likewise heavy substances should not be taken.

In Ayurveda, Vihara involves activities that need to be undertaken and which need to be avoided. For example, bathing with warm water; gentle pressing of the painful area; sleeping on the ground; sunlight exposure are essential activities that should be done in LBP. Whereas excessive exercise; lifting heavy weight; suppression of natural urges; use of uneven bed should be strictly avoided. According to Ayurveda literature, in case of LBP, travelling by cart; camel and direct exposure to cold air should be avoided as this may aggravate Vata doshaand may increase pain.

Moreover, yoga and meditation are an integral part of Ayurveda treatment regimen. Thus, Ayurveda treats LBPin a holistic manner by correcting the diet and lifestyle along with other procedures and medicines, if needed.

6. Acupuncture: It is a form of Chinese medicine though quite prevalent in India nowadays. According to acupuncture, the body contains patterns of energy force referred to as qi (pronounced as 'chi'). To maintain health proper flow of qi Is essential. The theory of acupuncture is there are 2,000 points on the human body. These are connected with 20 pathways which create flow of qi.

With acupuncture, hair-thin metallic needles are inserted into specific combinations of these 2,000 points. This is an attempt to correct and/or maintain a normal flow of qi.

7. Acupressure: This works on the principle of acupuncture.Acupressure involves changing the flow of energy by applying pressure with just hands or fingers and thumb on the same points used in acupuncture. A single point or multiple points are pressed in a specified order as needed to treat low back pain.

Nowadays various books are available in the market on the same. Moreover, people tend to practice acupressure by watching health shows on television. This may increase the pain and cause other problems as well. This is because in-depth knowledge of the energy pathways is required to actually practice this medicine. Therefore, a trained expert should be consulted for getting acupressure treatment.

There are varieties of treatments available for LBP. However, the actual cause of pain should be known and accordingly the choice of treatment should be made. It is important to look for non-medicinal/non-surgical cures for treating LBP if the condition is not life threatening. This is because medicines and surgery in the long run have side-effects. Various alternative remedies are also available fortreatment ofLBP. Not believing in alternative treatments is not a good option just because it did not prove beneficial for someone else. May be these treatments under supervision of experts prove beneficial and positive. Moreover, individual should choose the treatment that 'best suits them' or 'whichever works'. This is because one kind of treatment cannot be generalized to be 100% effective for every patient of LBP.

Myths and facts

1. Myth: Bed Rest is the best cure for LBP

Fact: Bed rest can help an acute back strain or injury. But staying in bed for long is not true. Sometimes remaining immobile in bed makes back pain worse. It makes the back more prone to injuries as a result of lack of flexibility. Thus, bed rest should be taken only for 3-4 days. After this the patient should try to go back to the normal routine.

2. Myth: Don't lift heavy objects

Fact: When lifting, it is just not the weight but also the way it is that is being lifted. When lifting, try to be as close as possible to the object and squat while lifting. Use your legs to lift and don't torque your body.

3. Myth: Skinny (being thin) means pain free

Fact: People who are too thin can also be at risk for back pain.

4. Myth: Exercise is bad and makes back pain worse

Fact: To stay healthy, the spine needs a regular regimen of stretching, strengthening and aerobic exercises. Start with mild exercises and slowly increases the intensity of exercises. Infact, patients must be advised to continue with back exercises regularly.

Do's And don'ts /General precautions for prevention and Treatment of low back pain

1. Discuss about your pain freely with your doctor and also about the treatment options available.
2. Follow all the instructions diligently.
3. Choose the treatment and best suits you or whatever works for you.
4. Keep a phone contact number of your doctor.
5. Go for second opinion also (esp. if surgery is advised or there is no relief).
6. Avoid sudden bending or lifting or any other jerky movements.
7. Be conscious about your posture.
8. Avoid sitting or standing for long hours. Always get up from your seat every 20-30 minutes.
9. Do not join gym or go for vigorous treadmill exercises.
10. Avoid getting massage from untrained house maids.

Dietary suggestions for healthy lifestyle and easing low back pain

'Healthy mind in a healthy body'

This is a famous saying that a healthy mind resides only in a healthy body. Thus, if we are physically healthy there are chances that we will feel more happy and energetic. Similarly, when we are not healthy we feel lazy, irritated and sad at times. The condition of LBP is not different.

However, to have a body i.e. free form pain and aches such as LBP, we need to exercise regularly, maintain correct body postures and eat a healthy diet. Exercises and body postures have already been discussed. This chapter deals with discussion about diet and food that help in reducing LBP.

Research has suggested that a proper and healthy diet helps in building muscle and bone strength. Proper diet along with regular exercise helps in reducing weight which is also important for preventing as well as reducing LBP. The Scottish guidelines on management of chronic pain have recommended that when proper diet along with exercise helps in reducing weight and also LBP. As such there is no specific diet plan for LBP, but there are certain foods that can help lessen the effect of risk factors associated with this condition. Certain foods and supplements that can help prevent and ease LBP are discussed below. However, always consult your doctor and/or dietician for its dosage and frequency before administering them in your diet.

Foods to eat to help ease LBP

Fruits & vegetables:These contain all the essential vitamins and minerals such as Vitamin C, B12, K2, calcium, magnesium, potassium that combat low back pain and swelling. These should be incorporated at every meal. Vegetables such as carrot, radish, lettuce, broccoli, spinach and fruits such as cherries, blueberries, red grapes, pineapples, pomegranate (annar in Hindi), strawberries are few examples that are pain reliving and also boost immunity. Foods such as tofu, soya, eggs and fish are rich in proteins that help in muscle building and strengthening. The American college of occupational & environmental medicine has suggested the use of capsicum for temporary relief from LBP. Eat a fruits and vegetable every day.

Omega-3 fatty acids:Fish such as salmon, or fish oil and other foods rich omega-3 fatty acids such as walnuts, flaxseeds(alsi in Hindi) and olive oil should be taken to reduce aches and pains in the lower back. At least one serving per day of omega-3 fatty acids should be included in the diet. The Scottish guidelines for management of Chronic pain have recommended with strong evidence that use of omega-3 fatty acids reduces joint pain

Milk and milk products:These are rich in Calcium which is essential for healthy and strong bones. It also helps to maintain necessary level of bone mass. Lack of calcium can cause weak and brittle bones.

Vitamin D: Foods such as eggs, mushrooms, cod liver oil and fortified food (e.g. fortified orange juice and breakfast cereals) are important for string and healthy bones. It also helps in managing LBP. This is also known as the sunshine vitamin as it can be optimized in the body through regular and appropriate sun exposure. Try to spend 10 to 20 minutes in sunlight daily.

Herbs and spices: Ginger, turmeric, cinnamon, dried chili pepper, basil, oregano, etc. help reduce LBP symptoms. These help in relieving stiffness and inflammation, if any. These spices and herbs add flavor to the food so can be added in every meal.

Moreover, the following fat burning foods can also be taken by everyone:

- Lemon
- Cinnamon
- Garlic/methi seeds
- Soya nuggets/granules
- High fibrous foods such as fruits and vegetables

Foods to be avoided: Some foods are perceived to increase LBP. These should be avoided regardless of whether you suffer from LBP or not

- Processed foods, fast foods, saturated fats: all these lead to inflammation. These include pasta, white bread, rice, sugary drinks and snacks, fried foods such as puri,parantha, samosa,namkeen mixture, pakoda, etc
- Preservative packed food: These include chips, crackers, pastries, etc.
- Certain vegetables like aalo, arbi, kachalu, kathal, etc
- Sugar, gur, honey, shakkar,
- Canned juices, sharbat, squashes, cold drinks/soda
- Alcoholic drinks

General Recommendations

- Eat a well-balanced diet, including, fruits and vegetables, proteins, cereals, grains, milk and products.
- Have regular meals. Skipping meals will not help in reducing weight. Avoid fasting, feasting and crash dieting.
- Drink plenty of water. Try drinking at least 2-3 litres/day.
- Keep a record of your weight. Weigh yourself every 15 days on the same scale with similar clothing and approximately at the same time. Excess bodyweight increases stress on the joints, esp. weight bearing joints like spine and knees.

Take home message/For future generations

In the modern day world, low back pain has become very common. Earlier it was thought to be a disease of the elderly. However, nowadays people in their 20's and 30's complain of LBP. Moreover, women are seen to be the most sufferers. This is because women over exert themselves. They run after other members of the family the whole day, this leaves them with no time to think about themselves. As for having a healthy diet, they often offer fruits to their children and force them to eat it. But they themselves will hardly eat one. They do not have any time to exercise also. In fact in our Indian society, exercising is not considered important for women.

Many women themselves think that running here and there after children, looking after the family, working in office the whole day is enough exercise for them. They consider this kind of lifestyle as equivalent to exercising. Then why would they ever suffer from low back pain? However, I must share this that there is a difference between exercising and over exerting!!!!What women do is over exert themselves. They do not exercise. As a result the muscles and bones become weak. Now as they adopt wrong postures while working in the kitchen, cleaning the house, washing clothes, etc. they complain of LBP. This is because they strain the already weak and loose muscles due to bad posture.

However, in search of relief they often visit the doctor who prescribes medicines and supplements. They take medicines and feel OK when the pain is relieved. But again after few days the cycle of pain begins. The catch here is to identify the underlying cause of pain. If it is because of some underlying pathology or deficiency, medicine or other available treatments should be taken from qualified and trained physicians or specialist as the case may be.Even in cases of pathology or deficiency, exercise and posture correction are suggested for treatment and reduction of LBP. This is because; the nourishment our muscles and bones get from exercising and stretching is more important than any supplements or medicines. However, exercising is also an art. It should also be done carefully. Many a times, LBP develops because of wrong and vigorous exercising. Thus, exercises should be done under the guidance of trained experts like physiotherapists /yoga experts, etc.

The kind of sedentary lifestyle we have adopted is also being passed to the future generations. Our children are adopting a similar lifestyle. Nowadays children have indulgence in gadgets like phones, computers, laptops, i-pads, etc. They hardly go out in the open to play. As a result they have weak muscles and bones. Moreover, they eat junk food. This is leading to childhood obesity. This is weakening the bones and muscles. Imagine if they have weak bones and muscles now, their condition will be worse than ours when they grow up. Moreover, even for simple pain they resort to medicines. This is weakening their tolerance threshold.This is also further weakening their bodies.

Thus, there is a need to change our lifestyle and inculcate a habit of exercising regularly. We should be conscious of our postures while working. Moreover, we should try inculcating these habits in our children at an early age so that they do not suffer ill-health and pain like us!!!

LBP is a lifestyle disorder. It is preventable provided we take care of our bodies.

Research on Low Back Pain by the authors

A Ph.D. thesis related trial was conducted by Dr. Neha to see the impact of two intervention strategies on occurrence and severity of low back pain in 400 non-teaching women employees of Panjab University Chandigarh. The employees were divided into 3 groups. In group 1, the women were distributed a booklet on various aspects of back pain prevention and management. They were also given one to one/ group training through lectures/demonstrations on exercise and posture; videos/ pictorial messages were sent through watsapp messenger (social media application) on phones and meditation technique was also taught to them. In group 2, only the booklet was distributed and videos/ pictorial messages were sent through watsapp messenger (social media application) on phones. In group-3 no intervention was given. Follow up visits were made up to 6 months to see the effect.

Results: Prevalence of low back pain was 51%, i.e., out of 400 women employees interviewed 202 were suffering from pain, stiffness or discomfort in the lower back. Only

28%of them had taken treatment. Majority preferred Allopathy as first choice of treatment. Most women took back pain as routine and ignored it.

As a result of our interventions (exercise and posture training), reduction in pain was reported by most women. This decrease was more in group -1 where training/demonstration of exercise and correct posture was given along with booklet provision.

Review of various guidelines on management of LBP

To have an update on management of LBP, 15 guidelines of various countries were reviewed for acute, sub-acute, chronic and prevention of low back pain (table 3-5).

Table 3 shows that exercise was recommended in half of the guidelines. Similarly, superficial heat, psycho-social interventions and education (about various aspects related to LBP) have favourable evidence in management of acute and sub-acute LBP in majority of the reviewed guidelines. Bed rest was not recommended in majority of guidelines.

Table 3: Review of guidelines on management of acute & sub-acute LBP (n=15)

Intervention components	*Comments on evidence in the guidelines for various components*			
	Favourable evidence/ Recommended	*Unfavourable evidence/ Not recommended*	*No clear evidence/ Conflicting recommendation*	*No mention of evidence*
Exercise	7	4	0	4
Massage	4	1	1	9
Superficial heat	8	0	0	7
Lumbar support/Belt	1	1	2	11
Self-care	3	0	0	12
Acupuncture	3	2	1	9
Psycho-social	6	0	1	8
Interdisciplinary	1	0	2	12
Back school	1	0	3	11
Education about various aspects of LBP	9	0	0	6
Bed rest	0	8	0	7
Mattress	0	0	1	14
Alteration of sleep posture	1	0	0	14

Exercise was recommended for chronic low back pain in all the reviewed guidelines. Favourable evidence was also cited for pyscho-social and multi-disciplinary interventions in most i.e. 13 and 11 guidelines respectively. Education (about various aspects of LBP) and self-care strategies through education booklets were recommended by almost 50% of the reviewed guidelines (table 4).

Table 4: Review of guidelines on management of chronic LBP (n=15)

Intervention components	*Comments on evidence in the guidelines for various components*			
	Favourable evidence/ Recommended	*Unfavourable evidence/ Not recommended*	*No clear evidence/ Conflicting recommendation*	*No mention of evidence*
Exercise	14	0	0	0
Massage	4	0	0	11
Superficial heat	1	1	2	11
Lumbar support/Belt	0	2	4	9
Self-care	7	0	0	8
Acupuncture	6	0	0	9
Psycho-social	13	0	0	2
Multi- disciplinary (physical + psychological)	11	0	0	4
Back school	5	0	0	10
Education about various aspects of LBP and its management	8	0	0	7
Bed rest	0	3	0	12
Mattress	0	1	1	13
Alteration of sleep posture	1	0	0	14

Table 5: Review of guidelines on prevention of LBP (n=15)

Intervention components	*Comments on evidence in the guidelines for various components*			
	Favourable evidence/ Recommended	*Unfavourable evidence/ Not recommended*	*No clear evidence/ Conflicting recommendation*	*No mention of evidence*
Exercise	4	0	0	11
Lumbar support/Belt	0	1	1	13
Education about various aspects of LBP and its management	3	0	0	12
Ergonomics	1	0	2	12
Back schools	0	1	0	14
Multidimensional intervention (education+ ergonomics+ physical activity)	1	0	0	14
Mattress	0	0	1	14

Exercise and education had favourable effect on prevention of LBP (table 5).

List of guidelines reviewed

- American college of Physicians (Feb 2017)
- Michigan quality Improvement Consortium guidelines (March 2016)
- Evidence informed primary care management of LBP – Clinical practice guidelines (December 2015)
- National program for disease management guidelines, Germany (August2011)
- Colorado division of workers compensation
- Institute of clinical systems improvement (Nov 2012)
- KNGF guidelines- Royal Dutch society of Physical therapy (2013)
- KNGF guidelines- Manual therapy for LBP (2013)
- Healthcare Improvement Scotland National clinical guidelines – Management of Chronic pain (December 2013)
- American Physical Therapy Association (2012)
- National Health Committee: LBP pathway to prioritization New Zealand
- American college of Occupational & environmental medicine (2007)
- Chronic LBP KCE report, Belgium (2007)
- Evaluation & management of LBP(acute, sub-acute and chronic) by American Pain society (2007)
- Evidence based clinical practice guidelines for management of persistent non-specific LBP (Saudi Arabia 2013)

References

1. Gest TR, Schlesinger J. MedCharts Anatomy [monograph online]. New York: ILOC, Inc.; 1995.
2. Kenyon J, Kenyon K. The Physiotherapist's Pocket Book- Essential facts at your fingertips. New Delhi: Elsevier ; 2007.
3. Hochschuler S, Reznik B. Treat Your Back Without Surgery- the best nonsurgical alternatives for eliminating back and neck pain. New Delhi: Rupa Publications India Pvt. Ltd.; 2012.
4. Hage M. The Back Pain Book- A Self-Help Guide for Daily Relief of Neck & Back Pain. Delhi: Pustak Mahal.
5. Kraus H. Backache Stress And Tension- Their Cause Prevention and Treatment. London: George Allen & Unwin Ltd.; 1966.
6. Saunders ES. Backache In Women. Bristol: John Wright & Sons Ltd.; 1966.
7. Mahtani R. The Power Of Posture- Mindful Alignment for a Pain-Free Life. Mumbai: Jaico Publishing House; 2016.
8. Kisner C, Colby LA. Therapeutic Exercises- Foundations and Techniques. 5th edition. Philadelphia: FA Davis Company; 2007.
9. Hawley G. The Kinesiology of Corrective Exercise. 2nd edition. Philadelphia: Lea & Febiger ; 1949.
10. Williams M, Worthingham C. Therapeutic Exercise for Body Alignment and Function. Philadelphia: W.B. Saunders Company; 1957.
11. Dongaonkar D. Yoga Application for Low Back Pain. New Delhi: Jaypee Brothers Medical Publishers (P) Ltd.; 2013.
12. Ramdev S. Yog Sadhna va Yog Chikitsa Rahasya. Haridwar: Divya Prakashan; 2005.
13. Singh AJ, Goel S, Senjam SS, Goel S,editors. Mantras for Healthy Lifestyle- A Salutogenic Approach. New Delhi: Century Publications; 2012.
14. Chaudhari A, Singh A; Dhaliwal LK. A Simple Solution To Painful Menses- A training manual for adolescent girls. New Delhi: Century Publications; 2011.
15. Singh AJ, Walia I, Dhaliwal LK, editors. Demedicalizing Women's Health. New Delhi: Gyan Publishing House; 2010.
16. Singh AJ, Goel S, Kathiresan J, editors. Health Promotion: Need for Public Health Activism Vol I and Vol II. Germany: Lap Lambert Academic Publishing; 2013.

Chapter - 4

Non Surgical Interventions and Exercises for Knee Osteoarthritis (KOA) Patients

— *Meenakshi Sharma,*
MS Dhillon, S Kaur, AJ Singh

In India, knee osteoarthritis (KOA) has been reported to be one of the common cause of disability among more than half of the people aged above 50 years. Intractable pain is the most common symptom of KOA. Quality of life (QOL) of KOA patients is seriously compromised because of the resultant loss of mobility. All this leads to dependence and disability.

Currently, there is no cure for KOA. Treatment is aimed primarily at symptom relief. Focus is on optimizing the QOL through improvement in joint mobility and function. Long-term effects of early to moderate KOA can be managed through non surgical interventions. This includes a combination of non-pharmacological interventions (comprising of patient education on a set of exercises and weight reduction etc) and a regimen of painkillers etc. Joint replacement surgery is a costly option mainly for people with severe KOA who are unresponsive to non surgical management.

In western countries, many RCTs have been done on non-pharmacological KOA treatment. Many treatment guidelines have been prepared and are being used. In fact, many countries have their own well established and elaborate KOA management protocols which are regularly updated. Even evidence grade of various components of recommended interventions are systematically documented. All such information including exercise videos is available in public domain on the internet. However, surprisingly, such an effort is lacking in India. No standard operating procedures (SOP) have been developed for KOA management. Even there is lack of consensus on the set of exercises to be done by KOA patients. Different consultants prescribe different set of exercises to KOA patients. There are many gaps in evidence base of non surgical care provision to KOA patients in India.

For example, it has been documented that KOA may result in changes that accelerate the deterioration of body balance system. KOA affects our proprioception (a sense or individual perception of body position, movement, and acceleration; a sense of how our bodies are positioned; a sense of the relative position of neighboring parts of the body). Impaired proprioception adds to functional insufficiency by generating impairment in walking rhythm, shortening step distance. It also leads to a decrease in walking speed and total walking time. There is less focus in India on inclusion of patient training in KOA management based on balance, postural stability, and proprioception. Incorporation of agility and balance training in intervention packages has been shown to facilitate more effective management of patients with KOA. KBA (Kinesthesia, balance, agility) techniques are designed to improve dynamic joint stability using a series of physical activities which challenge a participant's neuromuscular system to maintain balance and coordination. Improved joint stability has a potential to provide relief in the symptoms as well as to slow the progression of KOA.

Exercise therapy is well established as an important part of clinical management for people with KOA. But systematic reviews have shown that effects of exercise on pain and function are moderate.Hence there is a room for improvement in designing OA exercise therapy programs. Exercise therapy should not only focus on impairments associated with KOA such as lower-extremity joint motion deficits, muscle weakness, and reduced aerobic capacity but also need to provide the patient with exposure to other challenges of motor function (eg, quick stops, turns, and changes in direction; challenges to balance; negotiating obstacles) that may be encountered during daily functional activities. This can be accomplished if they are exposed to KBA training.

However, a pilot study done by us in PGIMER in 2013 has revealed that orthopaedics surgeons and physiotherapists are not using the concept of KBA in management of KOA. In contrast to western countries, where research has been regularly conducted to evaluate the relative impact of combining a variety of non pharmacological interventions on KOA, there has not been any systematic effort in India on these lines.

As of now, a lot of time of doctors / physiotherpists in apex medical institutions like PGIMER Chandigarh is utilized / wasted in explaining the exercises and other therapies to KOA patients.Instead, their time and resources can be devoted to other patients with more complications.In addition, use of laptop / video / brochure / booklet / posters based for training the KOA patients exercises etc. This will also can reduce the patient load on doctors / physiotherpists by saving their time.

Against this background, we conceived the idea of this text. We decided at the outset that its content has to be for lay people. We sought to make it different from other technical writings on KOA available hitherto. Here, it is clarified that in 21st century, surgery has come to occupy a definite place in KOA management. This has been made possible through advances, not only in development of better quality prosthesis (artificial knee joint structures), but also in the better surgical techniques. Many people have benefitted through this progress in orthopaedics discipline. Now, we have many super-specialists handling mainly TKRs. Their success rate is also high. However, this is for severe KOA cases only. Here, we have tried to address the problems pertaining to early to moderate KOA cases. This deals with the issues beyond the usual surgical or pharmacological aspects usually highlighted in other books. We have also attempted to instill a patient empowerment appeal in the text.

Aim & Audience

The aim of this text is to provide user- friendly reading material for Knee Osteoarthritis (KOA) patients and their caregivers on various aspects of conservative (non-pharmacological) management regimen with special focus upon exercises by -

- defining the major components of conservative care
- offering them sound advice based on best published clinical evidence
- taking into account their preferences to promote informed decision-making
- providing customized guidelines for a variety of situations faced by them

What this text is not about: A disclaimer

This text does not deal with the details on medicinal / surgical treatment of KOA. It also does not give any advice about the injections used (PRP or others) for these patients. Here, it needs to be understood that the KOA patients should follow a proper channel of referral and treatment for their problem. First, they should get a clinical evaluation done for their knee joint related problem. After a proper diagnosis of KOA has been done by the orthopedist (with X ray etc. done), they need to have a clear instruction from them about the line of treatment to be followed. Only those patients where the orthopedist has advised about physiotherapy may consider the contents of this text. In case of any doubt, once they start on physiotherapy, they need to consult the concerned experts.

Also since, as of today, there are no universally accepted and fool proof (with full guarantee) treatment options (failures are reported with each regime!), patients are also advised to seek and find what works for them and what does not. They may even consult trusted internet sites on this issue. Also, they need to watch out for side effects of medicines used by them, esp. pain killers! And last but not the least, choose an orthopedist / physiotherapist who is 'willing to listen to the patient'!

The text is intended for use by the following people or organizations:

- people with KOA and their care-givers
- patient support groups
- all healthcare professionals and service providers.

Introduction

For deriving proper benefit from this text, it is essential that the KOA patients and their care-givers first understand the **structure of the knee joint-**

Knee is one of the largest and most complex joints in the body. In any joint, there are bone, muscles, tendon, ligaments and cartilage. Also there is joint space between the bones. This space is filled with lubricating fluid (people call it GREASE in common language). Cartilage covers the bone edges / ends as a cushion. The knee joint links the thigh bone (femur) to the shin bone (tibia). The smaller bone that runs alongside the tibia (fibula) and the kneecap (patella) are the other bones that make the knee joint. Tendons connect the knee bones to the leg muscles that move the knee joint. Ligaments join the knee bones and provide stability to the knee. Two C-shaped pieces of cartilage called the medial and lateral menisci act as shock absorbers between the femur and tibia. Numerous bursae (> 10 fluid-filled sacs) act as cushion to help the knee move smoothly. These are located where muscles and tendons move over bony joint areas. Their function is to reduce friction caused by muscles and tendons moving against skin and bones, as well as to facilitate movement. These help with movement when we walk, run, stretch, or even cross our legs. These are located on the inside of each knee, between the muscles, tendons and the shin bone.

Cartilage (meniscus) is a firm rubbery material that covers the ends of bones in normal joints. It is primarily made up of water and proteins. The main function of cartilage is to reduce friction in the joints and serve as a "shock absorber". This quality of normal cartilage comes from its ability to change shape when compressed. It can do this because of its high water content.

What is Knee Osteoarthritis (KOA)?

KOA develops when the cartilage (meniscus) is damaged. For example, in a joint stressed by abnormal weight bearing loads - attempts by the immune system (body's defense system) to repair the damaged cartilage cause it to swell. The cartilage becomes thin, soft and cracked. It exposes the underlying bone. It may also lead to the formation of small cysts. Also new outgrowths of bone are formed (osteophytes or bone spurs). This further disrupts the way the joint works. All this aggravates the damage which has already occurred in the joint. The space between the bone ends gets narrowed, further altering the joint mechanics. This adds to the stresses within the knee joint. Other tissues in the joint such as the surrounding membrane (the synovium) ligaments and tendons may also be affected. Often, it is said that bone spurs need to be removed in KOA patients. But, some experts opine that not all bone spurs are bad. These may serve a useful purpose by providing an adjustment for the changed joint structure (e.g. displaced meniscus).

Osteoarthritis (OA) refers to a clinical syndrome of joint pain accompanied by varying degrees of functional limitation. It vastly affects quality of life of patients. It is by far the most common form of arthritis. It is also one of the leading causes of pain and disability worldwide. Knees, hips and small hand joints are most commonly affected by OA. This text primarily deals with KOA only.

KOA occurs more commonly among older people. Doctors call it a degenerative joint disease. It mostly affects cartilage which is the hard but slippery tissue that covers the ends of bones where they meet to form a joint. In healthy people, cartilage allows bones to glide smoothly over one another. It also absorbs energy from the shock of physical movement. So, it acts like a cushion. In OA, the surface layer of cartilage breaks and wears away. This causes bones under the cartilage to rub together. This leads to pain. Swelling may also develop. Because of pain there may be loss of motion of the joint.

This may lead to non- use of related muscles. In KOA, patients stop or reduce the use of thigh muscles. This weakens the muscles.

This happens quite commonly in cases of injury to our knees (post-traumatic KOA cases).This weakness, which may set in even within 2 days of reduced use of the muscles, disturbs the joint structure. Over a period of time, the knee joint may lose its normal shape. Alignment of the knee is altered. This also disturbs our walking pattern. Pain forces patients to walk slowly and awkwardly. Also, small deposits of bone—called osteophytes or bone spurs—may grow on the edges of the damaged joint surface. Bits of bone or cartilage can also break off and float inside the joint space. This causes more pain and damage. Hence, the condition of KOA patients gradually worsens with time.

Signs and Symptoms of KOA

Some of the signs and symptoms associated with KOA include:-

- Dull, aching joint pain

- Pain worsens with activity and gets relieved with rest
- Stiffness of the knee joint, often for a short time in the morning or after a period of inactivity
- Loss of flexibility
- Reduced range of motion (i.e. knee cannot move in the normal range of movements which other normal people can do)
- Crepitus (crackling sound movement)
- Effusion - increase in quantity of synovial fluid leading to swelling of joint
- Deformity (of knee and later of the leg)
- Cyst (a swelling behind the knee - sometimes painful)

And in case patients remain confined to bed (due to injury), situation may get more complicated. This is due to the fact that immediately after the trauma many patients go in to a phase of inactivity due to the pain (non-use of thigh muscle). This leads to muscle weakness and atrophy, particularly of quadriceps femoris (the muscle on front of thigh). This causes more deformity, further damaging the knee joint.

Impact of KOA on Quality of Life of patients

The discomfort due to symptoms of KOA affect the life of the patients in totality. All the following aspects of their health are affected -

Physical: Pain, tenderness, stiffness, loss of flexibility, grating sensation, bone spurs, joint stiffness and loss of movement of knee joints through full range of motion affect KOA patients' physical health.

Mental: Patients feel discomfort and tension due to pain, which does not get relieved even by routine painkillers.

Social: Patients have to curtail their social lives to quite an extent; problem is more pronounced in those living in multistory buildings / skyscrapers as use of stairs is troublesome. Their social participation is grossly affected. They may shun attending family functions.

Psychological: All the above problems lead to loss of self-image / esteem. Patients of KOA may feel depressed and left out. Even their sleep may be disturbed (due to pain / stiffness in various parts of the body or due to the psychosocial implications of KOA impacting their social life).

All the above dimensions influence each other. Thus, the overall impact of KOA is compounded. For example, social impact is dependent on physical impact (pain / discomfort /inability to negotiate stairs) and both of these adversely affect the psychological implications of KOA. Whole mindset and way of thinking of the patients may be affected due to their suffering.

Another aspect of KOA is that it is a self-perpetuating disease. Thus, initial pain of KOA restricts use of thigh muscles. This leads to atrophy of muscles. It further destabilizes the knee joint. As a reaction, there is stiffness in hamstring muscles (behind the knee) also. This causes more discomfort. All this affects the gait / walking pattern of the patient. Even shoulder and back muscles are affected. Alignment of bones of legs, torso and shoulder is affected. This also leads to deviation in the symmetry and the line of weight bearing. Whole body balance is disturbed. This further adversely affects the overall knee joint stabilization. Weakness of muscles also leads to unequal pull on patella. This also aggravates alignment problem. So, the symptoms keep worsening. In essence, unless the whole system of body balance needs to be addressed through correctional maneuvers.

In many cases, it is quite commonly seen that KOA patients keep trying different regimen of treatment without apparently getting a worthwhile relief from their symptoms. They do take painkillers. Some temporary relief may be there. But the pain tends to persist. They are advised exercises for muscle strengthening. But either they forget the correct way of doing these (due to overcrowded OPDs – getting not more than 3-4 minutes with the doctor). Often, they do not have enough motivation or enthusiasm to continue with the exercises. This is particularly true of women, who just do not consider these as a part of their culture or daily routine.

Quite often, when they present in OPD with a history of pain in knee joint area along with their other (vague) symptoms related to neck/shoulder/back, the orthopedist / physiotherapist have no patience to listen to them. As a consequence, musculoskeletal problems in other areas of their body remain unresolved. This aggravates the pain and problems in knee joint area and structures.

Treatment options for KOA - What works and what does not?

As indicated above, when KOA patients consult the orthopedics experts, the focus of treatment remains on quadriceps exercises. No attention is given on correction in the altered symmetry. So, the KOA patients may develop related symptoms in other body parts which are not attended to. This indirectly affects the knee joint structure. Thus, KOA symptoms remain unresolved. This leads to a general sense of dis-satisfaction among the patients with the treatment.

Hence, there is a major role of physiotherapy in management of KOA cases. However, even for exercises a lip service is given in most of the hospitals that too in a piecemeal manner. Reason is the overburdened orthopedists. In any orthopedics OPD, there are too many patients vying for their attention. But because of manpower and time constraints due attention is not given to systematic training of the patients for various exercises. Often, they forget whatever is told to them in a hurry in crowded OPDs.

Most of the patients are told by the orthopedists that the operation is inevitable. This demoralizes them. They are not told that much benefit can be obtained through physiotherapy. They are not told about the vital role of restoring the body balance and muscle strength. The ever-increasing disconnect between the disciplines of orthopedic and physiotherapy has not helped the situation. Even physiotherapy OPDs are now quite crowded. Even there, long waiting time due to manpower constraints and the need to come to the OPD for repeated sessions of exercises / diathermy etc. discourages patients from full compliance with the instructions. Moreover, the way these sessions are handled does not encourage patients or their escorts to come back! Hence, there is a definite need to empower the KOA patients about self-care.

The very fact that KOA patients keep trying a variety of treatment modalities, implies that an effective remedy of KOA is not available. In fact, many complementary and alternative system medicine (CAM) regimes are in vogue across the globe, e.g. rolfing, chiropractice, acupressure, Feldenkrais method or neuropathy. Even in allopathy, short wave diathermy, ultrasound therapy, taping, TENS (trans-electric nerve stimulation) etc are tried. Many nutraceuticals are also prescribed to KOA patients.

There is no definite evidence for efficacy of most of such regimes. Still, many patients claim benefit from these. There are many success stories. But again, even here, a clear picture fails to emerge. This is because, quite often, these patients resort to multi - modal therapies. For example, Mrs Baljit Amarjit Singh, (a 60 + teacher in a private school), a sufferer and a successful writer of the famous book on KOA, "I Can You Can - Resurrection!" concludes her book by giving the regime followed by her as – Yoga, pranayama, massage, light weight training in the morning; ankle weight training knee/foot presses in the afternoon / evening; Glucosamine and calcium tablets; one tablespoonful Flaxseed (ground) with meals twice a day. She has also emphasized the importance of weight maintenance and of keeping a positive attitude. In fact, as per the lead author's opinion, all KOA patients should read this book wherein the author has told her story as to how she successfully handled her KOA related problems.

In the preface of her book she has mentioned that she was advised total knee replacement (TKR) in 2005, eleven years after she was diagnosed as a KOA patient. She had severe pain in her knees. She had developed a limp with deformity in legs. X-ray revealed gross reduction in joint space with worn out cartilage. However, the discussions within her family led to deferment of any decision for surgery.

Many vital clues emerged from her book as to why the KOA patients get disillusioned by the advice given by the orthopedics / physiotherapy experts in OPDs. She writes," I did the exercises for a couple of days with the help of my husband. And then it fizzled out – partly due to inherent dislike for exercise and partly because I couldn't do them alone". (This aspect is mostly not addressed by the therapists).

About the addition of lateral wedge in shoes usually advised to KOA patients, she writes, "...I walked with the new pair for a few days, but very awkwardly and could walk only a kilometer instead of three. I gave up the shoes sooner than expected; they were damaging my self-esteem". (In fact, it has been seen that in many cases the shoes just lie unused after sometime).

Now, this narrative gives an insight in to the viewpoint of the KOA patients, which is usually never taken in to account by the orthopedists / physiotherapists. All the same, this aspect is important in understanding the factors affecting the adherence of the patient to the prescribed regimen. This may help the concerned doctors for devising appropriate counselling strategies for ensuring the same.

Some of her utterings in the book highlight the predicament of KOA patients.

"I had become an object of pity at home and at work. Pity can be so demeaning." "I refused to buy a walking stick (recommended by a doctor)"." I thought of giving up my job". "My principal helped me by shifting my class to the ground floor"." I went in to deep depression"." I lost confidence in myself. My self-esteem was at its lowest" "I saw myself as a cripple". "I had become totally negative"

She writes that she once went to an orthopedic surgeon with an aim to get clarifications to a list of 22 questions related to KOA / TKR etc. However, the doctor only devoted 3 minutes for the consultation. This shook her belief / faith in doctors. She dropped the idea of TKR. Thereafter, she resorted to CAM. Mrs Baljit reported an equivocal effect of various home remedies (*Giloy,mulethi,haldi,methre*). Ayurvedic remedies also did not have any specific impact!

The book elaborates about her victory over her KOA problem. Within 7 months she could reduce her suffering to a great extent through 'her experiments' with non-surgical treatments. She has attributed her success to faith, family support, focus on positive thoughts and neuropathy treatment.

However, our text mainly focuses upon the role of exercises and lifestyle changes in management of KOA patients. Other aspects and modalities may also need to be considered by them as per the need.

Conservative therapy for KOA

Patients usually consult the specialist doctors when the situation becomes worse. Once the problem starts, the KOA remain there with patients for lifetime. None of the available treatment regimens is 100% effective. There is no cure for OA. This means that the disease, once started, will persist. Often we are made to believe that the pain and disability in KOA patients will invariably worsen over time and that the process of damage is always progressive. However, there is evidence that relief can be obtained through adoption of suitable promotive (weight reduction/meditation/pain coping etc), preventive (avoiding use of stairs/ sitting cross-legged) curative and rehabilitative (physiotherapy maneuvers- exercises etc) strategies.

In view of the chronic unbearable nature of symptoms, KOA patients keep trying different treatment agencies and regimes. They consult orthopedists, physiotherapist and even lay bone setters. In any case, all patients are not benefited by such consultations. They keep on using drugs available over the counter (OTC).Often they indulge into unnecessary medication and adopt practices that don't have any scientific rationale. Many patients suffer numerous side effects due to indiscriminate use of pain killers. Even kidneys may be damaged by such medicines.

Surgical intervention is not indicated for all the patients of KOA. Even otherwise, all subjects cannot afford the expenses of surgery. Injection treatment may also not suit every patient. But is possible to relieve pain and improve joint function through conservative methods (without using any medicine or surgery). Proper treatment can slow down the progression of the disease. This book deals with this aspect only.

Why discussion on non-surgical management of KOA is important

KOA is one of the common cause of disability after fourth decade of life. In India, its prevalence has been reported to be in the range of 20 – 60 % among people aged above 50 years. Intractable pain is the most common symptom of KOA. Quality of life (QOL) of KOA patients significantly deteriorates with pain and loss of mobility causing dependence and disability.

There is currently no cure for KOA. Treatment is aimed primarily at symptom relief. Focus is on optimizing the quality of life through improvement in joint mobility and function. Nowadays, an impression has been created that all KOA patients need knee replacement surgery! However, this should mainly be an option (though costly) for people with severe KOA who are unresponsive to non-surgical management. The fact is that, long-term effects of early to moderate KOA can be managed through non-surgical interventions. Moreover, all patients may not be fit for surgery. Many may not agree for operation.

Even the latest findings on second opinion survey (published in a leading journal and carried in most national dailies, e.g. The Times of India, 4th Jan. 2015 48 % of knee replacement surgeries are not actually needed).

It is also seen that all patients who undergo surgery may not get complete relief. Many are definitely benefitted by TKR. However, some may even worsen. Apart from it, these days, there are many other interventional therapies are being advocated for KOA patients, e.g., intra-articular injections (by putting needle inside the joint), stem cell therapies. Again their results are variable. Some patients may benefit. Some have reported worsening. So, the situation remains unclear.

These days for any kind of medical treatment, doctors have come up with a system to judge which treatment is the best. On the basis of research they assign evidence grades to all therapies/regimes. In general, 6 grades are there. Grade A - Level I evidence is awarded to the BEST proven treatment as per the research proofs available. For example, grade B, level II evidence is accorded to the role of weight reduction in management of KOA. Grade A, level I evidence is given to low-impact aerobic fitness exercises; Grade B, level II evidence to quadriceps strengthening while Grade C, level V evidence is given to range of motion/flexibility exercises. Reduction of weight with an appropriate program of dietary modification and exercise removes the load from the knees. In addition, exercises strengthen the muscles. This helps in regaining the balance of the knee joint preventing further damage to the knees.

Dr MS Dhillon Professor Orthopaedics and Head of the department of Physical and Rehabilitation Medicine, PGIMER, Chandigarh gave following views regarding KOA Management —

"Our knee is a weight bearing joint. It helps in walking, running and sitting. Unfortunately with age, cartilage covering of knee degenerates. In some people, it degrades early because of genetic factors. For example, if your parents have KOA you have more chances of developing KOA. It is also commonly seen that KOA may get manifested due to some other reasons like fractures or injury. For example, in many cases, the diagnosis of KOA comes to the surface when x-rays etc are taken for a patient reporting to a hospital after a fall or accident. In such cases, it is incidental to find joint space reduction typical of KOA. Such post-traumatic cases result in mal-alignment and knee gets deformed from one side. Because of obesity also, degenerative changes occur early in knee joints of some patients. Hence, weight reduction has an important place in the management of KOA. Simple things can help a lot in such cases.

Some of the causes of knee joint degeneration are inevitable when we get old. For example, with aging we get graying of our hair and wrinkles on our skin. All this is normal. But if we don't take proper care and let it worsen then it progresses to full blown KOA. By 40 yrs. of age we may feel slight pain in knee. We should not be scared of it. This is a signal from our body that if we had not been performing any exercises till now, we should start doing it.

Some of our habits related to squatting worsen KOA. Like our praying habit which is a part of our culture. We generally squat for praying, while eating food and also for defecation. When we squat too much pressure comes upon our knees. So, degenerative changes related to KOA cause pain in our knees. Rather, squatting aggravates KOA. In addition to other precautions, we should avoid squatting. We should also stop using Indian toilet as it increases pressure on knee.

There are many types of osteoarthritis. Most common is KOA. Usually it affects both knees. One knee is slightly less affected than the other side. But ultimately it affects both knees. In layman language, in cases of KOA, 'grease' in our knee (which is useful for optimum mobility) gets reduced. Secondly, sponge covering of knee joints, i.e., cartilage develops cracks. The worn out part inside knee causes inflammation (redness/swelling) and causes pain. We commonly see that in cars also poor alignment causes degradation of tyre from one side. Overloading further increases the damage to the car parts. Similarly, eventual mal-alignment in KOA leads to further degeneration of knee joints. Obesity causes more aggravation of KOA. In fact, it becomes a vicious cycle. KOA leads to mal-alignment of knee joints, which causes aggravation of KOA.

KOA patients need to meet a doctor if the pain lasts for more than 10-15 days. If there is small injury or wound it heals and pain subsides .But if pain persists and there is inflammation and pain is felt at night, then there are chances of developing KOA. Pain reflects that the disease process has started. So, at this time your contribution for controlling disease should be maximum. Doctors will just advise exercises and other therapies. They will give you necessary instructions and directions. But you have to do the exercises yourself, '*karna toh aapko khud hai*'.

At this time, we generally don't recommend any medicines. You have to understand your problem, reduce your weight and perform exercises. Try to rectify your body instability and mal-alignment.

If grease /synovial fluid is reduced we can have injections for knee. These days we have a new technique of stem cell injections. Minor operation can be done by arthroscopy for small wounds, to remove loose pieces of cartilage / meniscus so that KOA doesn't progress further. So, at an early stage you should understand your problem and cooperate with your doctor and the medical counselor.

In case, it worsens further or if you have consulted doctor at a late stage then knee replacement may have to be done. But, this stage should be considered only when other methods have failed. Hence, operation should not be done at an early age. Generally, life of knee replacement is 15-20 years or less. So ideally, operation should be done after 65 years of age. Accordingly, after initial diagnosis, in the age group of 40-60 years, KOA patients should perform exercises, reduce weight and follow all necessary precautions. That is, for all practical purposes '*aapne ghutne ki situation ko apne haath main le lain*', i.e., we need to take control of the situation. Main dictum is that in KOA we should not neglect or ignore exercises. These are mandatory."

Post - traumatic KOA

This issue needs special discussion since in many middle aged patients, the KOA situation is worsened when proper care or immediate guidance is not available to them after they sustain an injury (leg, hip or back). The usual story is that after the fall, they develop pain, stiffness and aches in various parts of the body. Quite often they may delay consultation with an orthopedist. In case, they fail to do immediate cold fomentation (with ice etc), the pain worsens. They may choose to just take the rest. They may avoid using the leg. This creates problem as described above. The thigh muscles develop weakness, which may set in even within 2 days of reduced use of the muscles. It disturbs the joint structure. Over a period of time, the knee joint may lose its normal shape. Alignment of the knee is altered. This also disturbs our walking pattern.

When they reach hospital, X-ray may not reveal any fracture. It may just be a case of soft tissue injury. Mild KOA may also be diagnosed. Painkillers, glucosamine and exercises may be prescribed. Many sessions of hot pack/ ultrasound/short wave diathermy and tractions may follow. Still, the pain and discomfort may persist. This is because, quite often, the stiffness and alignment problem is not addressed by the therapists. This way the KOA problem keeps getting deteriorated. Hence, in injury cases both immediate and late stage proper and systematic care is needed. This will surely avoid mush suffering and disability among the patients.

Catch 22 situation in evidence creation for CAM (Complementary & Alternative Medicine) in KOA management

It is often commented by Allopaths that CAM are ineffective in KOA patients. Their logic is that there is no fool proof evidence (no RCTs) on this aspect. And the situation is that CAM people may not go for RCT (Their logic is that, "our patients get relief, we have been practicing it for long with good results, so, for us, there is no need of RCTs); Allopath also do not go for RCT on CAM (They say we don't know about CAM and we do not recognize this system, so we will not do any such RCT). Consequently, no evidence ever gets created for CAM. Though in the field of hypertension or diabetes treatment role of herbs, naturopathy, yoga and CAM is being tried even in Institution like AIIMS, New Delhi, there has not been any initiation of a dialogue between Allopaths & CAM practitioners for KOA. So, the status quo persists and patients suffer...since Allopath do not have answers for all of KOA patients' problems (though they are happy to prescribe evidence-less glucosamine / diacerein; PRP injections or even debridement ... they scoff at any suggestion for CAM. And as indicated above, even the TKRs, so rampant now, have been questioned).

What are non-pharmacological interventions for KOA?

Non-pharmacological interventions (NPI) are the mainstay management strategies for knee and hip OA. These often involve the clinical input of the multidisciplinary health care team. Components of NPI include –

(i) Patient education: In modern era, doctor patient equations have changed. Now, the KOA patients need to be actively involved in their self-management. Books/ brochures/videos/ one to one discussion/demonstration/training may be used for this purpose

(ii) Aerobic, resistive and KBA exercises: These have an important place in management of KOA patients. This helps in regaining the thigh muscle strength. (Details of basic exercises are enclosed later).

(iii) Lifestyle changes: Because of the activity limitation in KOA patients, they have to restrict some of their activities (in particular squatting / using stairs / jumping). This helps in preventing further damage to the knee joint. In addition, KOA patients also need to change their lifestyle for effective weight reduction.

(iv) Weight loss: A high grade evidence is available to support the strong role of weight reduction in management of KOA patients.

(v) Focus on symmetry & body balance

(vi) Various physical therapies.

These interventions generally have low or no side effects. Often these are used in conjunction with a pharmacological regimen to decrease pain and promote restoration of / improvement in functioning and quality of life. In western countries, a lot of research has been done on NPIs for KOA treatment. Many treatment guidelines have been prepared and are being used. In fact, many countries have their own well established and elaborate KOA management protocols which are regularly updated.

However, surprisingly, such an effort is lacking in India. No standard operating procedures (SOP) have been developed for KOA management. Even there is lack of consensus on the set of exercises to be done by KOA patients. Different consultants prescribe different set of exercises to KOA patients. There are many gaps in evidence base on NPIs for KOA patients in India.

Confidence building measures for KOA patients

One common observation in Indian set up in such patients is that they are a demoralized lot. Most of them are told that knee replacement is the only option. They are told that conservative therapy will not help. Surprisingly, this happens even at first consultation. However, even internationally, the standard guidelines clearly mention that at least 6 months of trial should be given to conservative therapies before even considering the surgical option. Generally, it is seen that no orthopedist tells KOA patients with conviction that they would get relief through conservative regimes like exercises. In doctor-patient interaction this matters a lot. If their doctor is not confident or convincing enough about the role of exercises, the patient get demoralized. Adherence of KOA patients with the prescribed regime is definitely affected by the degree of faith they have in their orthopedists.

There is a definite need to instill confidence in the KOA patients about the scope and potential of conservative therapies. Sincere reassurance of the KOA patients by the therapists can help a lot in this regard. However, in crowded OPDs of Indian hospitals it is a wishful thinking.

An anecdotal feedback (A case study of post traumatic KOA)

Recently, I discussed the condition of a post traumatic KOA patient (one of my personal acquaintance) with two of my colleagues (one a practicing orthopedist and the other a neurosurgeon; both in private sector in Delhi). The patient had a fall in mid-2012. She had her knee bruised. She developed pain, stiffness and aches in various parts of the body. She consulted the orthopedics department of a leading apex level medical institute of north India. X-ray revealed no fracture. It was told to be a case of soft tissue injury. Mild KOA was also diagnosed. Bone density scan revealed mild osteopenia. Painkillers were taken for few weeks. Vit. D and calcium were taken. Glucosamine was also started. It was discontinued after sometime due to the disturbed blood glucose control (she was a known type II diabetic). She had coccydynia also.

She underwent many sessions of hot pack fomentation /ultrasound and short wave diathermy. There was some relief in symptoms. Still, the pain and discomfort persisted. She was unable to descend stairs. She stopped sitting cross-legged. She also reported change in his gait. She also complained of a feeling of rotation of her legs. Her social life was seriously compromised. She was told by orthopedists / physiotherapists of a leading medical institute that total knee replacement (TKR) was the only option since the condition of joint would keep on deteriorating. She then consulted some lay bone setters / masseuse also. Surprisingly, they could judge alteration in her gait as well as asymmetry in her shoulders (about which no orthopedist / physiotherapist in the institute commented or even bothered about!). Still, after more than 4 years, symptoms have persisted even in Dec. 2016.

However, my colleagues from Delhi clearly told me that they saw many such cases regularly. They said that the issue in the given case was likely to be of musculo-fascial pain. They told that in such cases proper charting of the condition of trigger points/nodules needs to be done (this aspect is sadly missing in most government hospitals). Thereafter, specific exercises/diathermy, manipulation/massage is to be done to resolve the same. They clearly told that without this, even the exercises will not help. Pain may also has to be sorted out through judicious use of analgesics. They clearly told that if we consult some private physiotherapy facility the problem can easily be sorted out! Contrary to the bleak picture painted by other specialists, they guaranteed complete relief after requisite number of sessions. However, the strange thing here was that in the apex level medical institute, neither anybody talked about musculo-fascial aspects or trigger points/nodules nor they guaranteed any relief. No encouraging words were ever spoken. A doctor even commented, "These things are common in women. My mother also had similar problem. Like her you should also learn to tolerate it. It will not go away."

Rather, when she reported reduction in symptom severity through fomentation they dismissed the idea straightaway. They told that the perceived relief was only psychological. (Here, it seems that they focused on the theoretical concept that heat therapy would not help KOA symptoms. They failed to realize that it might have helped reduce the secondary stiffness etc, which, in any case, is required to provide any worthwhile relief and is a pre-requisite for complete recovery).Their interest seemed to be on interventionist approach of TKR or PRP injections! They focused more on KOA per se, rather than on the immediate problem of soft tissue injury. Being experienced orthopedists / physiotherapists, it was expected that they would understand and know the early as well as late effects of soft tissue injury in leg region, viz. trigger points / myo-fascial relief etc. They were expected to discuss with the patient about the role of various exercises in such cases. They should have also discussed the issues related to body balance and symmetry. However, none of this was done. Now, this kind of attitude in treatment is sure to lead to worsening of the condition of the patients (and eventually their turning up at OT for TKR!)

In this case, the patient again consulted another physiotherapist of the same institute in mid-2014. He told on the day one," your one shoulder is higher than the other. Also some stiffness is there in the back!" Now, in earlier sessions nobody paid any attention to this aspect! He advocated another series of sessions of ultrasound / short wave diathermy and tractions (not recommended so far by anyone!). He also told that he would give more emphasis to posture and traction. He said that only light exercises were required (no pain eliciting exercise was prescribed. Surprisingly, she got much relief with the tractions. Still, she had a feeling that her right leg was medially rotated. He also asked her for correction of posture and some simple shoulder exercises, which she did. Definite relief was there.

About a month later, a re-evaluation requisitioned by him (and done by a female student) revealed that she still had adductor spasm and some trigger points at the back. So, SWD and tractions were repeated. Ultrasonic diathermy (USD) was then advised. Yet again, when incidentally, one day the junior girl therapist was changed, her way of resolving stiffness in the back was much better. So much so that the patient said, "I slept soundly today. This session was miraculous. My leg position is also feeling much better!" The patient clearly told that she had a definite feeling of correction in the rotation of the leg, i.e., through shoulder stiffness resolution, the defect in the leg positioning improved on its own.

The girl therapist told that there were a lot of stiffness in the back. Many nodules were there! Surprisingly, except for one physiotherapist (the latest on the list...and a better one...who listened to the patient!), no one had discussed it ever. She also advised her to continue these USD sessions for 10 days and to use hot packs at home. These USD sessions were done in hospital physiotherapy room, with full baring of back, which was not possible in OPD setting. She also asked the patient to avoid lifting weight or heavy objects with the affected side hand. Her sessions improved the condition significantly. She then advised her to go for a session of tractions and then come back for USD.

Here also, one day when, incidentally she was on leave, the manipulations by another therapist, were not of much help. Rather the symptoms worsened. Similar unpleasant experiences (following the change of therapist) were shared by other patients also undergoing therapy in the same room. Even the results of intervention may depend upon which therapist attends to them! This highlights the importance of one therapist – one patient for the whole set of prescribed sessions. (This problem was witnessed by the case in question also when the therapist was changed in between the sessions).

However, in December 2014, when she travelled ~ 200 km in a taxi, the symptoms worsened. She went to a senior physiotherapist in OPD. Besides tractions he also asked her to do some exercises. However, these precipitated acute pain in her groin region. But he advised her to continue with the exercises. Here again, the quality of tractions varied with the physiotherapist who applied it. One day the traction would be helpful, the other day it would just seem to be a wastage of time. This was continued for 3 days. On day 3 the symptoms worsened. She discontinued the exercises / tractions and sought an appointment for USD sessions. After one session, the junior physiotherapist expressed her inability to continue with the sessions without an approval by her senior (who insisted on the exercises which aggravated the pain). Such intense discomfort was witnessed earlier also by her when a junior physiotherapist asked her to do an exercise involving medial rotation of thigh. There was also an instance when a female patient told a researcher that she cursed the physiotherapist when she experienced severe pain while doing the prescribed exercise. Surely, there is some problem with this exercise. However, the therapist community's attitude is too rigid to accommodate patients' perspective in their management plan!

Now, here the issue is that presently, the problem with management of KOA patients in government set up is the lack of empathy on the part of therapists. They just do not listen to the feedback given by the patients. There is no attempt at all for a customized approach. If an exercise does not suit a patient, particularly if it aggravates the pain, it needs to be deleted from the regime. However, there seems to be a fixed mindset among the therapists. They always insist on a defined set of exercises, oblivious of the fact that the patient may be having intense pain because of this.

There is a definite opinion among the saner experts that the physiotherapy interventions, including the exercises, will not be effective unless the trigger points are resolved (see below). But, the therapists insist upon the exercise much to the discomfort of the hapless patients. The result may be non-compliance, for which again they blame the patients! In the present case, all the relief obtained through myo-fascial release and ultrasound diathermy sessions was undone by the 'wrong' exercise prescribed by the senior physiotherapist! She could not sleep the whole night due to the pain. Result, naturally, was her loss of faith in the set of exercises as well as in the concerned physiotherapist. So much so that she commented that she was back to square one after so much of improvement in the symptoms. There seems to be no scientific effort on the part of the therapists to explain this situation to the patients or her escorts. Also as indicated above, empathy is entirely missing.

Above details indicate that much scope is there in improving the way women KOA patients are handled in physiotherapy department.

Piriformis imbroglio

In mid-October 2014 again, she consulted a Physical Medicine and Rehabilitation (PMR) specialist of a leading medical institute. She assessed her condition and diagnosed that quadriceps strengthening exercises were not being done to the desired extent leading to muscle weakening. She agreed that trigger points in upper and lower back needed to be addressed. She also diagnosed that she had a piriformis problem, which may require expert manipulation (or injection) by an orthopedist. However, another physiotherapist was also consulted the same day. He said that piriformis problem was definitely not an issue. He even demonstrated this through a test. Now, this difference of opinion is all too common in orthopedics / physiotherapy department. However, the sufferers are the patients, as they may not get the correct treatment.

There are other similar examples also, which indicate that, not infrequently, wrong treatments are prescribed to KOA patients, due to misdiagnosis. One such instance is the advice for quadriceps strengthening to each and every case suspected to be KOA, without realizing that the case might have been of ilio-tibial band syndrome or of patella-femoral pain syndrome. Also there seems to be an over-emphasis on a fixed set of exercises. Some patients may report worsening of symptoms on doing a particular exercise, esp. medial / internal rotation of thigh. Still, the therapists continue with the list of exercises, without properly explaining or reassuring the patients. The result is non-adherence of KOA patients with the advice. The dialogue between them and the therapists gets vitiated. Sufferers, of course, are the patients.

These examples only highlight an issue that many questions still remain unanswered in management of KOA patients. The irony of the situation is that there is no serious effort by the Indian Orthopedists / Physiotherapists / PMR specialists to settle the debate. Research based systematic effort to seek a solution to these questions is lacking among orthopedics / physiotherapy fraternity. There is a serious lack of any documentation of the impact of variation in physiotherapeutic techniques. Patients' feedback is given a go bye! They seem to be happy with the existing regimes.

The debate on trigger points in KOA patients

Another issue in KOA patients is that quite often the late effects of their injury / fall (which might have brought to the surface their diagnosis in the first place) are not adequately diagnosed or even addressed. This may be responsible for eventual worsening of their condition. They may have referred pain from trigger points (laypeople may call it knots /nodules in muscles). Studies estimate that in 75–95 percent of cases, myo-fascial pain is a primary cause of regional pain. This is the muscle tenderness that arises from trigger points. These may present at multiple sites (> 600) in muscle / fascia.

This aspect is not covered in traditional medical education. Consequently, the physicians/orthopedists rarely consider a myofascial source of pain in KOA patients. Hence they fail to deal effectively with pain. However, other specialists (physiatrists, osteopaths, chiropractors, acupuncturists, occupational therapists, athletic trainers, massage therapists) include trigger points in their practice.

Trigger points are diagnosed by examining signs, symptoms, pain patterns and manual palpation. Usually there is a taut band in muscles containing trigger points, and a hard nodule can be felt. Often a twitch response can be felt in the muscle by running your finger perpendicular to the muscle's direction. Pressing on an affected muscle can often refer pain. Clusters of trigger points are not uncommon in some of the larger muscles, such as the gluteus group. Often there is a heat differential in the local area of a trigger point. An expert practitioner can sense that.

Myofascial release for managing trigger points

A successful treatment protocol relies on identifying trigger points, resolving them; and if all trigger points have been deactivated, elongating the structures affected along their natural range of motion and length. In the case of muscles, which is where most treatment occurs, this involves stretching the muscle using combinations of passive, active stretching to be effective. Fascia surrounding muscles should also be treated, possibly with myofascial release, to elongate and resolve strain patterns. If this is not done muscles may return to positions where trigger points are likely to re-develop.

The results of manual therapy are related to the skill level of the therapist. If trigger points are pressed for too short a time, they may activate or remain active. If these are pressed too long or hard, they may be irritated or the muscle may be bruised. This will result in pain in the area treated. This bruising may last for a 1–3 days after treatment. This may feel like, but is not similar to, delayed onset muscle soreness. Here the pain is felt days after overexerting muscles. Pain is also common after a massage if the practitioner uses pressure on unnoticed latent or active trigger points. This often happens if (s)he is not skilled in myofascial trigger point therapy.

Myofascial release is a soft tissue therapy for the treatment of skeletal muscle immobility and pain. This alternative medicine therapy aims to relax contracted muscles, improve blood and lymphatic circulation, and stimulate the stretch reflex in muscles.

Fascia is a thin, tough, elastic type of connective tissue that wraps most structures within the human body, including muscle. Fascia supports and protects these structures. Osteopathic theory proposes that this soft tissue can become restricted due to psychogenic disease, overuse, trauma, infectious agents, or inactivity, often resulting in pain, muscle tension, and corresponding diminished blood flow. Although fascia and its corresponding muscle are the main targets of myofascial release, other connective tissues may be addressed as well.

It is also said that the physiotherapy interventions including the exercises will not be effective unless the myofascial release and trigger point issues are adequately resolved (through massage or pressure). Another reason for the failure of physiotherapy interventions is that not enough attention is paid to the associated aspects like joint stability or the muscle – nerve link. It is said that when a part of muscle gets shut down by nerves, it will not respond to the strength training. These shut down muscle areas are the 'trigger points'.

However, the underlying theory is not supported by medicine, i.e., myofascial release has not been demonstrated to be effective through any RCT for any condition. Yet, CAM practitioners use this technique. Many people claim to get benefitted by this! The 'Catch 22 situation' described above applies here also. Surely, there is a need to settle this debate also.

Ligament and muscles: Both are necessary for joint stability. Muscles provide micro level stability while the ligaments work for macro level joint stability. If ligaments are damaged, strength training through exercises will not be effective. Even this aspect is not given due importance in KOA patients' management. Approach in OPDs is rather casual. The lead author is witness to many cases where the diagnosis of ligament damage (or even of minor fracture) was confirmed after months of wrong line of management. So, KOA patients should go for second opinion, if there is no / less relief.

Symmetry: Damage to joint structure and stability is often uneven in KOA patients. It affects body symmetry. Upper neck has a special role in this aspect. Unless it is duly addressed, the wear and tear will further speed up. Simple tests are available to check which body parts have tightness and which movements are causing the trouble in KOA patients. After localizing the defect it is vital to get the symmetrical and balance motion back. This will require simple stretching exercises and attention to trigger points.

Often in injury cases, our musculoskeletal system rearranges the body balance forces. Adaptation process is initiated. One part of muscles compensates for the injury in the other. For example, we start using left hand more when our right hand is injured. In due course of time, we may complain of pain and soreness in left arm muscles. This is because, from the very beginning we have been using our right hand more. This kind of rearrangement of forces and functions may affect the body alignment. Similarly, KOA patients may complain have pain and aches in various parts of the body. Such symptoms should neither be trivialized nor ignored. Rather, the root cause / origin of the complaints should be traced and rectified. For example, KOA patients may have one shoulder higher than the other; head may be seen tilting to one side; one hip may be higher than the other or one side of shoes be wearing faster. All these defects reflect body alignment problems secondary to the original issue of KOA.

In this context, the lead author witnessed following interaction between a KOA patients and her physiotherapist. He told her," Your hip joint is also affected now. It happens in most KOA patients. Didn't anybody tell you to take care of your hip movements by not using it too much while walking? It could have been prevented if proper guidance had been given to you along with giving proper attention to the knee pain issue." This dialogue makes it clear that in KOA patients, due consideration needs to be given to avoidance of compensatory adjustments made by them in their gait or posture. If it is not done, secondary changes in the body musculature set in. This in turn, adversely affects body balance and symmetry. And since knee joint bears the whole body weight, eventually, initial damage in it is further compounded. This way the vicious cycle goes on. Ultimately, the patient is declared a case for TKR operation. Hence, the focus should be on correcting the balance, symmetry and alignment problems. Usual mistake is that almost exclusive attention is given on quadriceps strengthening. It needs to be noted that unless abovementioned aspects are taken care of, all exercises would be futile and patients will keep on suffering. Of course, all this need time and patience of the therapists as well as of the patient themselves. Sadly, these have become a scarce commodity, much to the detriment of the patients' welfare.

In fact, certain newer forms of unconventional therapies have emerged that deal with body alignment problems, e.g. Feldenkrais method, Rolfing technique (deep massage to release muscle tightness) and curve restoration etc.

Spine involvement: Quite often, vertebral column is also involved in some way or other in KOA patients. However, due attention is not given to this aspect either. It has been documented that small problems in spine can affect the shoulders, arms, legs, hips or feet of the KOA patients in a big way.

Lordosis (backward stretching of the spine, where shoulders also tend to be thrown back; this also causes the hollow in the lower back) is often seen in KOA patients as a compensatory mechanism. It has been seen that if due attention is paid to the altered spinal curve, there is a definite benefit to the KOA patients. It is also said that in many KOA patients, the problem is precipitated because of the initial pain and discomfort following some injury (as they say," Pain causes arthritis - arthritis does not cause pain"). Even some spinal nerve impingement in the back may eventually manifest as KOA.

Resolving all this requires a thorough check up. This, of course, is not possible in crowded OPDs and patients suffer.

Role of Hip joint in KOA patients: Often the therapists focus only at quadriceps strengthening exercises when they prescribe nonsurgical management for KOA patients. They tend to ignore the primary or secondary changes in hip joint or spine (whether these caused the problem or are a result of KOA changes). It is a fact that in KOA patients whatever happens at hip joint affects the knee joint structure and function. And if it is not attended to, the KOA symptoms will not subside. Rather the situation will keep on aggravating. Such cases tend to complain of groin pain / discomfort. This is more common in women. Due importance needs to be given to resolve it.

Team effort: Thus, management of KOA patients requires a comprehensive approach involving expertise of a team of physicians / orthopedists / physiotherapists and others who can correctly identify the defects in the joint structure, e.g. stability, alignment, trigger points, muscles and ligaments. Correct diagnosis and attention to all affected systems is required, otherwise as explained above, the problem will persist. Also due attention needs to be given to non surgical / non-pharmacological interventions, e.g., exercises and weight reduction. Here, it also needs to be realized that the team concept should incorporate the patients themselves. It is common to see that orthopedists / physiotherapists do not give any importance to the feedback given by the patients.

Actually, as is the trend now in other countries, focus should be on customized therapy. During and after each session of exercises, short wave diathermy (SWD), pulsed short wave diathermy (PSWD), microwave diathermy (MWD), ultrasonic massage and electrical stimulation, the feedback from the patients need to be taken about the relief obtained, any deterioration or discomfort. In this context, the lead author has personally witnessed that in some cases the patients were put on SWD for 10 minutes and the therapist went away (as is the usual case). Some of them developed burns! There was nobody to attend to them. Even there are arguments as to where to put the electrodes. Clear instructions are not there. In one case, the patient asked the therapist to put the electrodes in a particular position, which she perceived as the 'trouble spot'. Without listening to her, the therapist insisted on putting the electrodes his own 'fixed' way (as was taught and told to him). There was no relief. And when the patient, somehow, got her way the next day (through another therapist), the changed position of the electrodes provide good amount of relief. She even said that such relief has not been there ever during past two years' therapy. This highlights the need of involving the patients directly in their treatment. This, of course requires patient listening skills on the part of orthopedists / physiotherapists through a regular dialogue with the patients. They should respect the feedback from the patients and modify the therapy accordingly.

Co-morbidities: KOA patients with diabetes / metabolic syndrome are more likely to have cartilage damage and delayed or problematic recovery. This aspect needs to be kept in mind while evaluating the impact of interventions in KOA patients.

Cholesterol lowering drugs (like statins): These may also affect the recovery in KOA patients. These also interfere with blood sugar control in diabetes cases.

5. Physiotherapy/exercise regime; Routine vs. KBA: (pl. see annexures for details)

Physiotherapy is a conservative treatment option in the management of KOA. There is strong evidence for beneficial effects of exercises on pain relief and improvement in function in KOA cases. Adherence to the prescribed exercises helps in deriving better outcomes. Strengthening exercises for quadriceps and hamstring have been recommended in most KOA cases. Knee extension, knee flexion, hip abduction, hip adduction, hip internal rotation, hip external rotation, leg press (hip and knee extension) etc also have a role in KOA management. Some basic exercises are prescribed to all KOA cases. For others, there is a difference of opinion among the experts. In Indian setting, though desirable, there is scant focus on customization or individualization of exercises. Also, not enough time is devoted by the therapists on correctly teaching the way to do these exercises. This adversely affects the response to the treatment.

KBA training

KOA patients suffer from impaired postural stability. KOA has been shown to reduce walking speed, shorten stride length and prolong the stance phase of the gait cycle. Patients with KOA also have less range of motion of the hip, knee and ankle joints. KBA training has been shown to improve gait and balance, and decrease falls and associated fall-related injuries in the general elderly populations. While traditional exercise programs have not been well-tolerated in persons with KOA (due to pain) many studies have been conducted to evaluate the effect of KBA in addition to strengthening exercises in KOA patients. Some promising evidence suggests that programs incorporating knee-stabilizing kinesthesia, balance and agility (KBA) techniques with traditional therapeutic resistance training exercise (RT) may improve knee OA symptoms and function more rapidly than RT alone. KBA technique is widely used among sports-persons in routine fitness training as well as to rehabilitate and prevent knee ligament ruptures. It has been established that proprioceptive acuity, i.e. the awareness of joint position, joint movement (kinesthesia), and sense of resistance, declines both with age and as a result of KOA. KBA exercises help to restore it.

6. Other physiotherapy modalities & assistive devices for KOA patients

There are various physiotherapy modalities for KOA, viz SWD, PSWD, MWD, ultrasonic massage and electrical stimulation. Cryotherapy and hot packs are also prescribed by Orthopedists and physiotherapists. Heat therapy is applied to reduce pain. It also decreases muscle spasm.

Ultrasonic massage: Therapeutic ultrasound therapy has been widely used for many years in the treatment of KOA. Ultrasound energy gets converted into heat as it passes through tissues of varying resistance. It also reduces pain & muscle spasm through thermal effect.

Short wave diathermy: It is used for the treatment of soft tissue injuries and also for KOA related pain. It involves the application of deep heat to the affected area. This treatment has been reported to have a beneficial effect on patients with KOA. SWD is used to reduce pain and swelling. It is said to accelerate the healing in tissues with stiffness following injury. SWD increases temperature and circulation in the body part where it is applied. This accelerates the inflammatory process by increasing nutrition and oxygen supply to the affected area. It also helps in symptom relief by removing metabolic and waste products from the local site of pain and spasm.

While prescribing and applying these modalities, it is vital to watch out for various contraindications so that no harm is done to the patient.

Following are the common contraindications / precautions for diathermy:-

(i) Dermatological conditions (e.g. eczema, dermatitis)

(ii) Allergy to the electrode or contact material (tape / gel)

(iii) Patients unable to understand or respond to the instructions of the therapist

(iv) Patients with pacemakers

(v) Female patients with metallic uterine implants, such as an IUD, should avoid treatment in the pelvic area

(vi) Clothing containing metal to be removed viz earrings, buttons or zippers that contain metal. Watches and hearing aids should be removed because the therapy may affect their function.

(vii) It should be avoided during pregnancy as it can lead to abnormal fetal development

(viii) Patients with metal implants should not undergo diathermy treatment because the metal can act as a conductor of heat and result in serious internal burns. Diathermy should not be used in joints that have been replaced with a prosthesis or in those with sensory impairment who may not be able to tell if they are burning.

(ix) Patients with hemophilia should avoid the treatment because the increased blood flow could cause them to hemorrhage.

Hot packs or cold packs

Heat or cold therapy awakens body's internal healing forces. Heat reduces muscle spasms and stiffness of joints. It loosens the tissues. Heat dilates the blood vessels and stimulates the blood circulation. Hence, hot pack is not advisable for cases with swelling. It is only to be used if there is no swelling. There is no protocol for heat, which is typically applied with a heating pad or a hot, wet towel. Recommended application time is for 15 consecutive minutes.

So, if there is swelling in patients with KOA then ice pack is recommended. Ice reduces swelling by slowing the rush of blood to the affected area. For this, we can use cooling gel packs, a re-sealable plastic bag filled with ice, or a bag of frozen vegetables. Standard protocol for injuries calls for 20 consecutive minutes of ice every two hours over 72 hours after an injury. Some therapists advise lesser duration.

Many doctors recommend both heat and cold treatments to ease the pain and stiffness. Patients may go for "trial and error" to learn which therapy works best for pain. They may find the right combination of hot packs and ice packs to get the most relief from pain to manage arthritis. If it does not help, doctor need to be consulted. In addition to hospital based sessions of hot packs, it is always better to have a similar arrangement at home. This will help the patients with KOA to have hot packs in the comfort of their bedrooms. This may preferably be scheduled at night, so that there is no exposure to temperature variation after the fomentation.

Taping: It is said to be a controversial mode of therapy for KOA patients. The reason is that there is no research evidence of its effectiveness. As mentioned earlier, there are many alignment related issues in KOA patients. Here taping may be helpful theoretically. But the results of various studies do not support this.

However, anecdotal evidence is there. In the abovementioned case of post traumatic KOA patient (one of my personal acquaintance) she complained of difficulty in falling asleep (+ disturbed sleep) due to a feeling of bulging of abdomen to one side. When she reported this to the therapists, they just ignored it. They told that it was not possible to have such an after effect of a fall! Yet again, this symptomatology is endorsed by one of the expert in his book on OA. He mentioned tear of (injury to) rectus abdominis. Only one of the therapists empathized with her. He advocated taping of lower back for pulling back the sagging part of the abdominal surface. Surprisingly, the patient reported relief. She told that she was able to have a sound sleep after the taping.

Patient feedback is necessary to modulate the therapy

Quite often it is seen that above mentioned modalities (Ultrasonic massage / Short wave diathermy) provide only a partial relief. The reason for this is that in physiotherapy departments a fixed set of modalities is prescribed. For example, diathermy is usually prescribed as "" SWD shoulder region X 10 sessions". This does not specify or imply any discretion on the part of the persons managing the therapy room. The electrodes are applied by them on fixed sites every day (as has been taught to them). Even when the patient gives a feedback that a particular position of electrode (or that a particular session) was better than the other, there is no system of customizing the therapy. Flexibility is missing! This happens when the person applying the electrodes keep changing every day, with some minor changes in the site of application.

But the trend is not uniform, in many cases, opposite scenario is also seen. This happens because there is no documentation diagrammatic or otherwise as a guidance to the person applying the electrodes etc. The lead author has witnessed it many a times that the junior therapist asked the patients themselves, "Kahan *lagana hai aap ko* (tell me the site of application!).This indicates three things, i) an element of flexibility, ii) lack of uniformity in the approach in SWD room and iii) a lack of clarity in the written instructions! In such a scenario, relief in symptoms is a casualty. The therapists just fail to realize how difficult it is for the patients and their escorts to come to an apex institution just for a 10 minute session of SWD!

Assistive devices

When advised, and as per the need, KOA patients may (and should) use walking stick / cane etc. Of course, many patients may find it damaging to their self-image and dignity. **Knee braces / knee caps etc.:**

Similarly, they need to use knee caps. These will protect further damage to the knee joint. They also need to watch out for fitness of the caps (as these come in different sizes). Also these need to be changed when these get loose. In particular, these should be used whenever patients go out or use stairs.

Lateral wedge in shoes

KOA patients should also take special care of their shoes. Women, in particular may have to abandon many of their earlier shoes / sandals, particularly the high heeled ones. They may be advised to wear well-padded sport shoes. Lateral wedge may also be advised in their shoes. They need to get themselves familiar with their new foot wear. They also need to be careful while going outdoors. Special precaution need to be taken when they walk on uneven ground.

In nut shell, KOA patients often have to use an approach of "whatever works" as none of the regimens is 100% effective.

Pain coping skills for KOA patients

Increased stress and negative emotion can increase in perceived pain through a variety of mechanisms in KOA patients. This includes physical reasons like increased muscle tension or a psychological one like social isolation (avoiding daily activities).

As discussed earlier, initial severe pain is the dominant symptom in KOA patients. It is the trigger point for precipitating subsequent series of catastrophic events in their lives. Pain restricts use of thigh muscles which get atrophied. There is resultant stiffness in hamstring muscles. It further destabilizes the knee joint. Whole body mechanics and balance, gait / walking pattern of the patient is seriously disturbed. So, if the pain is controlled in some way or other, we can reduce the impending damage to the body alignment, the knee joint structures and related muscles.

Hence, given the fact that pain is more of a perceived phenomenon with a definite role of tolerance threshold, there is a need to teach KOA patients about the pain coping skills. They need to be provided an educational rationale for this pain. This will help them better understand how their thoughts, feelings, and behaviors can affect pain perception. They can also be trained to manage pain through their own efforts. This will favorably influence their pain experience.

For this, they need to be exposed to relaxation training. Goal setting and activity pacing are other strategies for altering their negative thoughts related to pain. This also involves regular practice at home. They need to learn to apply those skills to challenging pain-related situations. (e.g. managing pain aggravation).

Relaxation/meditation

For this, patients should learn to use deep breathing technique. This will help them to relax the body. This requires practice. This way they will be able to release muscle tension throughout the body. This is attained when they remove their attention from the pain. Meditation session can help them to practice relaxation.

Coping techniques for chronic pain begin with controlled deep breathing, e.g, Patient may sit in a relaxed, reclining position in a dark room. They should shut their eyes.

Then they need to begin to slow down breathing; breathe deeply, using the chest. Then they need to repeat or chant in their mind a word (such as the word "Relax-Relax" or "Aum- Aum" or "Shiva-Shiva"), and try to synchronize in order to time it with their breathing. If the mind wanders or is distracted, they need to let it wander. They should think whatever thoughts come to their mind. They should let the thoughts take their course. When they realize and remember that they were chanting, they need to start again. Like a session of transcendental meditation this may be continued for about 20 minutes of controlled breathing. Such sessions may be done once or twice a day. This may even be done during travelling in a bus / train. This will have a definite impact on releasing tension.

Cognitive restructuring

These techniques allow patients to decrease pain by helping them to identify and subsequently correct distorted conceptualizations. For many KOA patients, negative thoughts can begin to feel realistic and cause a worsening of anxiety and depression. This results in more pain. Cognitive restructuring techniques teach patients to -

- Identify negative ,automatic thought process
- Realize the relationship between thoughts, feelings, behaviors ,and pain
- Judge the evidence both for and against negative thought process
- Formulate a more realistic interpretation of the pain experience
- Simply stated, here the patients with chronic pain are taught to monitor negative thought processes. They are helped to develop positive coping skills (thought processes) to counteract the negative thought processes.
- As an example, a patient with KOA may have a pain flare up while shopping and subsequently have a negative, automatic thought like, "this pain is getting worse and may well rip me off before too long". This triggers the vicious circle of anxiety. This in turn leads to worsening of pain condition .With cognitive restructuring, the patient is taught to challenge this negative thought with a coping statement. "This pain has always waxed and waned in the past and will do so again. Thank God I can at least still walk and that I am not wheelchair-bound."

In this context, a very good account has been given by Mrs Baljit Amarjit Kaur, a sufferer and a successful writer of the famous book on KOA, "I Can". She writes," I shifted from — I have a lot of pain to — I am getting better". She continues, "By constantly worrying about my knees and talking about them I was actually affirming and assisting that negative thoughts to materialize. I merely changed it to positive thought ...in other words I took action...and the result is positive."

Activity pacing

One thing which is (and should be) clear to KOA patients is that their lives are never going to be the same. The speed with which they used to do all their work will be a thing of the past. They will have to readjust and convince themselves mentally that they need to do everything slowly, deliberately and tentatively. They will have to pace themselves according to their revised capacity and capability. Pacing an activity enables a KOA patient to consistently carry out activities without causing extra pain. It helps them to enable themselves to gradually increase the amount of work they can do at a stretch. This also helps them to prevent having bouts of over or under activity. This will definitely prevent any further damage to the knee joint.

A common cycle for KOA patients with chronic pain is that they tend to push themselves until the pain tells them to stop. Women, in particular are prone to this trap. They become greedy as far as domestic chores are concerned. On a pain-free day they may try to do all pending work! So, they get tired and may even precipitate pain again. This is invariably followed by a period of rest, taking painkillers and feelings of frustration and despair. In times of prolonged rest, the body starts to get out of condition. Joints may become stiffer and muscles become weaker. Consequently, they cannot cope with a higher level of activity. Over a period of time, their work threshold becomes less and less. Rest periods tend to become longer and activity levels, including fitness and function, tend to reduce.

This happens because despite the pain the KOA patients have to continue with their routine lives. Every such patient has to some odd bit of household or other job. This is particularly true with women, especially the housewives, for whom we usually say, "Their job is never done"! They have to look after kitchen, the housemaid, the grocery shopping and management etc. Even if they have pain while bending down, they may have to pick up things from the floor (or from bottom shelves of the cupboard/fridge). Actually, amount of activity we do as KOA patients is often based on how we feel on a particular day. When we have a 'good day' (less or no pain) we find that we want to make the most of this and get extra tasks done. This is detrimental to the body alignment, knee joint structures and related muscles.

Apart from this, another peculiar and bizarre problem has been witnessed by the lead author in the so called modern day women. In one such case (October, 2014), a female doctor (pediatrician; husband also a doctor) twisted her leg. She was diagnosed as post-traumatic KOA. She had intense pain. Over a period of 6 month treatment involving cold / hot packs, exercises and analgesics she recovered. However, after that, inexplicably she went on to join a gym and aerobic classes. She was a bit overweight. Eventually, she landed up again in OPD having twisted her leg with severe aggravation of her symptoms! Many such cases have been seen by the lead author, where women suffer the after-effects of a sudden urge to do aerobics of gym!

For example, in the next week, co-incidentally, he saw another lady doctor (MD Pathology) with a similar story reporting at orthopedics OPD. After an episode of acute KOA related pain, she successfully recovered through exercises etc. Yet, she went on to start vigorous treadmill exercises, only to precipitate knee joint injury with severe pain! The issue here is that the woman should have gone in to a 'knee joint protection' mode. As indicated above, once a diagnosis of KOA has been made, we need to change our lifestyle, in particular, the range, level and pace of our physical activities and exertion. The time of overenthusiastic indulgence in fancy exercises is over! Women need to watch out here. Particularly those for whom doing exercises regularly has not be a part of their routine. (This applies to most women in Indian setting)

Lifestyle changes for KOA patients with special focus on weight management and other dietary prescriptions /nutraceuticals/home remedies/Ayurvedic regimes

Obesity is said to be the biggest risk factor for developing KOA. Also once developed, obesity aggravates the condition to its worst. Weight loss can reduce the pain as well as risk of aggravation of KOA. Being overweight increases the load placed on the knee joint. This increases the stress and hastens the breakdown of cartilage, since our knees bear the most of our body weight. Being overweight has a direct (disproportional) effect on the stress on the knee joint. For example, for every 1 kg of extra body weight a person carries there is around a 4 kg increase in the pressure that is put on the knee joint. Hence, weight reduction has an important role to play in management of KOA. So, due emphasis should be given to this by the concerned therapists.

However, KOA patients often find it difficult to reduce weight. Some, who are successful in weight reduction, may not be able to maintain the same. Due to the difficulty they face in moving about, KOA patients frequently have trouble losing weight through exercise or walking. Moreover, weight loss through dieting has been associated with a potentially deleterious loss of nutrients, muscle mass, and bone in obese individuals. Therefore, for safe weight loss in obese KOA patients, strictly controlled diet is needed. During any such effort it is also important to ensure supply of key nutrients. This will help in maintenance of total content and density of bone mineral.

Obese KOA patients generally complain that they cannot do exercises for long duration because of pain. Hence, prescription of a diet for weight reduction therapy is very important. The focus of KOA management in obese patients is quite often on eating a balanced diet and on maintaining optimal weight.

Besides this, the matter may be complicated by other lifestyle diseases faced by KOA patients. This is because majority of such patients may be above 40-50 yrs age when diabetes and hypertension are also common. In these disorders also, dietary management has to be resorted to. This will, of course affect KOA management. Even otherwise, some of the nutraceuticals or other medicines prescribed to KOA may aggravate diabetes etc.In this context, the lead author witnessed an interaction between a KOA patient and an orthopedist. The patient posed a question regarding nutrition and supplements. *"Doctor sahib main kya khaun ki mera bhaar ghat jaye* (What should I eat to reduce weight)".In response to this the surgeon referred the patient to dietary clinic .On the follow up visit when researcher asked the KOA patient if he visited the dietary clinic, his reply was " *eh parcha phadaya hai unha ne, ehde vich likhya hai, ki khana hai"*(they handed over this paper which explains about what to eat). However, most of the dietary instructions mentioned on the paper were not relevant to Indian context .For example, 'eat salmon fish / tofu for protein diet'. So, for all practical purpose, it was a cut -paste job. It was not at all useful for patients. Rather, it was a lip service. No sincere effort was there. Even otherwise, the handouts are useless for illiterate or semi-literate patients! Clearly, 'salmon fish / tofu' are not a part of our routine diet. There is a serious need of providing practical and useful dietary advice to KOA patients. Referral to dietetics department is often futile. Rather in Indian set up (and elsewhere also) establishment of a dialogue between the counselor and the patients is essential. As they say, half of the patients' problem are relieved by talking to doctors. Our practical experience also endorses this. But, the issue is of lack of sufficient time with orthopedists/ physiotherapists.

Apart from this, many queries are posed by KOA patients regarding various food supplements widely marketed through departmental stores. Many of these claim to help KOA. Numerous internet websites are also devoted to food and nutrition aspects in management of KOA patients. There are also many publications in market on this issue. So, a clear and sound dietary advice need to be devised for KOA patients.

Tips that may help to reduce weight

Before making any dietary changes it is important to ascertain whether one is obese or not. For that, KOA patient weight and height can be compared with ideal height and weight chart and then BMI can be calculated.

(i) Table 1 shows the ideal weight for male and female (adults).

(ii) To calculate BMI, take your weight (in kg) and divide it by the square of your height in meters. For example ,if height is 1.6m (5 ft 4 in) and weight is 65 kg then BMI = 65 divided by 1.6 meters * 1.6 meters (2.56) = 25.39

(iii) Check BMI ratings : Less than 18.5 = underweight;18.5 -24.9 = healthy weight;

(a) 25.0 -29.9 = overweight; 30.0-39.9 = obese; 40 and above = morbid obesity

(b) A BMI of 25.39 would indicate the need to lose a little weight .But it is important to remember that BMI is only a guide. A muscular person with little fat may still have a high BMI, as it measures weight, rather than fat, in relation to height.

(iv) Another indicator to check weight is waist size. For woman, an 88 cm (36 inches) or above and for men 102 cm (40 inches) or above waist means risk of ill health.

(v) Dietary plans can be prepared in consultation with dietician. Various studies have recommended for a diet consisting of eight weeks of protein shakes and soup followed by adding low-calorie, high-protein foods. This can help people with KOA lose weight and lessen joint pain .This in turn will improve their quality of life. Such diet helps KOA patients whose obesity makes it impossible to exercise.

Dietary plan for 60 years old KOA patient with BMI >30 (Table 2): A case study

Radha: Aged 60 years, is an overweight woman with mild KOA. Currently she has mild pain at the end of the day which aggravates in winters. She has been advised to lose weight. Apart from her mild KOA Radha is well. She came for an advice from dietician about losing weight. She has been advised physiotherapy also. Radha says "***mujhe kuchch karna padega***" (*I need to work out something)*... "***Bhaar kaise ghatayun***" (*How to lose weight*). "***main din main exercise kar sakti hun par kitni exercise karni hai ?.... par dard main toh exercise nahi kar sakhungi aur dieting kaise karun ?***" *(I do have time during the day to exercise but I'm not sure how much I should exercise and I'm afraid it will be too painful with KOA. What should I do with my dieting plan)*

Table 1 : Standard Height and Weight for Indian Men & Women Men Women

Height (Feet & Metres)	*Weight (kgs)*	*Weight (kgs)*
5'-0" (1.523 m)	*50.8 - 54.4*	*50.8 - 54.4*
5'-1" (1.548 m)	*51.7 - 55.3*	*51.7 - 55.3*
5'-2" (1.574 m)	*56.3 - 60.3*	*53.1 - 56.7*
5'-3" (1.599 m)	*57.6 - 61.7*	*54.4 - 58.1*
5'-4" (1.624 m)	*58.9 - 63.5*	*56.3 - 59.9*
5'-5" (1.650 m)	*60.8 - 65.3*	*57.6 - 61.2*

(Contd...)

5'-6" (1.675 m)	*62.2 - 66.7*	*58.9 - 63.5*
5'-7" (1.700 m)	*64.0 - 68.5*	*60.8 - 65.3*
5'-8" (1.726 m)	*65.8 - 70.8*	*62.2 - 66.7*
5'-9" (1.751 m)	*67.6 - 72.6*	*64.0 - 68.5*
5'-10" (1.777 m)	*69.4 - 74.4*	*65.8 - 70.3*
5'-11" (1.802 m)	*71.2 - 76.2*	*67.1 - 71.7*
6'-0" (1.827 m)	*73.0 - 78.5*	*68.5 - 73.9*
6'-1" (1.853 m)	*73.3 - 80.7*	*73.3 - 80.7*
6'-2" (1.878 m)	*77.6 - 83.5*	*77.6 - 83.5*
6'-3" (1.904 m)	*79.8 - 85.9*	*79.8 - 85.9*

Question: What are dietary changes required for weight loss?

Answer: Main requirements for weight loss through dietary adjustments are:

- reducing total energy intake
- sustaining reduced energy intake over time
- providing all essential nutrients in sufficient quantities

Key eating strategies:-

- restricting saturated fat intake
- adopting energy controlled eating plan
- recognizing poor nutritional choices and reduce hidden sources of empty calories and saturated fat
- consuming high fiber, increased protein and low glycemic index foods
- other dietary changes to consider include reducing consumption of energy dense foods and drinks / portion sizes.

Table 2: Indian diet chart for Radha

Early morning	Tea/lemon tea/ lemon water/Herbal tea/Green tea/(Without sugar)
Breakfast	2 Stuffed *chappati* /parantha(without ghee) with veg./curd Or 2 whole bread (sandwich/patty) Or Wheat porridge/cornflakes/oats (20-25gm.)
Mid-morning	1 fruit/ salad veg/ sprouts (25g)/plain *nimbu pani* (without sugar)/tea/*lassi*
Lunch	2 *Chapati* (no ghee), *Dal* (One *katori*), Vegetable (seasonal) (One *katori*), *Raita*/curd (One *katori)*, Salad
Evening	Tea (without sugar); Sprouts/boiled or roasted *chana* (25g) Biscuits (2)/plain *poha/suji upma* (20g)/*idli* (1 pc.)
Dinner	Soup (home made) *Chapatti (-ghee)*
Any one	Dal/soya nutri-nuggets (15g)/*paneer* (25g)/fish (80g)/chicken (100g)/curd (125g)/salad – note : many people advise no curd at night !

KOA patient may also take following fat burning foods:

- Honey(in warm water)
- Cinnamon powder
- Berries (Strawberry/blueberry etc.)
- Cabbage
- Garlic/*methi* seeds
- *Alsi* seeds = Omega fatty acids
- Nutri(soya) nuggets / granules
- Fibrous foods

General instructions

- Keep a record of your weight every 15 days. Weigh yourself on the same scale in similar clothes at approximately the same time.
- Incorporate some amount of exercise in your daily routine - walking is the best form of exercise.
- Have regular meals. Skipping meals will not help you in reducing weight. Avoid fasting or feasting.
- Do not starve yourself; choose from free foods listed below.
- Using double toned/skimmed milk instead of full cream milk has a definite advantage.
- Stopping sugar completely has no adverse effects as long as you are consuming the prescribed balanced diet.
- Less oil is good for health. Use nonstick pans to reduce the intake of oil.
- Limit the use of processed convenience foods viz. instant mixes, dehydrated soup powder etc.

Foods which can be taken freely

Clear vegetable soup, plain tea/coffee, plain *nimbu pani*, plain soda, butter milk, thin salted *lassi*, green leafy vegetable, salad vegetables, tomato juice, *dhania podina chutney*

Foods to be taken in prescribed amount

Milk and milk products, *chapattis*, rice, *dalia*, pulses, fats and oils

Foods to be avoided

- Fried food like *puri, parantha, samosa, poka*da, *namkeen* mixtures, butter, *malai*

- Sugar, *gur, shakkar*, honey, *mithai*, puddings, ice creams, cakes, pastries.
- Cold drinks /soda, *sharbat*, squashes, juices.
- Alcoholic drinks
- Pickles in oil
- Banana, mango, *cheeku, litchi*, grapes and dates
- *Aloo, arbi, jimikand, Kathal, kachalu*
- Mutton, pork, ham and sausages

It is quite common to see that when patients are advised to reduce weight they may succeed initially. Immediate weight losses are greater with dietary restriction. It is also seen that obese people relapse back to their usual overweight situation after success in the beginning. This is a common feature with any attempt to habit / lifestyle change (e.g. in alcoholic people also we see this happening). It takes a lot of self-control, dedicated effort and courage of conviction to maintain the reduction in weight once achieved. Role of family members (esp. spouse) is important here. Adherence to the prescribed regime is the key. Long term weight loss is more likely to be maintained if patients participate in a regular level of increased, accumulated physical activity.

Pain is a major consideration in Radha's case described above. Her KOA may cause her pain if she exercises. And if she does not do exercises KOA may aggravate leading to more pain (due to weakening of muscles as well as weight gain). This paradoxical and rather a catch 22 kind of situation is all too common in KOA patients. However, weight loss may reduce the pain.

The key is to provide physical activity options that support her weight and protect her joints. Careful assessment of her joints may help to tailor a program suited to her needs, such as cycling or range of motion exercises.

Foods to Eat to Help Ease KOA Symptoms

Below mentioned foods may help ease certain osteoarthritis symptoms.

Fruits and vegetables: These contain vitamins, minerals, and phytochemicals (natural chemicals found in some plant foods) to combat joint pain and swelling. The more colorful the better. Fill breakfast, lunch, and dinner plates with as much color as one can—taste the rainbow. Red grapes, blueberries, carrots, and spinach are some examples of fruits and veggies that may have anti-inflammatory benefits. Eat fruits and/or veggies at every meal.

Omega-3 fatty acids: Fish, such as salmon, and other foods with omega-3 fatty acids (essential fatty acids that can help reduce inflammation and pain) can help ease sore, achy joints. If not a fan of fish, eat walnuts, flaxseed (*alsi*), and olive oil, or take an omega-3 supplement to get the same benefits. Eat a serving of omega-3s per day.

Vitamin D: Foods with vitamin D, such as eggs, mushrooms, and fortified foods (e.g., fortified orange juice and breakfast cereals), can help manage OA-related pain.

Spices: Ginger, turmeric, dried chili peppers, and cinnamon can help ease KOA symptoms: They may have anti-inflammatory effects on the body, helping to reduce swelling and stiffness. An added bonus is that these spices are brimming with flavor without adding any calories. When possible, sprinkle them in at every meal.

Foods to be limited by KOA patients

Some foods can exacerbate pain and other OA symptoms. It's actually a good idea to limit these foods—regardless of whether you have KOA.

Aspartame: This man-made sweetener contains certain chemicals that can increase pain perception. They do this by triggering neurons in your brain. It can be found in all types of foods—from soft drinks to ice cream to seemingly healthier foods like yogurt.

Processed foods: Eating enough foods that contain monosodium glutamate (MSG) or nitrates may eventually lead to inflammation. MSG is found in some frozen dinners, and nitrates can be found in hot dogs.

Trans fats and saturated fats: The packaged baked goods and fast food like French fries: These foods can promote inflammation and clog blood vessels also.

Should One Take Supplements for KOA?

Of course, the best way to get all of key nutrients is from what is eaten. But if our diet is lacking in any way, we need to take a supplement.Before considering taking any vitamins or minerals, a doctor should be consulted. He will let you know how much need to take and whether it will interact with medications or other supplements being taken.

Dietary Supplements

Dietary supplements are commonly known as nutraceuticals. These play a pivotal role in the KOA management. These functional ingredients are usually sold as powders, pills, and other medicinal forms not generally associated with food. However, scientific evidence is also insufficient for most of supplements as well as herbal plant remedies. For example, in many countries guidelines mention that glucosamine type medicines are **not** to be prescribed for KOA patients.

Quacks also take advantage of this situation of lack of an effective cure for KOA. They suggest various herbal remedies for KOA. Petty manufacturers also claim to treat KOA with a variety of their products .Publicity is also done for these through various media channels. When lead author asked a KOA patient about her experience of a supplement named ***** Sudha . She told " *pata nahi kya hai us main, maine toh dekha ki TV par dikha rahe the aur itna bada actor bata raha tha, toh ajma kar dekh leti hun ,par kuch paharak ni pada*"(I don't know what is in that product.I saw on TV that a renowned actor was doing publicity so I thought to try the product. But it has no effect".Dietary supplements have also been the subject of clinical trials on KOA (Table 3).

Table 3: Dietary supplements for KOA patients

S.No	*Dietary supplements*	*Examples*
1.	Nutraceuticals	Glucosamine, Chondroitin, S-adenylmethioniune (SAMe), collagen hyrdolysate, Diacerein, Oxaceprol, Avocado –soyabean, Vitamin C, D, E, K
2.	Ayurvedic Drugs and Indian Herbal plants	Boswellia Serrata; Curcum (Turmeic), Ginger, Withania somniefera, Camellia sinensis (green tea)
3.	Fruits and vegetables	Punica granatum (pomegranate), Annnas comosus (Pineapple), Red grapes, blueberries, carrots, capsicum, spinach

Glucosamine

Glucosamine has emerged as a sort of wonder drug for KOA. It is said to be capable of stimulating the regeneration of cartilage. It has further been shown to reduce pain. It is also claimed that glucosamine leads to a decrease in joint space narrowing. Overall result is improved joint mobility and function.

Also glucosamine generally has been reported to be drug well tolerated by patients; however, adverse effects have also been documented in about 10% patients. These were mainly gastrointestinal tract symptoms like dyspepsia, abdominal discomfort, and diarrhea. Most of these disappear on stopping glucosamine. There are also reports of insulin resistance and the development of diabetes mellitus in animal experiments with glucosamine. Surprisingly, an orthopedic surgeon told during an interview regarding prescription of glucosamine "kucchh *toh likhana hi hai. Yehi chalta aa raha hai; yeh theek hai ki evidence inconclusive hai."* (We have to prescribe something. This supplement is being prescribed for quite a long time; even though evidence is inconclusive on this medicine)"

Chondroitin

Chondroitin has received almost as much attention as glucosamine in both medical and lay circles. It often is marketed as a combined preparation with the latter. However, it is also available as a solo product. Like glucosamine, it is most widely available in its sulfate form. Glucosamine and chondroitin appear to act in a synergistic manner. Adverse effects have also been reported, like asthma, and interaction with anticoagulants such as warfarin and heparin, leading to excessive bleeding.

Evidence for utility of both glucosamine and chondoitin in KOA treatment is inconclusive. Many countries have not recommended the use of these for treatment of osteoarthritis.Once a renowned orthopaedics surgeon of PGIMER, told the lead author," Doctors prescribe these because patient ask for it; only for their psychological satisfaction. They tell KOA patients 'eh *grease vadhan wali goliyan hain*'(these are grease enhancing tablets)." Many patients reported taking nutraceuticals on their own for more than 4 -5 years. They learn about these through word of mouth publicity.

Collagen Hydrolysate

Hydrolyzed gelatin products have also been sold for many years by pharmaceuticals as nutraceuticals. This is said to help regeneration of cartilage/ collagen. It is associated with minimal adverse effects characterized by sensation of fullness or unpleasant taste.

Diacerein

It has been used extensively to treat KOA. It is an anti-inflammatory medication that works differently from the typical painkillers. It is also claimed to reduce joint space narrowing. Diacerein may be tolerated well by patients with impaired kidney function. Adverse effects include mild to moderate changes in bowel habits (diarrhea) at doses higher 50 mg twice per day. These disappear on stoppage of the drug.

Oxaceprol: This nutraceutical has been reported as an effective pain killer. Also it is tolerated better. It has no adverse effects on the gastrointestinal system.

Fish oils: There is some evidence that it may help preserve cartilage. In any case since most people after Vit D deficient it makes sense to take such supplements. Also anti-oxidants, in general, will help KOA patients.

Ayurvedic Drugs and Indian Herbal plants

Boswellia Serrata: It is a tree of intermediate height found in hilly areas of India. On stripping the bark, it yields a gummy oleoresin, which contains oils, terpenoids and gum. Since antiquity,dried gum resin (*guggulu*) extracted from Boswellia serrata has been claimed to possess good anti-inflammatory, anti-arthritic, and analgesic activity. Boswellia gum has been mentioned in ancient Indian Ayurvedic texts – the *Sushruta Samhita* and the *Charak Samhita*.

Boswellia has been claimed to assist in keeping articular cartilage in good condition. This is also said to be responsible for the recovery of the patients with osteoarthritis and to prevent progression of the disease. Boswellia also may decrease the severity of pain and swelling, as well as a return of function and range of movement. The frequency of joint swelling is also decreased. Adverse drug reactions of Boswellia therapy may include diarrhea, epigastric pain, and nausea. Evidence for Boswellia serrata's effectiveness in treating OA is still considered inconclusive.

Curcumin (Turmeric; *Haldi*)

Turmeric comes from the root of (*C. longa)*. Curcumin, an active component of *Curcuma longa*, commonly known as turmeric, is used as a spice, flavoring agent, food preservative as well as a coloring agent. Its potential in OA has been widely studied. During interview with KOA patients, many of them told the lead author that they used to take turmeric powder with milk twice a day to relieve the pain for healing the injury.

Ginger (Adrakh)

Zingiber officinale is commonly known as ginger, belonging to Zingiberaceae family, and is a very popular spice in cuisine. Ginger has been used traditionally in Japanese, Indian and Chinese medicine as an anti-inflammatory agent for musculo-skeletal disorders. Ginger has been proven to be effective in reducing the symptoms associated with osteoarthritis. Many KOA patients reported to researcher that they use *saunth*(dried form of ginger) for relieving the pain especially during winter season.

Camellia sinensis (green tea)

Green tea has been reported to have anti-inflammatory, anti-obesity and neuro-protective effects .Tea consumption in general has not displayed any acute or chronic toxic effects, and in fact, it is health promoting. Many overweight patients reported to lead author that they took green tea because they believed that it would reduce their weight .They also told that as they could not do exercises for longer duration for weight reduction, hence they took green tea. Most of them were from upper economic strata.

Adherence to Prescribed Treatment in KOA Patients

Efficacy of any treatment depends on the degree of adherence of the patient with the prescribed regime. Even a proven effective treatment, if not followed religiously, cannot bring the desired results. It has been observed that the level of adherence of patients to a treatment regime is directly proportional to its tangible success. Studies have found that globally, the overall adherence level to treatment is around 50%. Adherence to prescribed medicines has been seen to be better than that for lifestyle modifications. It is also a general observation that as the treatment gets complex and imposes more restrictions on the patients the rate of adherence drops further. Even the potential of latest advancement in field of medicine can only be realized if patients adhere to treatment. Almost every patient has varying degree of difficulty adhering to medical recommendations, especially when the advice entails self-administered care. In general, poor adherence to therapy results in medical, psychological and economic consequences.

KOA is a chronic condition. Patients find it hard to perform daily activities with constant pain and discomfort. The multi-modal treatment approach including medications, dietary supplementations / modifications, physical activity and following an overall healthy lifestyle can improve their condition. Despite such knowledge, KOA patients often fail to adhere to doctors' recommendations. Reasons for such failure are many.

Firstly, it is well known that none of the treatment for KOA is 100% effective even if the instructions are followed rigorously. Symptoms may subside temporarily but disease condition is not cured. When people take one regime, they may get some temporary relief. As a result, they may stop following the regime and / or get back to their old habits. This may cause the symptoms to reappear. This distress forces them to try a new treatment option, and again the same cycle repeats. Eventually, they lose faith in the treatment and doctors. Adherence is naturally affected. When the condition worsens beyond tolerance they may be forced to undergo surgery.

It has also been observed that the rate of adherence for different components of the prescribed regimen is different. Patients are most adherent in taking medication and less so for prescribed diet and exercise. The "pill for ill" mindset is deeply engraved in the minds of people. Popping pills looks far easier and convenient to patients than changing their lifestyle or daily routine. Generally, KOA is aggravated or is in part precipitated because people follow unhealthy habits. Most KOA patients find it hard to incorporate changes in their lifestyle as this requires a lot of effort and commitment.

Poor adherence to therapy results in worsening of their condition over time. As the pain and discomfort due to KOA increases, person's mobility gets restricted. Occupational, social and recreational activities are greatly hampered. This state of helplessness can also lead to stress, anxiety, tension and even depression. In desperation to get relief patients spend a lot of money on various therapies.

KOA regime requires a significant level of adherence. To achieve this, the focus should be on developing good adherence behavior. But before that it is imperative to understand the determinants that affect adherence. It is not just patient's responsibility. Their therapists as well as family members need to encourage them to adhere with the prescribed regimen. In fact, it is a complex behavioral process and is affected by following factors:

(i) **Patient-related factors** – These include the patients' socio-demographic profile:

* Age – This disease mostly affects people in middle age and old age. During these stages KOA patients have also to face family responsibilities and work pressure. Moreover, forgetfulness affects adherence to medicines and lifestyle prescription. As age progresses these problems multiply. Attitude of people also becomes more rigid. This also has an adverse effect on adherence.

* Stress – Continuous and lifelong management is required to stay healthy in KOA patients. They find it frustrating to incorporate too many changes in their daily routine. Even a slight amount of deviation may lead to relapse of symptoms. After putting so much of effort even a slight setback can de-motivate them. Such negative attitude and concern can make them stressed and more sensitive towards pain. This makes the treatment administration and continuation more complex.

* Knowledge – The knowledge and awareness regarding one's disease is an important factor affecting adherence. As this condition requires significant degree of self-management, a well informed and literate person can understand and manage his condition better. And thus, his chances of overall adherence will increase.

  However, at times, little knowledge can also become a barrier. Some well-read people are most difficult to convince and counsel. In modern era, easy access to vast and often incorrect/misleading information over internet results in more confusion. Many a times contradictory information from various sources perplexes the patients. This leads to loss of faith of people in treatment and adherence.

* Perception of control – Locus of control concept refers to the belief individuals have about the amount of control they have over their lives. Health locus of control is defined as a generalized expectation about whether one's health is controlled by one's own behavior or forces external to oneself. Individuals with internal locus of control are reported to be more likely to exert efforts to control their environment and to take responsibility for their actions. Such individuals listen to all the advice given

by doctors but follow what they think is right. Such patients with high perceived control (Rich / literate) have better health because they are more likely to take health-enhancing actions. That is, perceptions of control influence whether an individual will try to prevent and remedy his /her own health problems. They also believe that treatment outcomes are a direct result of their own behavior.

Individuals with external locus of control believe that treatment outcomes are a result of either chance or powerful other people, such as physicians. These individuals consider a doctor as God and comply with whatever the he says. Generally, illiterates and poor people have more external locus. Their compliance is likely to be better provided that they have the necessary resources.

* Expectations – Failure to meet the expectations of the patients from the treatment can also affect adherence. It is important to have realistic expectations from the treatment to stay motivated. The treatment takes time in improving the patient's condition. It would be wrong to expect the treatment to do magic in a day or so. The doctors are expected to explain the treatment regime thoroughly to the patients. And patients are also expected to get their doubts clarified. Doctor's busy schedule prevents them from properly explaining the details of the therapy to the patients or their caregivers. As a result patients suffer.
* Socioeconomic status - Poverty, illiteracy, low level of education, unemployment, lack of effective social support networks, unstable living conditions can make adherence to treatment difficult. Illiteracy and unemployment are major problems of our country. These conditions favor an external locus of control. It is seen among patients with low/unstable income and poverty. Lack of financial resources affects poor patients' access to good medical care. Many people can't even afford to purchase daily medicines. This seriously affects their adherence levels.
* Family - Support from family members plays a key role in adherence. Supportive and encouraging family members and friends can help motivate and encourage the patient to continue their therapy. Thus, it helps in improving adherence.
* Culture and lay beliefs - What one perceives about one's condition can play a critical role in adherence. Negative perception of disease will lead to further deterioration of health. Beliefs held by individuals about health, illness and diseases

also affect their adherence levels. In some societies, allopathic medicines are not widely accepted. Though Indians widely use allopathic medicines, majority of them still try and trust traditional health systems like Ayurveda. As a contrast, orthopedist promote surgery as the only treatment for KOA. Such a mindset adversely affects adherence to the advice.

* Money – In a country like India, it is an important factor as most citizens are not medically insured. The high cost of treatment makes it unaffordable and out of reach for lower and middle class sections of society. Therefore, poor financial condition directly decreases the treatment adherence of majority of KOA patients.

(ii) Health care team and system-related factors

Poor quality of health care services in India also affect adherence. Hospitals are overcrowded; doctor- patient ratio is not good. The time spent by a doctor with a patient is very less. Health professionals recommend the treatment regimens without addressing to patients' individual needs. Customization is usually not attempted by the doctors. No empathy is shown. Patients are also not adequately informed about their condition or about the treatment. In such a scenario patients feel de-motivated and do not adhere to prescribed regime.

Casual and callous behavior of doctors also has an important impact on compliance. Patients need sufficient time with a doctor in OPD to explain their condition. Ideally, even doctor should not only diligently listen to patients' problems but also explain them at length about the disease and the treatment. Doctor should educate the patient regarding the treatment options and what to expect from various regimens. A healthy relationship between patient and doctor can have a great impact on the adherence. However, in crowded OPDs in most Indian hospitals, this is more or less impossible. So, adherence level is seriously compromised.

(iii) Condition-related factors

- Severity of the disease or condition – The severity of disease, related complications and disabilities also affect adherence. The treatment for KOA patients is cumbersome. Due to this the patient feels a lot of stress. Moreover, the treatment requires a lot of self-management and self-care. This adds ups to the emotional burden of KOA patients. To make things worse, family and social support is also variable.

The level of adherence to prescribed treatment in serious and severe conditions is expected to be higher than the mild or moderately severe cases.

When symptoms are severe, patients often put maximum effort for fastest improvement. Often, it is seen that as the condition improves the patients gets relaxed. Further, as they engage themselves in daily chores, they forget about the disease condition and get irregular with treatment regime. This increases the probability of relapse.

Co-morbidities - If the patient suffers from other diseases or complications along with the osteoarthritis (which is quite common) then also the adherence become difficult due to too many restrictions and recommendations. As the treatment becomes more complex the chances of misunderstanding and confusion increases. In such cases, the recuperation is slow. Due to delayed outcome the person feels de-motivated. This further decreases the adherence. Thus, patients who suffer from multiple diseases (like hypertension / diabetes / heart disease) find it difficult to adhere to complex treatments. They are bogged down by too much medication.

(iv) Therapy-related factors

In the prevailing health culture promoted by medicalization of life, patients give more importance to drugs. Once medication starts they don't feel the need to follow any advice on diet or exercise. Both of these require lot of effort and self-control.

Distance from hospitals and cost of transportation also affect treatment adherence.

Loss of faith in medicine - If the degree and speed of relief obtained in the initial phase of the treatment is slow, then the person feels miserable, depressed and loses hope in his treatment. In such cases, the adherence is greatly affected. It is very important to have faith and optimistic approach regarding one's treatment. If a person has no faith in his doctor or the treatment then the chances of adhering with the prescribed treatment reduce. Thus, a good and healthy doctor-patient and relationship also plays an important part in treatment adherence.

Improving Adherence

Permanent relief from symptoms in KOA patients remains a challenging task. This can be achieved if patients follow the prescribed treatment sincerely. Improving adherence calls for a holistic health care approach. The mindset of patients also needs to be changed. Patients do not tend to follow life style modification because they have this concept in mind that they can control their condition by medicines alone. Doctor's should stress more on lifestyle modifications rather than providing an easy way out to patients in the form of medications.

The doctors should also acquire and improve their skills in communication for building better doctor-patient relationship. To improve adherence it is important for doctor to understand the patients, their health needs and all other related factors. This will help in providing treatment that best suits their individual needs. Better adherence can be achieved by supporting the patients, instead of blaming them (quite commonly resorted to by irritated and exasperated doctors in crowded OPDs).

Adherence is a dynamic process. To inculcate a desired level of adherence in patients it is important that they are regularly and properly counselled. Regular and timely health checkups, proper patient education, cheaper medical facilities, setting achievable health targets and continuous motivation can go a long way in improving treatment adherence.

Evidence base through research conducted in PGIMER, Chandigarh

In this context, Dr Meenakshi Sharma has conducted an RCT as a part of her PhD work with an objective to compare the impact of two non-pharmacological intervention packages on quality of life in KOA patients reporting at PGIMER Chandigarh. The trial was registered in the **Clinical Trials Registry-India (CTRI)** -REF/2013/09/005703 CTRI/2014/01/004270].Overall 123 patients (87 females and 36 males) were enrolled in the study. All except 4 patients (who had unilateral KOA) were diagnosed with bilateral KOA. There were 63 patients in mild grade group. Of these, 4 were lost to follow up. Most (n=49) patients complied with the instructions. Few (n=10) were non-compliant. Sixty patients had moderate grade KOA. Here lesser number (n=22) were compliant.

The response has been quite good. There was improvement in the condition of many patients as measured by VAS and WOMAC scale. In general, more of the compliant participants showed better improvement as compared to the non-compliant patients. The mean WOMAC scale decreased from 32.1 to 22.8 for the compliant participants. The mean VAS score decreased from 5.1 to 3.1.

The enhancement in quality of life of the patients as a result of our intervention is also reflected through their verbatim responses as under (difficulties/problems faced by them in complying with the instructions given in the hospital are also highlighted):

(a) Experiences of KOA patient (*JK*)at PGI Chandigarh —

I am a young man of 60 plus recently retired from State Bank of India. Notwithstanding my sedentary life style in office I used to balance with routine cycling and exercise almost daily and also with use of stairs at office as my office was on sixth floor. As such I was confident of having a healthy body. Inspite of all this, my confidence was shaken when I could not ward off the signals of aging as one day I notice some pain in my left knee. On getting examined from Ortho doctor at Panchkula I was diagnosed symptoms of Osteoarthritis, which was not digested by me although doctor said is normal in this age. Being in Panchkula I wanted to have a second seasoned opinion. So, I visited PGI as I had the impression that there would not be any commercial motive. Besides I was also searching and taking help from Google aunty for the exercises on the net for knee pain. But there was not any perceptible change till I was referred to physiotherapy section of the Hospital. The protocol advised by Dr. Meenakshi has really helped me in alleviating not only my pain in the knee (left one more in trouble) but with religiously following the set of exercises as advised it almost cured me. I would like to mention here that although one gets good amount of help from net but one ought to miss fine nuances, which one gets from personal attention by routine checkup intermittently at weekly / fortnightly intervals by Dr. Meenakshi and her team which has been really useful.

I feel happy to place on record my appreciation to Dr. Meenakshi and her team for devising this protocol of exercises and I must say that it is desirable not only to do these (exercises) regularly but to bring this regimen of exercises in one's lifestyle.

***PK** :- Bahut fark hai tablet chhod di bahut fark hai.Main tang ko last visit tak utha nahi pa rahi thi, abhi to bahut fark hai (With exercises there is a lot of improvement I have stopped taking painkillers. Till last visit I could not even raise my legs. Now I can)*

***BS**:-15-20% pharak hai. Dard di goli band kar di.pehle din vich do baar goli khanda si,pichhchle 25 dino se nahi khayi(there is 15-20% relief. I have stopped taking painkillers for last 25 days.I used to take 2 tablets per day earlier).*

***TS:**-50 percent aaram hai (there is 50% relief)*

***RB:**-Pehle farak tha chhodne par dard hota hai (With exercises there is improvement; pain reappears on leaving it)*

***RK**:-Mujhe adha fark hai(there is 50% relief)*

***VK**:-Pehle se dard kam hai ;car mai par baithne main problem hai (there is improvement in pain, but there is problem when I sit in the car)*

> **Mr X :** I was severely suffering from Knee Pain for a year. I was to get my Knee plates replaced. I had consulted many knee hospitals, such as Rajindra Hospital Patiala. Fortis, Mohali Chandigarh. They all had advised me to replace the Knee plates. But before going for it I felt to have some advice from PGI Chandigarh. So I came here and got my checkup done in the Ortho. OPD of PGI. They sent me to physiotherapy department. Hence, I came here. (I have been under treatment through physiotherapy / exercise sessions for two months. I did the exercises advised to me by the physiotherapy regularly. Now after two months, I felt 70% relief in my pain I have also stopped taking pain killers which I took regularly. So I am now really thankful to PGI authorities for initiating such a service. So as of now, I have postponed the decision to go for surgery.)

Dr Meenakshi Sharma's RCT (a part of her PhD work) has proved that there is a definite role of non-pharmacological intervention packages (lifestyle changes, weight reduction, meditation and exercises) in improving the quality of life of KOA patients.

Special problems faced by female KOA patients

It has also been observed that KOA problems of women are not given the due attention they deserve (by the orthopedists / physiotherapists). For example - one common symptom reported by women with KOA is – pain in the groin region. There is no reference to this in the mainstream literature. Some researchers have, of course referred to hip / sacro-iliac joint problem as a cause of such symptoms.

Quite often, the terminology used by women to explain their symptoms do not match with that of the doctors, who tend to trivialize their suffering. In fact, the lead author himself witnessed an interaction between a radiologist and a female post traumatic KOA patient in MRI unit of a leading apex level medical institute. While waiting for her turn to get the MRI done the radiologist commented," My mother also had a fall, she had similar problem. She is using a walking stick. You may also learn to live with your problem. Nothing will be gained in this hospital. Women have to face these problems"!

It seems that the orthopedists and physiotherapists do not take problems of women KOA patients seriously. It was also observed by the lead author that when a KOA woman complained about stiffness, pain or altered gait, the concerned physiotherapist did not acknowledge the same. Rather he commented that such symptoms are 'not anatomically possible'. Here, the issue is that, if a patient complains of something, there is definitely something wrong with her. Otherwise why would she go to a hospital? It is also not necessary that her vocabulary / terminology will match with that of medical fraternity. After all, they have not obtained a medical degree. They have not studied in a medical school. They will naturally try to explain their symptoms in their own language. Challenge is for doctors to make sense of it and fit the same in their medical conceptual framework. They are supposed to provide relief to KOA patients convincingly. They need to satisfy all the doubts and apprehensions of women patients. Sadly, this rarely happens and patients continue to suffer (at the hands of doctors)

Also when prescription is written for them there are no clear guidelines for restriction of household work in such patients (bending down; reaching up). They often report worsening of symptoms when they do household chores. Unless this is addressed, their condition may worsen. Often their symptoms are due to the altered body alignment. However, no visible effort is made by orthopedists / physiotherapists for correcting this.

It is a well-known fact that in KOA patients there is a definite impact on body alignment. Also there is compensatory posture adjustment. Hence, if the primary problem of KOA related pain is not solved, secondary problems aggravate the situation. Eventually, the painful condition and stiffness worsen. Patients keep visiting hospitals off and on. They are prescribed a mix regimen of SWD/hot pack/exercises etc. Compliance is often questionable. Relief is also variable. The result is that both patients and the orthopedists / physiotherapists become apathetic and casual about the issue. Rather they adopt a resigned attitude towards the problems of women KOA patients

Another aspect here is that exercises and weight control are not an 'in thing' in Indian women especially after 40 years age. And both of these interventions are crucial for obtaining relief in symptoms of women KOA patients. In general, most of the middle aged Indian women of this era might not have done any exercise in their childhood / adolescence. So, they may find it hard to start on a regime of regular exercise! There is a definite need to change this attitude. Behavior change theories need to be applied here seriously. The patients need to be clearly told that they would have to shed all inhibitions if they really want relief from the symptoms. They need to be exposed to successfully treated women through exercises & weight control. However, in the usual scenario of crowded OPDs in Indian hospitals, there is usually no scope or inclination to address these issues. This results in a general lack of motivation among female KOA patients for compliance with any advice for exercises or weight control.

A minor but important related issue is the clothing patterns among Indian women. They may not be willing (or may not like) to expose their body parts during examination, therapy or exercise training. This way, it may become difficult for the concerned orthopedists / physiotherapists to go for body measurements to check for alignment problems. This should be an integral part of any attempt at KOA management. It is also vital to ensure compliance by the women to the instructions given to them in the hospital. Here, they need to exercise patience with women KOA patients. Keeping in view the cultural aspects, they need to devise their own ways to diagnose, monitor and manage such patients.

Risk factors for KOA; who are more likely to get it?

It is a well-known fact that risk and chances of KOA increase with age. KOA is often labeled as a degenerative or wear and tear disorder. In addition many mechanical, metabolic, and genetic disorders can also enhance the chances of KOA. So, people who indulge in heavy physical work involving weight bearing and repeated injuries to knee are at risk of KOA. Basically, it can be regarded as joint failure just like any other organ failure. Factors associated with KOA are enlisted in table 4. Hence, if there is an evidence of more proneness for KOA, the concerned individuals should take anticipatory preventive measures to retain or enhance their quality of life. For example, in old age they need to be careful about their bone density as well as dietary intake of vitamins C & D.

Table 4: Risk Factors Associated with Osteoarthritis

Category	*Factors*
Constitutional factors	Old age Female gender Obesity Reduced bone density Muscle weakness Joint laxity
Mechanical Factors	Heavy physical activity Major joint injury Meniscal injuries
Endocrine factors	Disease which change cartilage structure-Hemochromatosis
Genetic factors	Mutations in the type II collagen gene
Occupational factors	Regular working in a kneeling or squatting posture, Lifting or carrying heavy weights
Dietary	Low dietary intake of vitamin C Low dietary intake of Vitamin D

Myths and misconceptions About KOA

Like other diseases, many layman's theories are associated with KOA also. People have many wrong notions about it.

(i) It only affects older people : While the risk of osteoarthritis increases with age, it can affect individuals of all ages. In India, it is the second most prevalent disease in the younger generation. It affects more than 12 % of the population in the age group of 25-30 years.

(ii) It cannot be treated: While there is still no cure yet for osteoarthritis, research shows that early diagnosis and appropriate management can help reduce the pain and disability associated with many types of arthritis.

(iii) Winter is the culprit: It is commonly believed that cold weather can cause osteoarthritis. The truth is that cold weather can only exacerbate joint pain and joint stiffness. Winter will not have any effect on the progression of the disease.

(iv) It isn't in your genes: KOA is linked to genes. It is more prevalent amongst women. They tend to develop it in the same joints and around the same age as their mothers.

(v) High heels are high risk: People tend to believe that walking in high heels will lead to long-term damage of the knee and back. This isn't true. Usage of inappropriate footwear (with or without high heels) in any way causes pain in the spine thus leading to back pain.

(vi) Using stairs is the best way to burn calories and reduce weight: People believe using the staircase is a good exercise. But unfortunately, it puts a load on the knees. This leads to pain which eventually aggravates KOA. So, it is not a good idea for KOA patients to go for this exercise for weight reduction.

Do's and Don'ts / General precautions for diagnosed KOA patients

- Discuss to your satisfaction frankly with your doctor about your disease and the available treatment options.
- Follow all the instructions diligently.
- Keep a phone contact number of your doctor.
- Go for a second opinions also (esp. if operation is advised or if there is no relief)
- Do not sit cross legged(use bench in temples/*gurudwaras*)
- Avoid climbing stairs (use lift)
- Avoid jumping, jerky movements or vigorous activities
- Avoid walking in areas / grounds with uneven surface
- Avoid high heels
- Use knee caps /canes as per the need
- Do not join gym or go for vigorous treadmill exercises

Stop press!

After the results of Dr Meenakshi's PhD thesis work and our UT – DST project on KOA started reaching the masses through word of mouth publicity, the idea seems to have been picked up by private sector as well as many other institutions (like AIIMS, New Delhi). Few news articles have appeared in national and local dailies which highlight the role of non-pharmacological intervention packages on quality of life in KOA patients. The article are now quoting figures like, "one third knee replacement surgeries are not required'. Statements are being issued that lifestyle changes, weight reduction and exercises can avoid the need of surgery! (Please see annexure 2 press clippings)

Moreover, there are now talks about improving doctor-patient communication and even about establishing an information kiosk for empowering the patients (The Times of Chandigarh, Dec.2, 2014). Here, it is not out of context to mention that this approach has already been pioneered by the authors through preparation of a multilingual brochure and a video CD on KOA management. Computer based patient education sessions are being imparted. Also, a Multipurpose Behaviour Therapy (MPBT) Room approach is already being implemented in Gynecology OPD of the same hospital (PGIMER, Chandigarh), through a DBT funded project awarded to Dr Amarjeet Singh and co-workers. It also focuses upon an approach of reducing load on doctors in OPD. Here also, emphasis is given on leisurely counseling of the patients on self-care. Results, so far, have been excellent.

References

1. Kellgren JH, Lawrence JS. Radiological assessment of osteoarthrosis. Ann Rheum Dis. 1957; 16(4):494–502.
2. Kulkarni C, Leena A, Lohit K, Mishra D, Saji M.J.. A randomized comparative study of safety and efficacy of immediate release glucosamine HCL and glucosamine HCL sustained release formulation in the treatment of knee osteoarthritis: A proof of concept study; J Pharmacol Pharmacother. 2012; Jan-Mar; 3(1): 48–54.
3. Recommendations for the medical management of osteoarthritis of the hip and knee: 2000 update. American College of Rheumatology Subcommittee on Osteoarthritis Guidelines. Arthritis Rheum. 2000;43:1905–15.
4. Jordan KM, EULAR recommendations 2003: An evidence based approach to the management of knee osteoarthritis: report of a task force of the Standing Committee for International Clinical Studies Including Therapeutic Trials (ESCISIT). Annals of the Rheumatic Diseases. 2003;62(12):1145–55.
5. Guideline for the non-surgical management of hip and knee osteoarthritis. Melbourne, The Royal College of Australian General Practitioners, 2009; 70.
6. Hoogeboom TJ, Mirelle JPM Stukstette, Rob A de Bie, Cornelissen J, Broeder AA, Cornelia HM van den Ende. Non-pharmacological care for patients with generalized osteoarthritis: design of a randomized clinical trial; BMC Musculoskeletal Disorders 2010, 11:142.
7. Stephen PM. Diet and Exercise for Obese Adults with Knee Osteoarthritis; Clin Geriatr Med. 2010; 26(3): 461–477.

8. Huang MH, Lin YS, Yang RC, and Lee CL. a comparison of various therapeutic exercises on the functional status of patients with knee osteoarthritis. Seminars in Arthritis and Rheumatism 2003; 32, 6 :398-406.
9. Diracoglu, D., Aydin, R., Baskent, A. and Celik, A. Effects of kinesthesia and balance exercises in knee osteoarthritis. Journal of Clinical Rheumatology 2005; 11: 303-310.
10. Fitzgerald, G., Childs, J., Ridge, T. and Irrgang, J. Agility and perturbation training for a physically active individual with knee osteoarthritis. Physical Therapy 2002; 82: 372-382.
11. Fitzgerald, G., Piva, S., Gil, A., Wisniewski, S., Oddis, C. and Irrgang J. Agility and perturbation training techniques in exercise therapy for reducing pain and improving function in people with knee osteoarthritis: a randomized clinical trial. Physical Therapy 2011; 91: 452-469.
12. Mikesky, A., Mazzuca, S., Brandt, K., Perkins, S., Damush, T. and Lane, K. Effects of strength training on the incidence and progression of knee osteoarthritis. Arthritis and Rheumatism 2006; 55, 690-699.
13. Rogers, M., Tamulevicius, N., Coetsee, M., Curry, B. and Semple, S. Knee osteoarthritis and the efficacy of kinesthesia, balance & agility exercise training: a pilot study. International Journal of Exercise Science 2011; 4:124-132.
14. Rogers, M., Tamulevicius N., Semple, S., Coetsee, M. and Curry, B.Comparison of clinic-based versus home-based balance and agility training for the symptoms of knee osteoarthritis. South African Journal of Sports Medicine 2011; 23: 80-83.
15. Sekir, U. and Gur, H. A multi-station proprioceptive exercise program in patients with bilateral knee osteoarthritis: functional capacity, pain and sensoriomotor function. A randomized controlled trial. Journal of Sports Science and Medicine 2005;4, 590-603.
16. Kumar S. Proprioceptive training as an adjunct in osteoarthritis of knee J.Musculoskelet ,Res 2013;16:10
17. Maggo A, saxena S, The effect of priproprioceptive and strengthening exercises in knee osteoarthritis.Indian Journal of Physiotherapy and Occupational Therapy –2011;5:144-148
18. Jawahar R, Yang S, Eaton CB, McAlindon T, Lapane KL. Gender-specific correlates of complementary and alternative medicine use for knee osteoarthritis. J Womens Health (Larchmt). 2012;21(10):1091-9.
19. Fransen M, Crosbie J, Edmonds J. Physical therapy is effective for patients with osteoarthritis of the knee: a randomized controlled clinical trial. J Rheumatol 2001;28(1):156-64.
20. Zhang W, Moskowitz RW, Nuki G, Abramson S, Altman RD, Arden N.OARSI recommendations for the management of hip and knee osteoarthritis, Part II:OARSI evidence-based, expert consensus guidelines. Osteoarthritis Cartilage 2008;16(2):137-62.
21. Zhang W, Nuki G, Moskowitz RW, Abramson S, Altman RD, Arden NK . OARSI recommendations for the management of hip and knee osteoarthritis: part III:

Changes in evidence following systematic cumulative update of research published through January 2009. Osteoarthritis Cartilage 2010; 18(4): 476-99.

22. Fransen M, McConnell S, Bell M. Therapeutic exercise for people with osteoarthritis of the hip or knee. A systematic review. 2002; 29(8): 1737-45.
23. Deyle GD, Henderson NE, Matekel RL, Ryder MG, Garber MB, Allison SC Effectiveness of manual physical therapy and exercise in osteoarthritis of the knee. A randomized, controlled trial. Annals of Internal Medicine. 2000; 132: 173–181.
24. Thomas K S.Home based exercise programme for knee pain and knee osteoarthritis: randomized controlled trial. BMJ 2002; 325.
25. Heuts PH, de Bie R, Drietelaar M. Self-management in osteoarthritis of hip or knee: a randomized clinical trial in a primary healthcare setting. J Rheumatol 2005; 32: 543–9.
26. Tak E, Staats P, Van Hespen A. The effects of an exercise program for older adults with osteoarthritis of the hip. J Rheumatol 2005; 32: 1106–13.
27. Hughes SL, Seymour RB, Campbell R. Impact of the fit and strong intervention on older adults with osteoarthritis. Gerontologist 2004;44: 217–28.
28. Felson DT, Anderson JJ, Naimark A, Walker AM, Meenan RF. Obesity and knee osteoarthritis. The Framingham Study. Ann Intern Med 1988; 109: 18-24.
29. Felson DT, Zhang Y, Anthony JM, Naimark A, Anderson JJ. Weight loss reduces the risk for symptomatic knee OA in women: the Framingham Study. Ann Intern Med 1992; 116: 535-539.
30. Haralson K. Physical modalities. In: Banwell BF, Gall V. Physical Therapy Management of Arthritis New York, NY: Churchill Livingstone Inc; 1988: 77–106. Clinics in Physical Therapy Series.
31. Goats GC. Continuous short-wave (radio-frequency) diathermy. Br J Sports Med23 1989 123–127.
32. Hecox B. Physiological response to local heat gain or loss. In: Hecox B, Mehreteab TA, Weisberg J, eds. Physical Agents: A Comprehensive Text for Physical Therapists East Norwalk, Conn: Appleton & Lange; 1994: 91– 114.
33. Kimmatkar N, Thawani V, Hingorani L, and Khiyani R. Efficacy and tolerability of Boswellia serrata extract in treatment of osteoarthritis of knee –A randomized double blind placebo controlled trial. Phytomedicine 2003; 10: 3–7.
34. Sahu R. Non drug non invasive treatment in the management of patellofemoral osteoarthritis. Indian J Med Sci. 2011 May; 65(5): 203-11.
35. Bee T A, Liew A. Dietary Supplements Used in Osteoarthritis. Proceedings of Singapore Healthcare, Volume 19, Number 3, 2010.
36. Ghanekar R K, PRaina P, Potential of Nutraceuticals and Medicinal Plants in the Management of Osteoarthritis. Review Article, Acta Biologica Indica 2012, 1(1): 27-46.
37. James J. Clayton Nutraceuticals in the Management of Osteoarthritis, Orthopedics August 2007 - Volume 30 · Issue 8.
38. How to Eat Well When You Have Knee Osteoarthritis.http://www.practicalpainmanagement.com/patient/conditions/osteoarthritis/knee/how-eat-well-when-you-have-knee-osteoarthritis.

39. AJ Singh (Editor), (Mrs.) Indrajit Walia, LK Dhaliwal (Co-editors)." Demedicalizing Women's Health". New Delhi, Gyan Publishing House, 2010.
40. Singh AJ, Goel S and Kathiresan J.(editors). "*Health Promotion: Need for Public Health Activism, Vol. I & II Germany* LAP LAMBERT Academic Publishing, 2013.
41. Singh AJ, Kaur S and Kishore J (editors). Comprehensive Textbook of Elderly Care, New Delhi, Century Publications, 2014.

Annexure - 1

Guidelines for Physiotherapy Of Knee Osteoarthritis Patients

SELF INSTRUCTION MANUAL

STRETCHING EXERCISES

A. Standing Quadriceps Stretch

Main muscles worked: Quadriceps

You would feel stretching of muscles in the front of your thigh

Step-by-step directions

1. Stand straight near a wall (on your side).
2. Put your hand at or above shoulder height on the wall.
3. Bend your knee (the one away from wall).Bring your heel up toward your buttock .Thus, trunk and lower extremity should be in same line.
4. Grasp the front of your ankle with your free hand. Gently pull your heel closer to your body.
5. Hold this position for 30 to 60 seconds. Breathe normally.
6. Come back to normal standing position .Turn around and repeat with the opposite leg.
7. Hold for 30 seconds and perform 5 repetitions at a time for 7 days a week.

B. Supine Hamstring Stretch

Main muscles worked: Hamstrings

You should feel this stretch at the back of your thigh and behind your knee

Step-by-step directions

- Put a mat on the floor. Lie supine on your back on a mat with both legs bent.

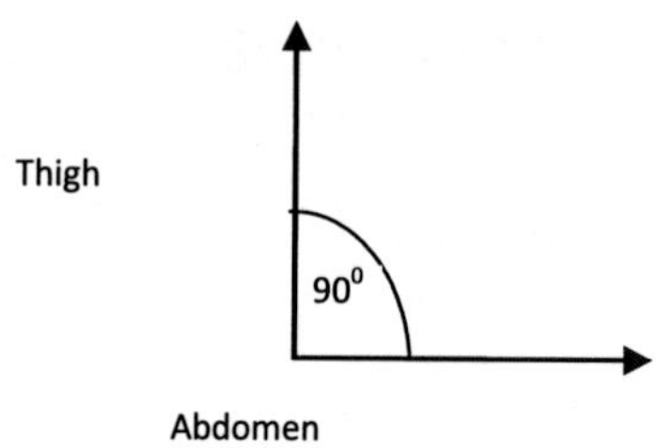

Fig. 1

- Lift one leg off of the floor. Bend it Clasp your hands behind your thigh. Bring the knee toward your chest up to 90° thigh abdominal position.
- Now, straighten your leg. Your foot should face the roof. Pull the toes it gently toward your head, until you feel a stretch. (If you have difficulty clasping your hands behind your leg, loop a towel around your thigh. Grasp the ends of the towel and pull your leg toward you.) Hip should be fixed by stabilizing thigh at 90°. Breathe normally.
- Hold this position for 30 seconds.
- Repeat with the opposite leg and perform 5 repetitions at a time for 7 days a week

Tip: Do not twist or arch your back while doing this stretch

STRENGTHENING EXERCISES

A. Short Arc Lift

Main muscles worked: Strengthens the quads muscles without much knee movement

Equipment needed: Towel

Step-by-step directions.

1. Lie down flat on your back on a flat surface
2. Fold one leg as shown in figure Place a rolled up towel (approx 10 cm diameter) under the knee of other leg.
3. Pull your toes towards you and contract/ tighten your thigh muscles.
4. Slowly lift your foot up off the bed until your knee is straight (fully extended knee).
5. Keep your knee resting on the towel.
6. Hold for 3-5 seconds and slowly lower the leg.
7. Repeat with other leg. Perform 10-12 repetitions at a time for 7 days a week.
8. If pain is not much progression can be done by increasing the size of the towel under the knee. Further progression can be done by adding light ankle weight or by wearing a shoe.

B. Isometric Quadriceps Exercise

Main muscles worked: Quadriceps

You should feel contraction (tightening) at the front of your thigh

Step-by-step directions

(i) Lie supine on a mat with both legs straight with hands by your side.

(ii) Bend your toes inwards (towards your head).

(iii) Keep your knee straight while bending the toes.

(iv) Tighten the muscle in the front of your thigh of both legs as much as you can, pushing the back of your knee flat against the floor. This will pull your kneecap up your thigh, toward your hip.

(v) Hold this position for 10 seconds, trying every second to pull even tighter and relax. Perform 10-12 repetitions at a time for 7 days a week.

Tip : Do not bend your knee.

C. Isometric Quadriceps (with medial rotation of hip)

Main muscles worked: Quadriceps

You should feel tightening of muscles at the front of your thigh

Step-by-step directions

1. Lie in supine position (on your back) on a mat with both legs straight with hands by your side.

2. Keep your knees straight.
3. Raise one leg (6-8 inches) and move your feet inwards (towards other leg) as shown.
4. Tighten your thigh muscle ; raise your leg while performing medial rotation (movement towards other leg) of hip.
5. For this rotate foot and legs towards inwards as shown in the picture Hold position for 10 seconds.
6. Repeat with other leg.

Tip: Do not bend your knee.

D . Quadriceps Isometrics (sitting position)

Main muscles worked: Quadriceps

You should feel tightening of muscles at the front of your thigh

Step-by-step directions

1. Sit comfortably on a mat with leg stretched together in a straight position.
2. Keep your knees straight and keep your hands under the knees. Bend your feet inwards and hold this position Press knees on your hands for 10 seconds.

E. Hamstring Isometric

Main muscles worked: Hamstring

Step-by-step directions

1. Adopt an inclined sitting position as shown in Photograph-13. Keep your palms behind your back on the bed for support. Sit in resting position.
2. Bend your knees slightly approximately 40-60°.
3. Tighten the muscles on the back of the thigh.
4. Bend your toes up towards your head.
5. Dig down with your heels on the bed.
6. Hold for 10 seconds and perform 20 repetitions at a time for 7 days a week.

Tip: Do not let your buttock come off the floor/mat.
Do not hold your breath

F. Hip Abduction

Main muscles worked: Abductors, gluteus medius

You should feel tightening of muscles at your outer thigh near buttock

Equipment needed: One kg weight or sand bag (1 Kg)

Step-by-step directions

1. Lie on your side with your one leg on top and the bottom leg bent to provide support. Hip is straight at exercise side(upper leg). Knee is also straight.
2. Straighten your top leg
3. Slowly raise the top leg it to 45°, keeping your knee straight, but not locked.
4. In mild KOA patients (when pain is less) gradually 1 kg weight (sand bag weighing-1 kg) can be attached to foot.
5. Hold this position for 5 seconds.
6. Slowly lower your leg and relax it for 2 seconds. Perform 20 repetitions at a time for 7 days a week. Repeat with other side also.

Tip : Do not rotate your leg in an effort to raise it higher.

Note:

(1) Patients should also keep in mind that besides these exercises they should also comply with other advice given by doctors – weight reduction, change in lifestyle etc.

(2) If you have any difficulty in doing these exercises consult your doctor/trainer.

(3) In such cases you can also start with lighter version of the exercise. Later full strength exercise may be tried.

KINESTHESIA, BALANCE & AGILITY EXERCISES

These exercise help to restore the confidence of patients regarding his/her balance maintenance in day to day activities.

General instructions

- Agility exercises **(A)** are done at walking pace; for safety's sake, do not attempt to 'run'. As you improve you should be able to do these at a faster pace. But please start slow.

(vii) Always stay near a wall during agility exercises, so that if you start to lose balance you can put your hand on the wall for support.

(viii) For all agility exercises, begin by standing with your feet shoulder width apart. Complete the number of steps prescribed.

- Balance exercises **(B)** should be done next to a sturdy, non-rolling chair or some counter at your home so that you can catch yourself if you start to lose balance. Do not forget that during one-legged balance, if you feel uneasy you can simply put your foot back on the ground to regain balance quickly
- It is important to ensure your safety during these exercises. It is preferable that someone watches you during these exercises. If this is not possible, ensure they are completed in a safe area (free from clutter) and in a position where you can be supported in case you lose your balance, i.e. in a corner of the room with a soft chair or by a bed. If you feel as if you are falling or losing balance, stop the exercise and regain your balance. Rest for a few minutes sitting on a chair before starting again.

Important note

1. Stop and rest if you feel you have had enough of a particular exercise.
   - If you are finding them difficult, carry out the exercises at a slower pace paying particular attention to one aspect of the exercise at a time.

(A) AGILITY EXERCISES

(i) Wedding march: *{Photograph - 17 (a, b, c)}*

1. Stand straight. Keep hands by your side
2. Step forward and slightly outward with right leg.
3. Bring feet next to each other by stepping forward with left leg.
4. Repeat by alternating the lead leg (i.e step out with left leg)
5. Step forward with right leg to bring together both feet.

(ii) Backward wedding march: *{Photograph - 17 (a, b, c)}*

1. Stand straight.
2. Step backward and slightly outward with right leg.
3. Bring back left leg and bring feet next to each other.
4. Repeat by alternating the lead leg.

(iii) High knees march: Walk forward while lifting your knees high as shown in picture (flexing hip about 90 degrees like Independence Day parade by soldiers. But one should not stomp the feet hard on the ground) *(Photograph - 18)*

(iv) Side stepping: *{Photograph - 19 (a, b, c)}*

1. Stand straight.
2. Step sideways to your right with your right leg.
3. Bring left feet with right feet. Walk 4-5 steps this way to the right.
4. Repeat for the given number of steps and come back to original starting point by leading with the left leg.

(v) Semi-tandem walk: Walk forward along an imaginary straight line, but slightly to the outside of the line with each foot. The heel of one foot should land just in front of the toes of the other foot. *(Photograph - 20a)* **(One foot ahead of the other as if taking a step)**

(vi) Tandem walk: Advanced version of above; heel lands directly in front of opposite foot. Tandem is a gait (method of walking) where the toes of the back foot touch the heel of the front foot at each step. Place one foot directly in front of the other, touching heel to toe and hold. Repeat with other foot in front. Progress to taking a step or two by placing your heel to your toe with each step. *(Photograph - 20b)* If you find difficult to balance avoid it first practice with semi tandem walk.

(vii) Cross-over walk: (Ramp Walk) Walk forward along an imaginary line by stepping over to the opposite side of the line with each foot. *{Photograph - 21 (a, b, c)}*. This is like a fashion model walks on ramp.

(viii) Toe walking: Walk forward on toes; try to keep heels from touching floor. *(Photograph - 22)*

(ix) Heel walking: Walk forward on heels; try to keep toes from touching floor. *(Photograph - 23)*

(B) Balance Exercises

Here the person closes eyes with hands, hanging by the side. This standing position is to be maintained for 10-30 seconds. (watch out for balance ask someone to supervise)

(i) Modified Romberg exercise (standing in balance with eyes closed).

(a) On hard ground *(Photograph - 23a)*

(b) On soft ground (on a mat) *(Photograph - 23b)*

(ii) Standing on one extremity for 30 seconds (To be alternated in both extremities). *(Photograph - 24)*. One foot should be held 3-4 inches above the floor level.

(iii) Wide /narrow circle exercises

Draw circles (one wide and one narrow) with chalk on the floor.

Patient should walk on the circle lines. The patient should first do 5 round of each type alternately, instead of drawing small circle patient may walk around a chair. For wider circle thy may walk around dining table.

(a) Walking slowly, wide circle

(b) Walking quickly, wide circle

(c) Walking slowly, narrow circle

(d) Walking quickly, narrow circle

Note:

(1) Patients should also keep in mind that besides these exercises they should also comply with other advice given by doctors – weight reduction, change in lifestyle etc.

(2) If you have any difficulty in doing these exercises consult your doctor/trainer.

(3) In such cases you can also start with lighter version of the exercise. Later full strength exercise may be tried.

Annexure - 2

Newspaper cuttings on role of conservative therapy in KOA

एक्सपर्ट की राय | डॉ. छाबड़ा ने बताया-एक्सरसाइज से घुटनों के दर्द से मिलती है राहत

27·11·14 DR

नी रिप्लेसमेंट से बचना है तो एक्सरसाइज करें

■ कहा- इस तरह की सर्जरी को फिजियोथैरेपी से ही टाला जा सकता है

भास्कर न्यूज | चंडीगढ़

कई बार जोड़-घुटने या हिप्स रिप्लेस करने की जरूरत नहीं, बल्कि फिजियोथैरेपी से ही ऐसी सर्जरी को टाला जा सकता है। घुटनों की रिप्लेसमेंट से बचने के लिए एक्सरसाइज और वजन कम करना जरूरी है। ऐसा करके दर्द और सर्जरी दोनों से बचाव संभव है। डॉ. छाबड़ा ने दावा करते हुए ये बात वीरवार को सेक्टर-7 में फिजियोथेरापी इन द करंट सिनेरियो पर हुई वर्कशॉप में कही। रोटरी चंडीगढ़ शिवालिक क्लब के मेंबर्स के लिए हुई इस वर्कशॉप में डॉ. छाबड़ा ने घुटनों और हिप्स के रिप्लेसमेंट से जुड़ी कई भ्रांतियों को दूर किया।

इस वर्कशॉप में डॉ. छाबड़ा ने कहा कि जोड़ों की सर्जरी से बचाव के लिए सबसे जरूरी है कि अपने जोड़ों में मदद करने वाली मांसपेशियों को मजबूत बनाया जाए। हमारे चलने फिरने या भागने से लेकर वजन उठाते हुए टांगों पर पड़ने वाले वजन का बोझ क्वाड्रीसिपस बर्दाश्त करते हैं। ऐसे में क्वाड्रीसिपस मजबूत होने से जोड़ों पर कम वजन आएगा। फिर भी अगर घुटनों के जोड़ों पर दबाव आ गया गया है तो जरूरी नहीं कि सर्जरी की जाए।

आम तौर पर ऐसे मरीजों को सर्जरी या स्टेरॉयड इन्जेक्शन लगाने का ही सुझाव दिया जाता है, लेकिन पीठ दर्द, कंधों में अकड़न या किसी भी दूसरे दर्द होने पर फिजियोथेरेपिस्ट की गाइडेंस लें। ज्यादातर केस में मरीजों को सर्जरी के दर्द और खर्च की जगह फिजियोथैरेपिस्ट ही इन बीमारियों को दूर कर देता है।

दूसरे लोगों को भी बताने की जरूरत

रोटरी चंडीगढ़ शिवालिक क्लब की सेक्रेटरी रोटेरियन मनजीत कौर ने कहा कि डॉक्टरों से मिलीऐसी जानकारी के बाद लोगों को महंगे इलाज और चीरफाड़ से बचाव में मदद मिलती है। लोगों को इस बारे में दूसरों को भी बताने की जरूरत है, ताकि लोगों को मदद मिले।

'35% knee replacements in India needless'

DurgeshNandan.Jha @timesgroup.com

New Delhi: Is total knee replacement justified in arthritis patients as young as 45? Or should it be done only on the elderly who have exhausted all options, including lifestyle modification and reducing weight?

These questions are being raised by medical experts in face of an exponential increase in the number of total knee replacements in India. Indian Society of Hip and Knee Surgeons reported 66,352 total knee replacements in 2013 compared to merely 9,951 cases in 2008.

While there is no study to assess how many of these total knee replacements were uncalled for, a new study published in Arthritis & Rheumatology, a journal of American College of Rheumatology, has called over one-third of such surgeries conducted in the US "inappropriate". Dr C S Yadav, professor in the department of orthopaedics at AIIMS, said, "Nearly 30-35% of knee replacements conducted in India are unnecessary. At AIIMS, we have been holding awareness programmes to educate patients about the need to focus more on lifestyle modification than be lured by the idea of a replacement surgeries pushed by private practitioners."

Say no to knee surgery with weight loss, therapy

TIMES NEWS NETWORK

Chandigarh: "Many times, there is no need to get your knees or hips replaced, as physiotherapy can help avoid such a surgery. Exercise and weight loss are actually the first line of defence in the case of a joint replacement. It may help prevent the pain and surgery," said Dr Harshneet K Chhabra, while speaking on 'The role of physiotherapy in the current scenario' to the members of Rotary Chandigarh Shivalik Club in Sector 7 on Friday. Over 35 members of the club and their guests attended the session.

Elaborating, Dr Chhabra said: "The main component of joint surgery avoidance is strengthening muscles that support your joints. The quadriceps and hamstrings are the key to knee strength. Every time you walk or run or do anything weight-bearing, the quads absorb the shock. The stronger your quads are, the lesser the load that gets transferred into the joint. I have many patients who either cancelled or postponed their joint replacement surgery," she added.

Physiotherapy can be your saviour in many other health problems too, where either surgery or steroid injections are routinely recommended. "Whether it is back pain, frozen shoulder, or any other sort of pain, do visit your physiotherapist, follow his advice, and you will find yourself getting better without the pain and possible complications of a surgery."

Following pictures illustrate the exercises to be done for Knee Osteoarthritis (KOA) Patients (to be read with annex 1)

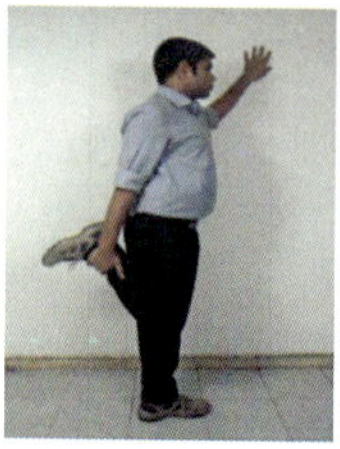

Photograph: 1

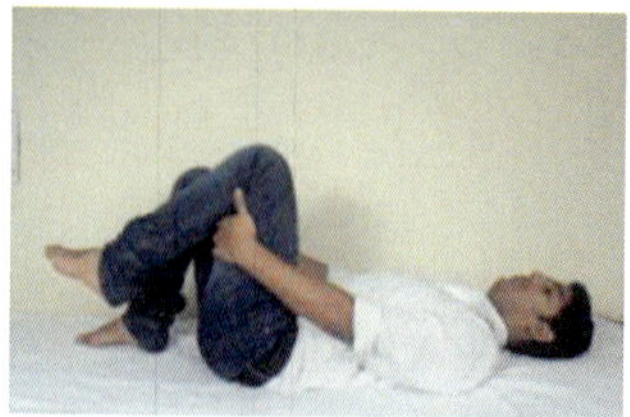

Photograph: 2

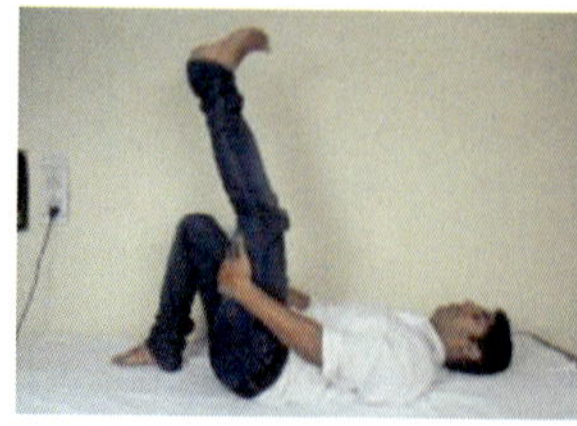

Photograph: 3

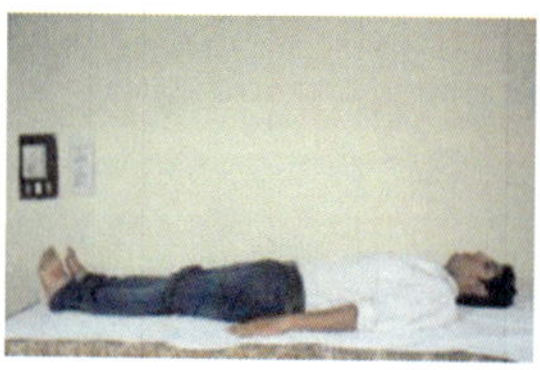

Photograph: 4

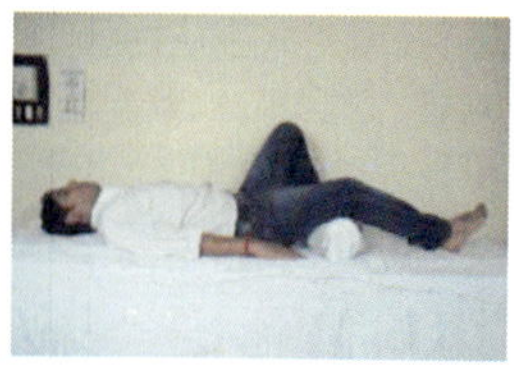

Photograph: 5

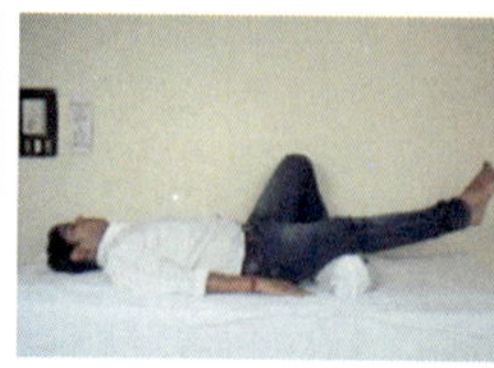

Photograph: 6

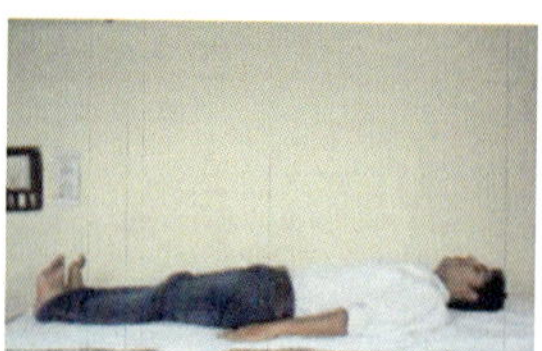

Photograph: 7

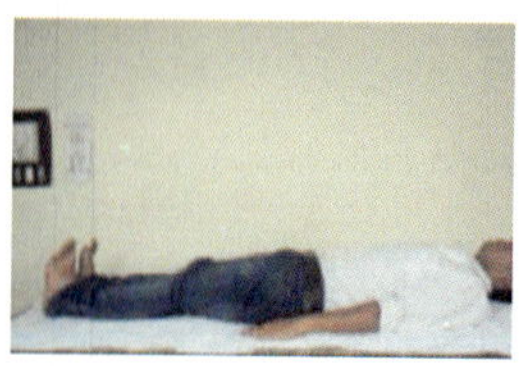

Photograph: 8

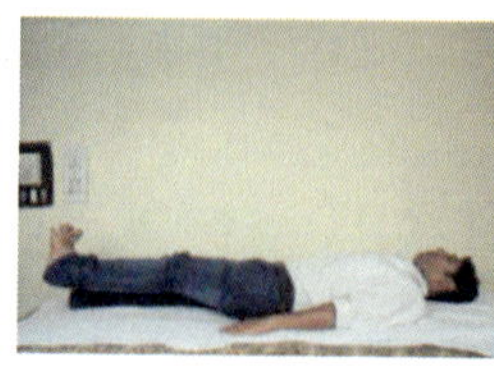

Photograph: 9

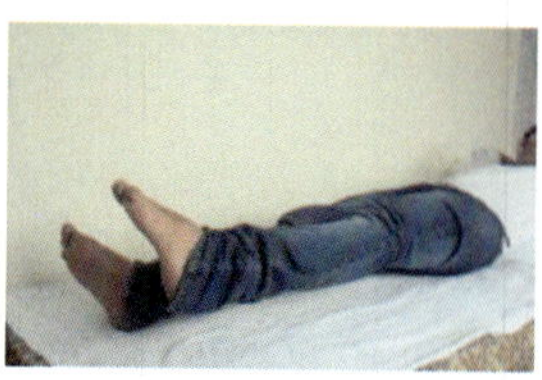

Photograph: 10

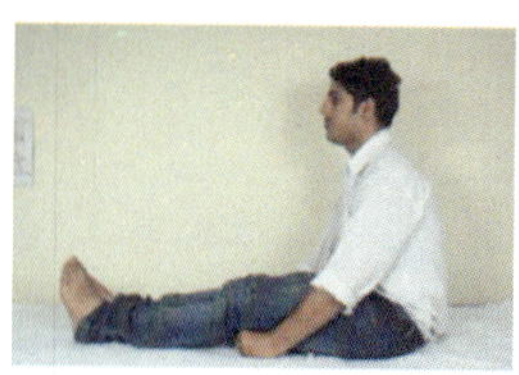

Photograph: 11

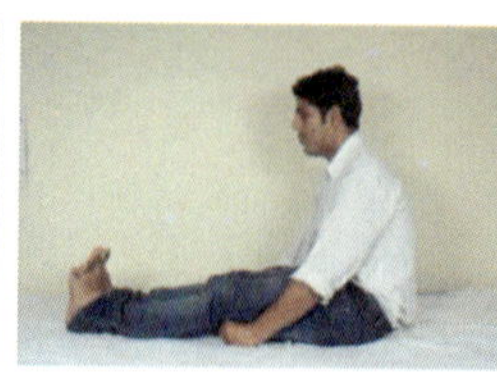

Photograph: 12

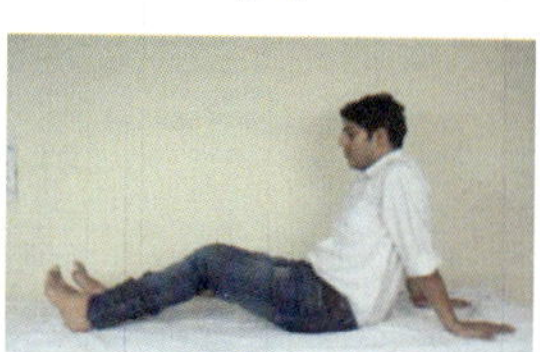

Photograph: 13

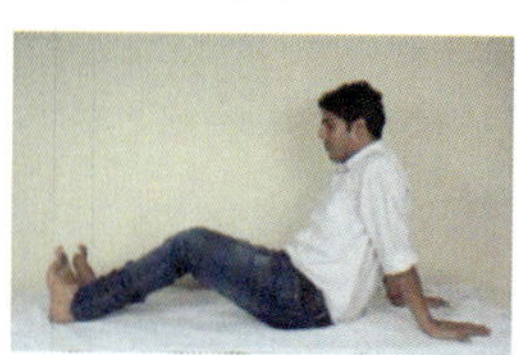

Photograph: 14

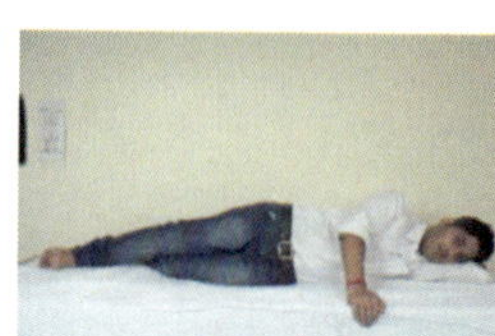

Photograph: 15

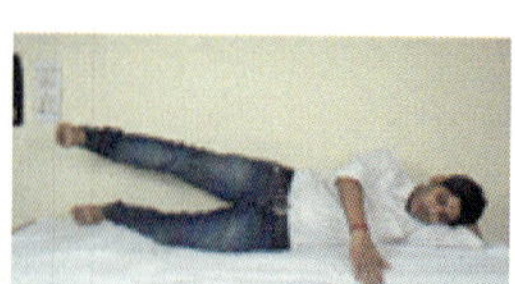

Photograph: 16

Guidelines for Kinesthesia, Balance and Agility Training of Knee Osteoarthritis Patients

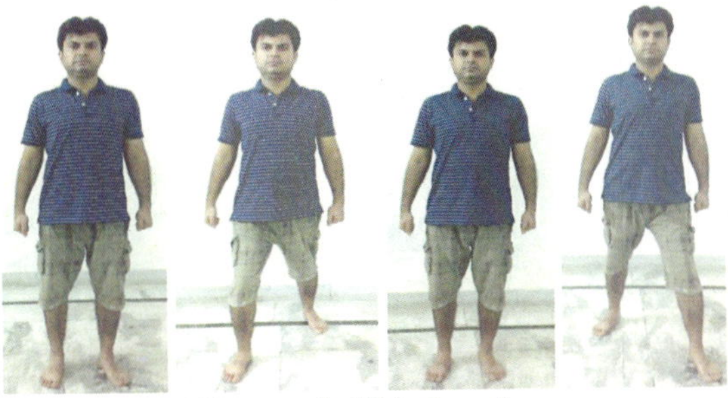

Photograph: 17 (a, b, c, d).

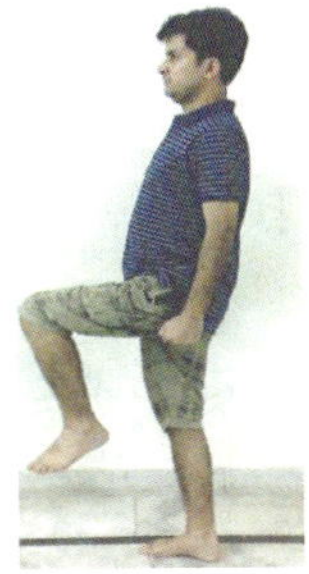

Photograph: **18.**

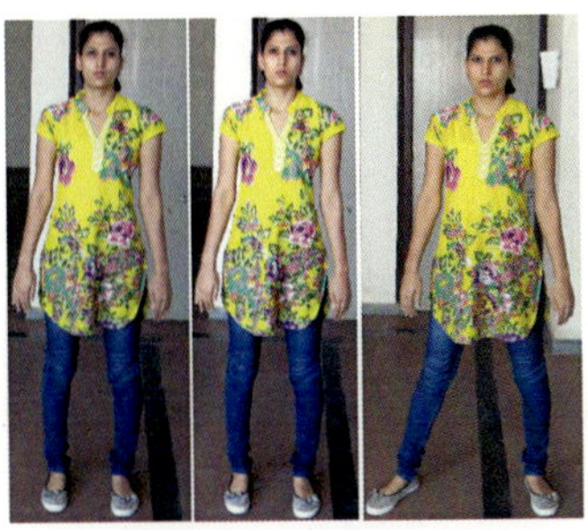

Photograph: 19.

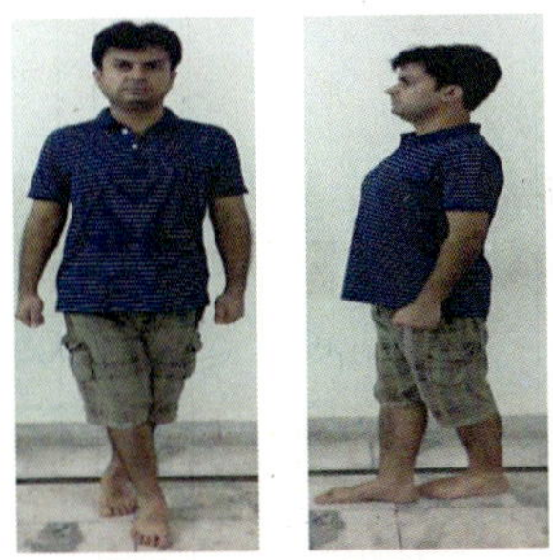

Photograph: 20 (a, b).

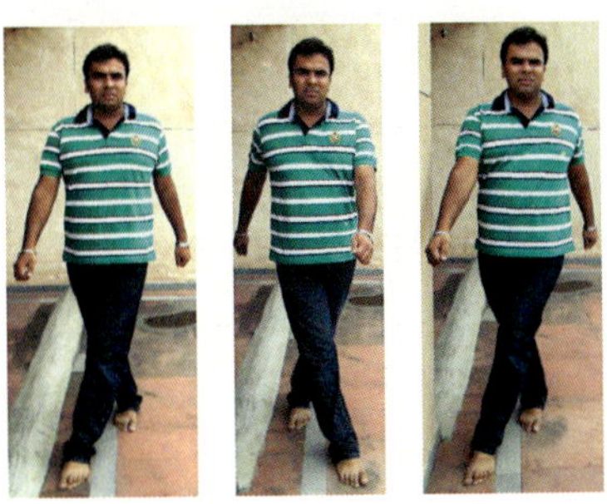

Photograph: 21 (a, b, c).

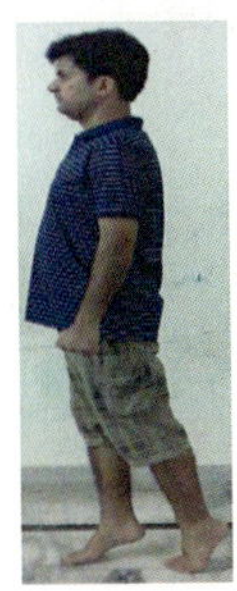

Photograph: 22.

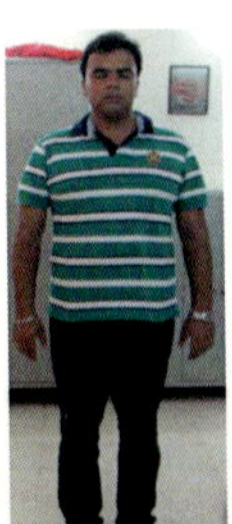

Photograph: 23a.

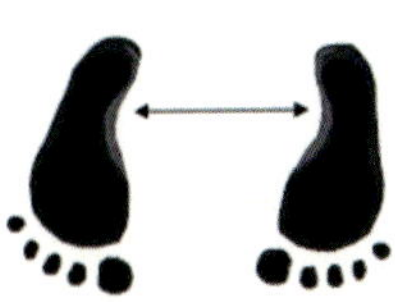

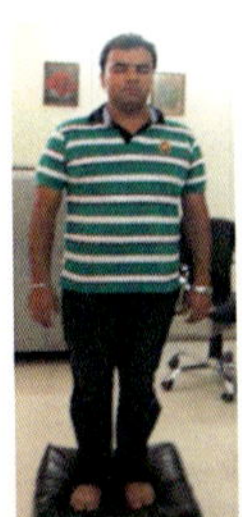

Photograph: 23b.

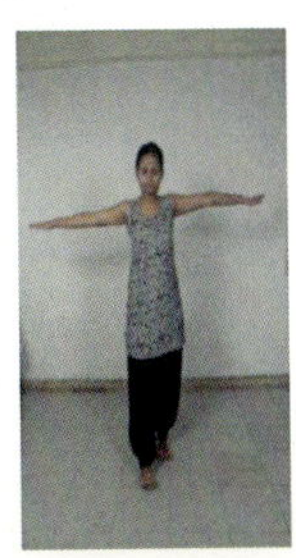

Photograph: 24.

Chapter - 5

How to Deal With Congenital Malformations & Genetic Disorders – A guide for caregivers/parents

—*Alka Rani, InushaPanigrahi, Neelam Aggarwal, Abhik Ghosh, Amarjeet Singh*

Introduction

Marriage is an important event in our society. It helps in the perpetuation of our lineage. A family is considered to be complete with the arrival of a child.Most couples have a normal healthy baby some have a baby with birth defect. After marriage, a couple may have problemslike -

Not having a child.

Abortion may occur in approximately 15 to 20% of pregnancies.

Some cases are diagnosed with birth defect in womb.

In some cases, pregnancy continues up to the 9th month, but sometimes serious problems (birth defect) ** arises, and a dead baby maybe born (still birth) due to anencephaly (no head is formed), spina bifida (gap in back bone).

Sometimesthe baby may die within hours or days, e.g., congenital heart defect (baby turns blue).

In some cases,baby survives for a month or years e.g. cleft lip/cleft palate (split in lips or *taloo*).

In other cases, child survives for a long time with treatment e.g. thalassemia.

Others survive for variable periods butthe quality of life is seriously compromised whereas in others it affects less, e.g., Down's syndrome (mental retardation).

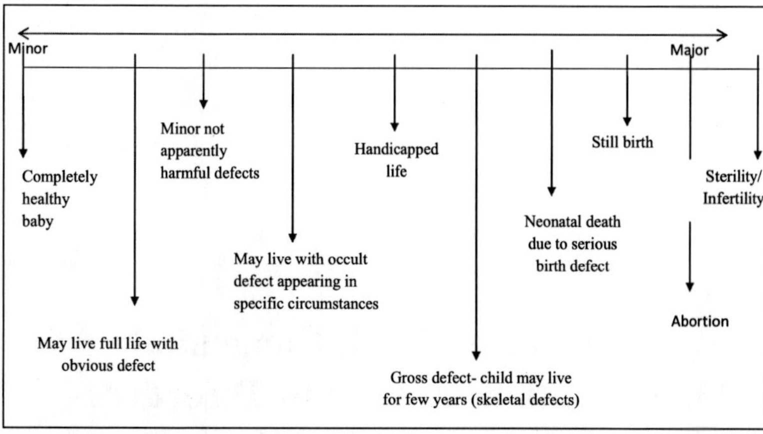

Thus, in the spectrum for the fate of any marriage with child bearing, on the one hand is the birth of a completely healthy baby & on the other hand is infertility (childlessness).

Understanding congenital disorders and related terms

Congenital disorders is a broad category that includes in itself a variety of conditions. The word congenital means ' since birth' and "disorders" means a group of diseases.

The terms congenital physical anomaly, congenital malformation, birth defects or genetic disorders are often used interchangably. However, they have different meanings.

Congenital physical anomaly: It refers to abnormality of structure of a body part" e.g. curvatures of 5th finger (clinodactyly).

Congenital malformation: It is a congenital physical anomaly that is harmful, i.e., a structural defect perceived as a problem.

Birth defect:It is a congenital physical anomaly. It happens while a baby is developing in the mother's body. It is recognized at birth. It is significant enough to be considered as a problem, .e.g, cleft lip,cleft palate.

Genetic disorders: These are caused by one or more abnormalities in our genes, e.g., haemophilia A In this book all these terms are used interchangeably.

Types of birth defects

Birth defects may be fatal (causing death) or non-fatal (does not cause death). Anencephaly is a serious birth defect in which a baby is born without parts of the brain and skull. It is a type of neural tube defect (NTD). Syndactyly (wherein two or more digits are fused together, like HRITHIK) is nonfatal.

Birth defects can be grouped in to Major/Minor and Structural /Functional related defects.

Major defects- They can have a serious, adverse effect on the physical health, development, or functional ability of the baby,e.g.,congenital cardiac defects.There are 8 externally visible major birth defects .e.g. neural tube defect including microcephaly, orofacial defects (cleft lip/cleft palate), talipes equinovarusclub foot), limb reduction defects, hypospadiasis, exomphalos/ omphalocele, gastrochisis, imperforate anus.

Minor defects- These include the minor variations of normal morphological features of little or no known medical, surgical, or cosmetic significance.But they can have significant psychological impact e.g. Preauricular tags, low-set ears, single transverse palmar creaseetc.

There are two other main categories of birth defects.

Body structure related birth defects

These are related to a problem with body part or body structure. In short in this a specific body part is defective.

Examples - Cleft lip or cleft palate, heart defects, such as hole of heart, Abnormal limbs such as a clubfoot; Neural anomalies such as spina bifida, and problems related to the growth and development of the brain and spinal cord.

Body Function or Developmental birth defects

These are related to a problem with working of a body part or body system. These problems often lead to intellectual and developmental disability

Type	***Explanation***
Nervous system or brain problems	Behavioral disorders,Speech or language difficulties, Seizures and movement trouble, Down syndrome, Fragile X syndrome.
Sensory problems	Hearing loss and visual problems (blindness or deafness)
Metabolic disorders	Biotinidase deficiency, Hypothyroidism
Degenerative disorders	Muscular dystrophy , X-linked adrenoleukodystrophy

Table -1 Some examples of body function or developmental birth defects

In some cases, birth defects are caused by a combination of factors. Some birth defects affect many parts or processes in the body, leading to both structural and functional problems.

Some examples of birth defects	*What happens in this birth defect*
CHD	An abnormality in the heart that develops before birth.
Down's syndrome	An extra chromosome 21 causing developmental and intellectual delays.
Cleft lip and cleft palate	Openings or splits in the roof of the mouth and lip.
Spina bifida	A birth defect in which a developing baby's spinal cord fails to develop properly.
Club foot	A birth defect in which the foot is twisted out of shape or position.
Phenylketonuria	A birth defect that causes an amino acid called phenylalanine to build up in the body.
Cystic fibrosis	An inherited life-threatening disorder that damages the lungs and digestive system.
Huntington's disease	A condition in which nerve cells in the brain break down over time.
Duchenne muscular dystrophy	A disorder of progressive muscular weakness manifests in children, typically in boys.
Sickle cell anemia	A group of disorders that alters shape of red blood cells.
Hemophilia	A disorder in which blood doesn't clot normally and bleeding in joints occurs (especially in boys)
Thalassemia	A blood disorder involving lower than normal amounts of an oxygen carrying protein, requiring blood transfusion.

The birth prevalence of congenital anomalies in the developing world is underestimated. This is due to deficiencies in diagnostic capabilities and lack of reliability of medical records and health statistics. As a result, recorded diagnoses in vital statistics focus on overt acute illnesses, rather than on pre-existing congenital conditions that increase vulnerability to infections and malnutrition (WHO, 1985). Every year 15 lakhs children (6% of total births) are born with birth defect in India. Major birth defects are diagnosed in nearly 6% of the infants. Congenital anomalies affect 1 in 33 infants. There are 3.2 million birth defect related disabilities.Birth defects associated deaths; predominantly occur in first 24 hours; up to 7 days of life.Every year approximately 2.7 lakh newborn die before 28 days of life due to birth defects.70% of the BD's are treatable and manageable if identified at birth. Most common serious congenital disorders are heart defect, neural tube defect and Down's syndrome.

Late Bollywood actress Madhubala suffered from congenital heart disease. She had a Ventricular Septal Defect (VSD), a disorder referred to as a "hole in the heart." At the time of her birth, there was no effective treatment available for VSD. If this woulld have been available she would have lived to celebrate her 80th birthday today with us. Bollywood star Hrithik Roshan has an unusual thumb: he has two thumbs on his right hand - and it concerns a rather complex combination of abnormalities: 'polydactyly' (= extra digits) + 'syndactyly' (= fused digits). In her recent post on facebook, actress Celina Jaitley on September 10, had talked about her twins and their birth. She revealed the bitter news of having to lose one child due to a congenital heart defect.

Risk Factors

Risk of having a child with birth defect increases under any of the following conditions:-

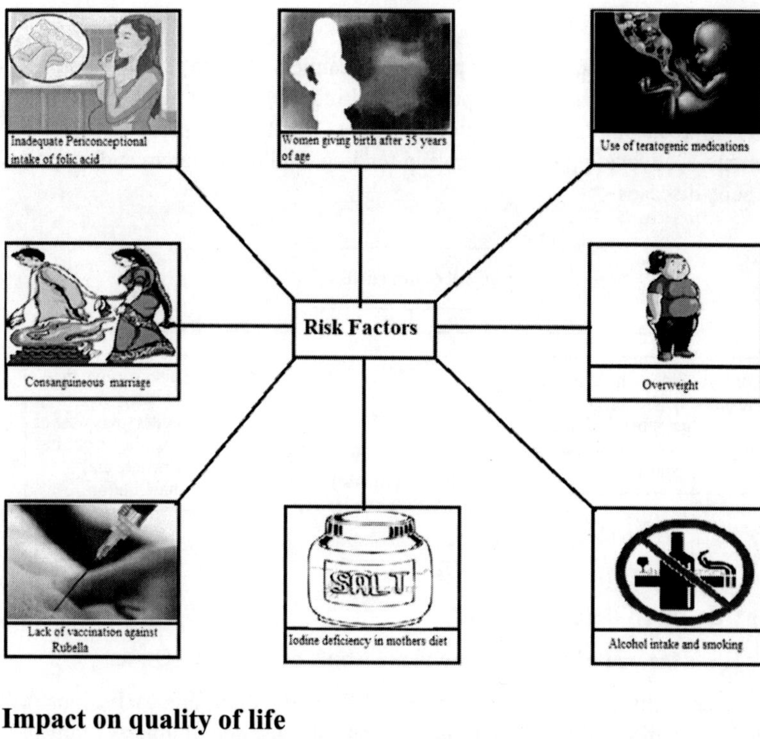

Impact on quality of life

Having a child with a birth defect impacts various spheres of life of children as well as family.Birth defects may lead to mental,social,medical, family problems due to long term suffering for the patient.

Parents of children who have birth defects face unique challenges and desire to make life better for their kids. They need psychological support.

They also want to understand the way that can help them to prevent birth defects in their future children. Some of the challenges parents face involve communication with healthcare professionals.

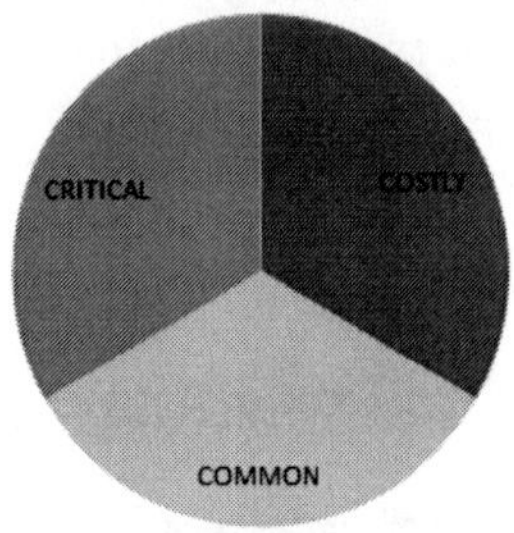

There are also quality of life issues the treatment of some genetic disorders or birth defectscan be quite expensive and requires government support or other sources of funding in selected cases. Health care providers create awareness, advocating for research and funding, finding resources and support for such diseases.

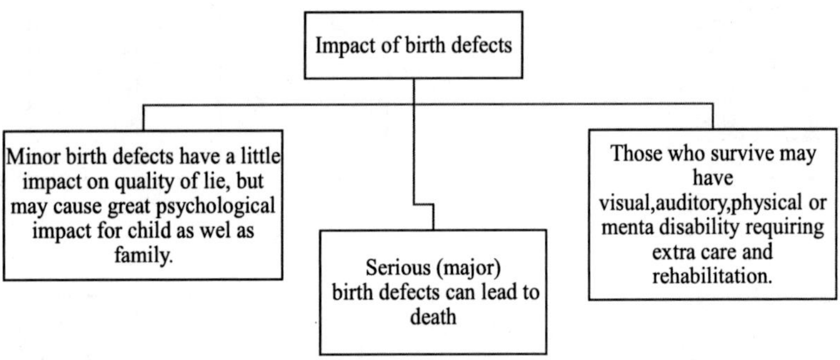

Why do birth defects occur?

HE is the one who shapes you in the womb as He Wills -Quran

Every culture views life experiences differently; therefore, each ethnic or racial group has different beliefs and theories of causation of illness. Many of the non medical causes of birth defects are attributed to maternal impressions, something the pregnant woman thinks or sees e.g. a child born with microcephaly or anencephaly is the result of his/her mother looking at a monkey during the pregnancy. Some believe that a cleft lip is caused by looking at or eating a rabbit, hence the name "hare-lip".

Some cultural groups believe persons with supernatural powers can also cause birth defects. In some cultures, individuals may feel that a family is "given" a child with a disorder as a punishment by God for parental sin. The "evil eye, is a force that gets much recognition in many cultures for being the determinant of bad fortune, including birth defects.

There are many other examples of superstitions such as : the effect of the moon, specifically a lunar eclipse causes cleft lip or palate, spina bifida can result from eating potato eyes during pregnancy, eating chili peppers in pregnancy may cause blindness in the fetus.

As per medical sciences the birth defects can be due to many factors, However, the exact causes of certain birth defects are often unknown.

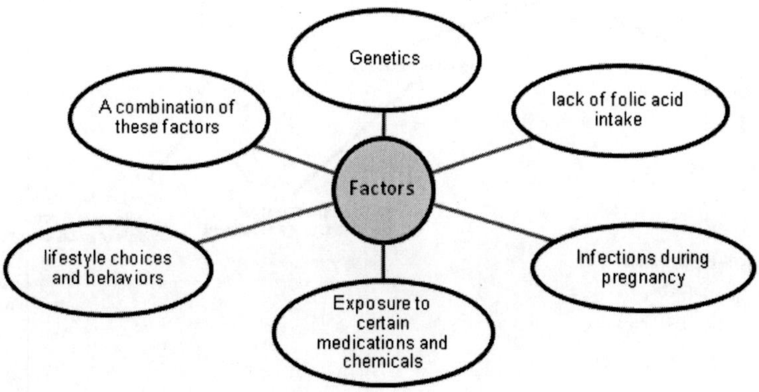

Causative factors

Birth defects may be caused by genetics or by environmental factors or a combination of both. In certain disease genetic element is so overwhelming that it expresses itself predictably without any need of environmental challenge.

Genetic (Hereditary)

The mother or father may pass on genetic abnormalities to a baby. These defects are caused by mutations or consanguinity and are unpreventable. There are three categories of genetic disorders: chromosomal disorders, multi-factorial inheritance and single-gene disorders.

Mutation

It means abnormality in the gene, leading to disease. It also includes the new mutations in one of the germ cells that gave rise to the fetus.

Consanguinity

This refers to marriage among close blood relatives such as first cousins and uncle-niece marriages. Endogamy (practice of marrying within relatives/ cousins or a specific social group, class or ethnic group) should be avoided and exogamy should be preferred. Such marriages increase the probability of mating between two individual heterozygotes for the same recessive gene. The offspring of consanguineous parents are at a risk of many diseases like cancer, mental disorders, beta thalassemia,hypertension, hearing Deficit, and leukemia, diabetes mellitus, and epilepsy, congenital heart diseases. The practice of preferential cousin marriages has been recorded as a characteristic feature of Muslims; in Some Hindu groups too and among the Gujjar also.

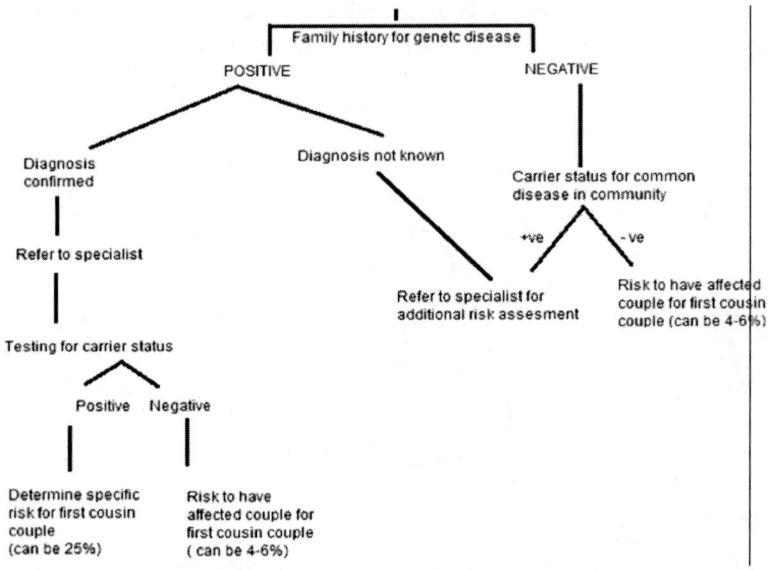

Environmental

Advanced maternal age

Risk of having a baby born with congenital malformations increases with increase in age of mother. E.g. Down's syndrome. (Age affects quality of sperm and ovum).

Alcohol use

Consumption of alcohol by the mother during pregnancy can cause many birth defects e.g. Heart disease, brain damage, kidney abnormality, Behavioral and cognitive disorders like hyperactivity including difficulties with learning and memory.

Paternal smoking

Smoking prior to conception can lead to some mutation in DNA of the parent. Hence there may be an increased risk of passing congenital abnormality in the offspring.

Maternal obesity

Obesity has been found to be linked with an increased risk of certain types of birth defects. This may include neural tube defects, shoulder dystocia, Macrosomia.

Toxic substances

Toxic substances that can cause congenital disorders are called "teratogens". These may include usage of certain drugs or exposure to many environmental toxins during pregnancy. Examples- intake of valpoic acid by pregnant lady in the first trimester may lead to heart defects, cleft lip, or a neural tube defect (an opening in the baby's spine or brain). Other examples may include use of Phenytoin (in epileptic women) and thalidomide (used to treat morning sickness during pregnancy). Even a single dose caused severe birth defects in first trimester, including amelia (absence of limbs), phocomelia (short limbs), incomplete or absent bone growth, ear and eye abnormalities, congenital heart defects.

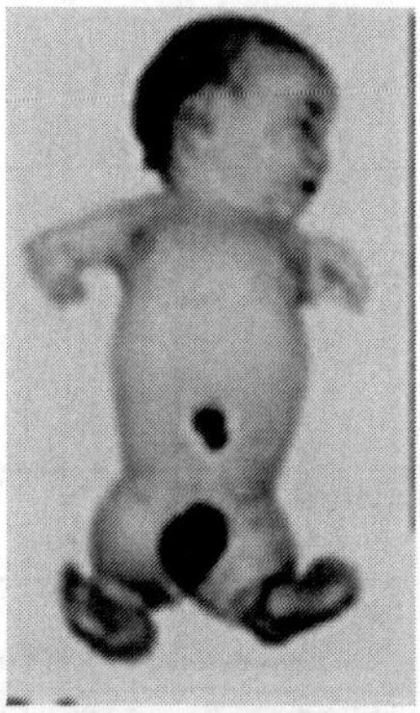

Baby born to a mother who had taken thalidomide in pregnancy for multiple myeloma

Infections

Infection caused by some virus ,bacteria, or, parasites get transmitted directly from the mother to the embryo, fetus or baby during pregnancy or after childbirth. Fetal exposure to rubella during 5-10 weeks of development (the sixth week particularly) can cause cataracts in the eyes. It can also cause abnormalities of the internal ear, heart, and sometimes the teeth also. Other infectious agents may be syphilis, herpes simplex virus, toxoplasmosis, etc.

Radiation

Excessive exposure to radiations can be harmful both the mother and her unborn baby. The mutations caused in the DNA by radiations, lead to birth defects e.g. reduction in height, mental retardation, small head size and retarded brain development. One of the well-known harmful environmental radiation hazards is Chernobyl disaster (reactor explosion) that occurred in Pripyat, Ukrainian SSR, Soviet Union on April 26, 1986. According to the Chernobyl Children International (CCI) lives of millions have been affected and many have been found to suffer from congenital heart defects and other disabilities too.

Lack of nutrients

Lack of folic acid in the diet of a mother can cause neural tube defect (NTD) and Spina bifida.5 microgram of folic acid, before the pregnancy and till 12 weeks of pregnancy can help in prevention of birth defect.

Unknown or multifactorial

Approximately 65% of the birth defects have no known cause. This shows their random occurrence regardless of maternal living conditions.

Some important chemicals that can lead to birth defects

Chemical	*Source*	*Effect*
Lead	Lead-based paint or occupational exposure	Premature delivery, abortion/ miscarriage Low birth weight Neurological damage, Developmental delays
Methyl **Mercury**	Fish and seafood	Effects fetal nervous system development
Pesticides	Unwashed vegetables and fruits, contaminated water	Increases the risk of birth defects
Toluene	Shoemaking, painting, printing, Varnishes, gasoline, glues.	Increased risk of abortion and low birth weight.
Carbon monoxide	Gas fumes, automobile and industrial exhaust, cigarette smoke	Low birth weight and premature delivery.
Organic solvents	Alcohols, paint and paint thinners, nail polish removers, paints, varnish removers	Spina bifida, heart defects, clubfoot, and deafness
Glycol ethers	Photographic applications, silkscreen printing, and dyes.	Increased risk of miscarriage
Chlorine	Chlorinated drinking water	Increased risk of miscarriage and poor fetal growth.

Use of desi –dwai during pregnancy to ensure birth of a baby boy is an important cause of birth defect. Consumption of indigenous medicines used for sex selection, also known as Sex Selection Drugs (SSD) during the first trimester of pregnancy is prevalent in certain northern parts of the country.

It is important to note that SSDs are consumed during the most critical period of development of the embryo, i.e., first trimester of pregnancy to have a male baby. Consumption of such drugs is dangerous and detrimental to the growth and development of the embryo. These contain phytoestrogens and testosterone.Shivlingi & majuphal are the herbs used for such purpose. These are often sold in tablet or powder forms. Often mothers in law or other relatives force the pregnant women to take such medicines to get a son.

Use of such medicines may lead to an unfortunate situation, where the baby is born which looks like male (external genitals male, but actually it is a hermaphrodite i.e. a hijra. So there is no benefit (rather harm).

Research from PGIMER, Chandigarh by Dr.Sutapa, Dr. Chinmayea and Dr. Amarjeet Singh (School of Public Health) revealed that more than 90% of the women were aware of the availability of SSDs. Fifty (45.5%) of them. reported to have used these. Of them, 48 (96%) reported giving birth to male babies after taking SSDs. Use rate of SSDs was significantly more in women who did not have a son as compared to those who didn't have.

What to do if parents have a baby with congenital disorder

Every child born with birth defect needs immediate neonatal screening. E.g. baby born with G6PD deficiency, neonatal jaundice and kernicterus may appear, affected infants are monitored for several weeks for bilirubin level. Early managent may help a child to lead a better life. E.g. a baby born deaf if not diagnosis early will have dealyed speech, as child wont be able to hear to learn to speak.They are following two situtions that arise when a couple already has a child with birth defect.

What to do in preconceptional phase?What to do in antenatal phase ?

Preconceptional phase- Before planning pregnancy parents should go for preconceptional counseling. During this the risk factors will be assesed and the tests required to confirm the diagnosis of birth defect in child will be done through neonatal screening. They may be refereed to geneticist in pediatrics for diagnosis.e.g If a couple already has a child represents features of down syndrome, karyotyping is must to confirm the diagnosis before planning for next pregnancy. Although neonatal screening generally plays a smaller role than antenatal screening, still it provides an important opportunity to identify birth defects early in the neonatal period. This way parents may be able to seek therapy or surgery early in life. Early, appropriate treatment can prevent or reduce some lethal or disabling sequelae of birth defects. For neonates born in hospitals, screening should occur before they leave. Even when little can be done to help the infant, accurate diagnosis of birth defects can alert parents to the risks they may face in future pregnancies.

Karyotyping report of father

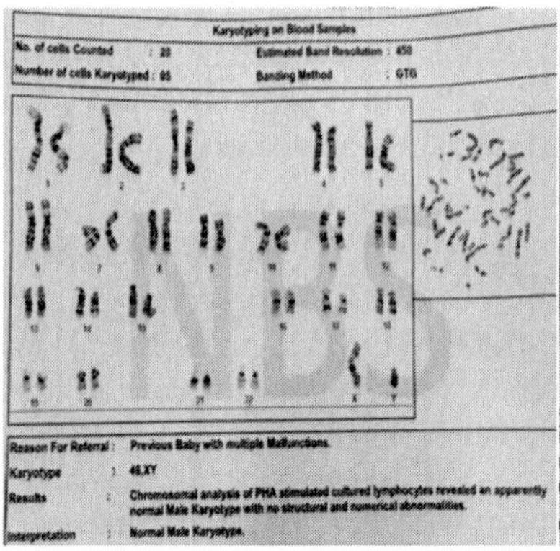

Karyotyping report of mother

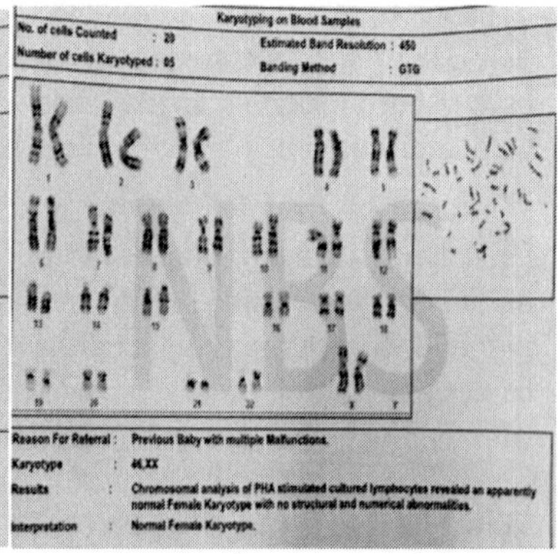

Antenatal phase- In case a couple has not gone for genetic counseling in preconceptional phase then in antenatal stage both neonatal screening and antenatal care/genetic counseling to rule out any CMF is must.

e.g. if couple already has a a thalasemic child then at 11-13 week current pregnancy they are advisedto go for chorionic villi sampling (CVS) to confirm the same in fetus. If needed thay are also referred to a genetic counselor. Depending upon the gestatonal age they are advised to decide regarding fate of fetus. (MTP/ Continautionof pregnancy).

Genetic counselor will help them to understand the

Available screening tests, diagnostic methods, and options for preventing or treating birth defects.

Limitations of screening tests are explained, along with the goal of identifying high-risk pregnancies.

Results of the screening process and answer their questions. Those who had a positive screening test will be provided information on the diagnosis, etiology, prognosis, and consequences.

Impact of that birth defect on baby's health.

Educate them about reproductive choices, thereby allowing them to make free and informed decisions.

Risk of having a baby with birth defect in the next pregnancy.

Investigations available for detection and diagnosis of birth defects

There are many birth defects that can be detected during pregnancy with early screening. Timely detection can give a chance for medical termination of preganancy(before 20 weeks of pregnnacy). But if it is detected after 20 weeks MTP cannot be done as per PCPNDT act in India. At this time a multidisciplinary approach should be followed. Pregnostication should be done. Parents must be completely informed about the diagnosis. They must be given psychological support and should be motivated for institutional delivery e.g. in case of diagnosed CHD if a baby is delivered at a tertiary care hospital ,immediately baby may be given cardiology care because he may need a pacemaker.

If a antenatal women who is at risk for birth defect somehow misses these detection tests baby may be born with a birth defect. However these tests does not give 100% surity of detection of all the birth defects some birth defects can only be diagnosed after birth of the baby.

Detection of birth defects during pregnancy (in fetus)

With early Prenatal Screening &detection it is possible to diagnose a birth defect as early as possible during pregnanacy. Two types of tests are available. Screening test and diagnostic tests.

Screening test

These provide individual risk assessment tests, examinations or other procedures, e.g., Down's syndrome or a neural tube defect. A positive report only hints at the possibility of occurrence of a birth defect. If needed , a diagnostic test is done to confirm the presence of a genetic disease.

For whom are prenatal screening tests recommended?

These are recommended for all expectant mothers.

How are screening tests performed for genetic disorders?

Both, Invasive and noninvasive (ultrasonography) tests are available for the screening. These clearly distinguishe between individuals who are at risk for the condition and those who are not.

What happens if screening tests show that there is a problem?

Positive test results usually indicate a higher chance of having a particular genetic disorder. This leads to consideration of further diagnostic tests.

Genetic screening of populations identifies clinically normal individuals who have genotypes associated with a birth defect or who are at high risk of producing offspring with a birth defect. It aims to identify as many affected individuals as possible, but screening alone does not detect all individuals at high risk. Diagnosis usually follows a positive screening test.

Diagnostic tests

Diagnostic tests are usually recommended when a screening test has shown an increased risk of a birth defect. These are the tests that definitively identify a defect if present,e.g, Chromosomal abnormality (aneuploidy), genetic mutation (Sickle cell), etc.

> For whom are prenatal diagnostic tests recommended?
>
> When a screening test is positive and also when couples already have genetic disorder (e.g. previous baby with down syndrome) that increase the risk of having a baby with certain birth defects.
>
> How are diagnostic tests for genetic disorders performed?
>
> Diagnostic tests are done on the cells obtained from the fetus (amniocentesis or chorionic villus sampling (CVS)). These cells are analyzed using different techniques, e.g, Karyotyping
>
> What happens if diagnostic tests show that there is a problem?
>
> If a diagnostic test shows a positive result, a multidisciplinary approach helps in making choices and considering the available option.

List of various tests

Screening test	Diagnostic tests
Thalassemia Screening	Chorionic villus sampling
Thyroid Screening	Amniocentesis
Nuchal Translucency (NT& NB Scan) +USG	
Dual Marker+ UGG	
Triple Screen / Quadruple Screening,	
NIPT	

Thyroid Screening

Thyroid problem can harm the baby as well as the mother in pregnancy. During pregnancy two pregnancy related hormones HCG and oestrogen increase thyroid hormone levels in blood. It is critical for normal development of brain and nervous system of the fetus. During first trimester, supply of thyroid hormone to fetus is through placenta of mother. Baby's thyroid begins to function at its own after 12 weeks of gestation.Hypothyroidism results in misscarriage, preterm births (in 7th or 8th month), intrauterine growth restriction, and fetal death inside uterus, problem with breathing or heart beat and increased perinatal mortality.

Pregnancy specific and trimester specific reference levels for TSH are as : Ist trimester - 0.1-2.5mIU/l; IInd trimester - 0.2-3mIU/l; IIIrd trimester - 0.3-3mIU/l. venous blood samples should be taken with other antenatal care (ANC) investigations in a single sitting

Thalassemia Screening

All the antenatal mothers are advised for thalassemia screening through Hb electrophoresis between 10-12 weeks of pregnancy. If the result of the test is positive, then the partner is advised to go for thalassemia screening. If the result of test is negative, then nothing is to be done. But if the result comes out to be positive in both the partners, a diagnostic test (Chorionic villus sampling) is done to confirm thalassemia in fetus.

If the baby is affected by alpha thalassemia major, couple is advised to go for MTP. The time for undergoing the test is crucial because if the fetus turns out to be thalassaemic, MTP has to be done within 20 weeks of pregnancy.

First trimester screening for birth defect

First trimester screening includes a test of pregnant women's blood and an ultrasound examination. Both tests are usually performed together at 11-13+6 weeks of pregnancy.

Nuchal translucency/ Nuchal bone (NT/NB) scan

This test involves a ultrasound scan of the collection of fluid under skin at the back of baby's neck. A Value of 2.5-3.5 indicates a normal result,whereas a value greater than 3.5 indicates some problem (Down's syndrome, trisomy 18, congenital heart defects, other genetic syndromes). Results can be obtained the same day. The measured value of NT on USG scan is assessed in relation to the period of pregnancy.

Advantages - Safe, Non-invasive.

Disadvantages- It detects only 80% of Down's syndrome cases.

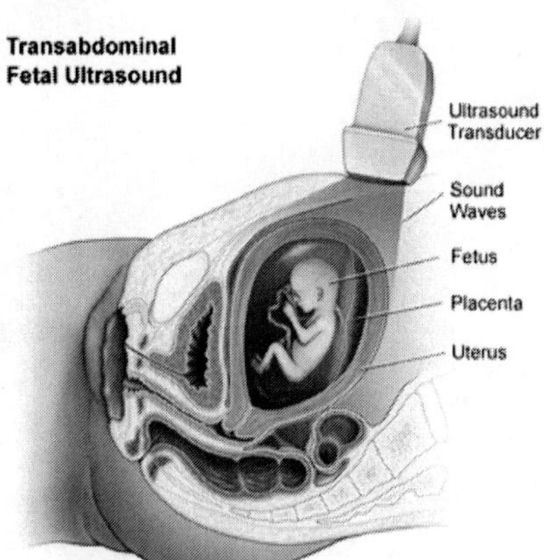

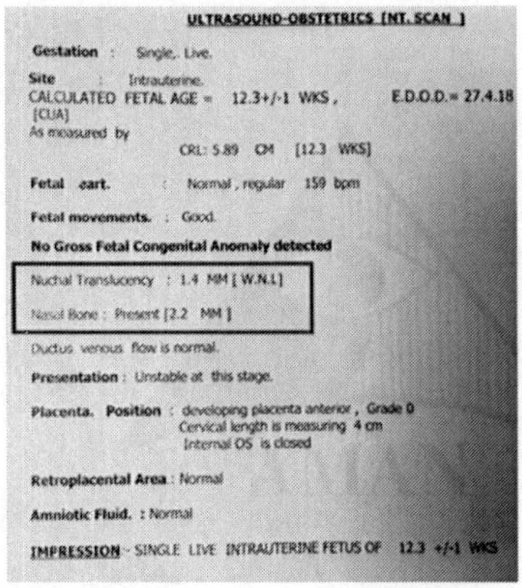

ULTRASOUND-OBSTETRICS [NT. SCAN]

Gestation : Single, Live.

Site : Intrauterine.
CALCULATED FETAL AGE = 12.3+/-1 WKS , E.D.O.D.= 27.4.18
[CUA]
As measured by
CRL: 5.89 CM [12.3 WKS]

Fetal eart. : Normal , regular 159 bpm

Fetal movements. : Good.

No Gross Fetal Congenital Anomaly detected

Nuchal Translucency : 1.4 MM [W.N.L]

Nasal Bone : Present [2.2 MM]

Ductus venous flow is normal.

Presentation : Unstable at this stage.

Placenta. Position : developing placenta anterior , Grade 0
Cervical length is measuring 4 cm
Internal OS is closed

Retroplacental Area : Normal

Amniotic Fluid. : Normal

IMPRESSION - SINGLE LIVE INTRAUTERINE FETUS OF 12.3 +/-1 WKS

Dual Marker(for 2 factors)

This test is performed on maternal blood sample. It detects free HCG and PAPP-A level in the blood. In first trimester, it identifies pregnancies that have a high risk of babies having the chromosomal abnormalities e.g. Trisomy

21 (Down's syndrome), Trisomy 13 (Patau syndrome),Trisomy 18 (Edwards syndrome). It is not a diagnostic test, hence it only identifies the risk of the baby being affected.

2nd trimester screening for birth defect

2nd trimester scrrening includes blood test (triple test, quadruple test), ultrasonography (level 2 USG) and if required ECHO.

Triple test (for 3 factors)

This is performed between 15 to 20 weeks of pregnancy. In this test blood sample is taken from mother, it measures level of AFP, HCG, Estriol.It can detect NTD, spina bifida, trisomy 21(Down syndrome), trisomy 18 (Edward's syndrome) or other types of chromosomal abnormalities.

AFP: a protein that is produced by the fetus.

HCG: a hormone produced within the placenta.

Estriol: an estrogen produced by both the fetus and the placenta.

Triple test has a 70% sensitivity and 5% false-positive rate.

The quadruple test (for 4 factors)

Thistest is performed between 16 to 18 weeks of pregnancy. This test is similar to triple test. Only difference is that it tests inhibin-A(a protein produced

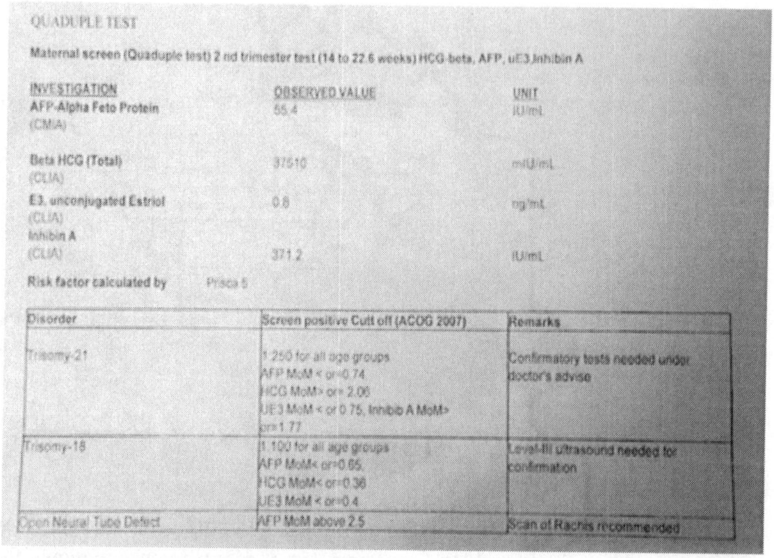

QUADUPLE TEST

Maternal screen (Quaduple test) 2 nd trimester test (14 to 22.6 weeks) HCG beta, AFP, uE3,Inhibin A

INVESTIGATION	OBSERVED VALUE	UNIT
AFP-Alpha Feto Protein (CMIA)	55.4	IU/ml
Beta HCG (Total) (CLIA)	37510	mIU/mL
E3, unconjugated Estriol (CLIA)	0.8	ng/mL
Inhibin A (CLIA)	371.2	IU/mL

Risk factor calculated by Prisca 5

Disorder	Screen positive Cutt off (ACOG 2007)	Remarks
Trisomy-21	1:250 for all age groups AFP MoM < or=0.74 HCG MoM> or= 2.06 UE3 MoM < or 0.75, Innibib A MoM> or=1.77	Confirmatory tests needed under doctor's advise
Trisomy-18	1:100 for all age groups AFP MoM< or=0.65 HCG MoM< or=0.36 UE3 MoM < or=0.4	Level-III ultrasound needed for confirmation
Open Neural Tube Defect	AFP MoM above 2.5	Scan of Rachis recommended

Sample of quadruple test

by the placenta and ovaries) in additional to other factors of triple test. This test can detect trisomy 21 and trisomy 18 and neural tube defects. Report of the test usually comes in 2-3 days. It can predict about 85% of open neural tube defects, problems with the development of the baby's brain and spinal cord. It predicts about 80% of fetuses with Down syndrome in women over age 35 and about 75% in younger women.

Level 2 Scan

This is a non invasive procedure (without inserting any instrumentinside the body).) this is performed at around 18-22 weeks of pregnancy. It detects any gross CMF(major physical defects in the brain and spine,facial features,abdoen,heart and limbs.). A TIFFA scan (Targeted Imaging for Fetal Anomalies) is also popularly known as fetal anomaly scan. It involves a detailed scanning and examination of the fetus for any abnormalities. It can be a 3-dimensional scan or 4 –dimension.

Advantage- USGs are noninvasive and have minimal risk for any complication to the fetus or mother.

Disadvantage- Unnecessary USG can put unnecessary exposure to radiation.

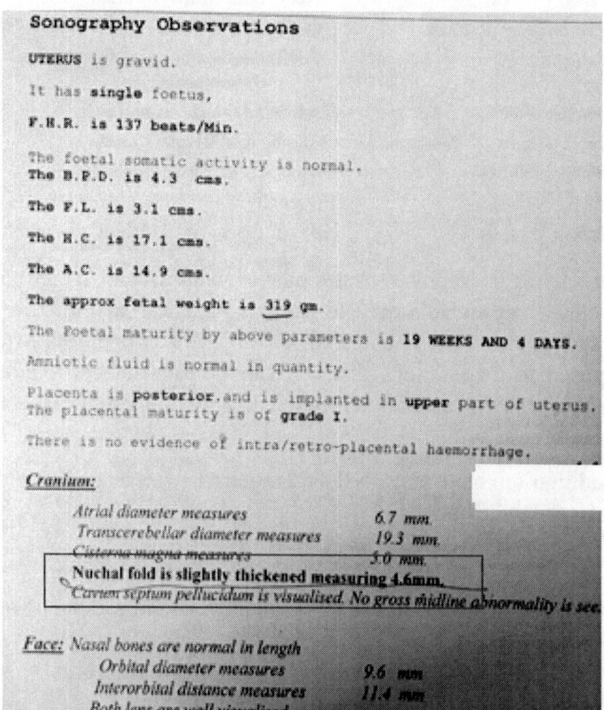

Sonography Observations

UTERUS is gravid.

It has **single** foetus,

F.H.R. is 137 beats/Min.

The foetal somatic activity is normal.
The B.P.D. is 4.3 cms.

The F.L. is 3.1 cms.

The H.C. is 17.1 cms.

The A.C. is 14.9 cms.

The approx fetal weight is 319 gm.

The Foetal maturity by above parameters is **19 WEEKS AND 4 DAYS.**

Amniotic fluid is normal in quantity.

Placenta is **posterior**.and is implanted in **upper** part of uterus.
The placental maturity is of **grade I.**

There is no evidence of intra/retro-placental haemorrhage.

Cranium:

Atrial diameter measures 6.7 mm.
Transcerebellar diameter measures 19.3 mm.
Cisterna magna measures 5.0 mm.
Nuchal fold is slightly thickened measuring 4.6mm.
Cavum septum pellucidum is visualised. No gross midline abnormality is see

Face: *Nasal bones are normal in length*
Orbital diameter measures 9.6 mm
Interorbital distance measures 11.4 mm
Both lens are well visualised.

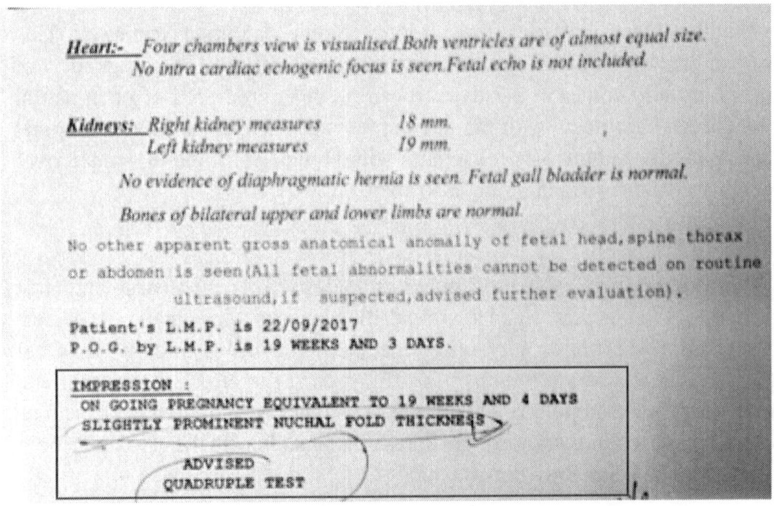

Heart:- *Four chambers view is visualised. Both ventricles are of almost equal size. No intra cardiac echogenic focus is seen. Fetal echo is not included.*

Kidneys: *Right kidney measures 18 mm.*
Left kidney measures 19 mm.

No evidence of diaphragmatic hernia is seen. Fetal gall bladder is normal.

Bones of bilateral upper and lower limbs are normal.

No other apparent gross anatomical anomally of fetal head, spine thorax or abdomen is seen (All fetal abnormalities cannot be detected on routine ultrasound, if suspected, advised further evaluation).

Patient's L.M.P. is 22/09/2017
P.O.G. by L.M.P. is 19 WEEKS AND 3 DAYS.

IMPRESSION :
ON GOING PREGNANCY EQUIVALENT TO 19 WEEKS AND 4 DAYS
SLIGHTLY PROMINENT NUCHAL FOLD THICKNESS

ADVISED
QUADRUPLE TEST

Some of the Problem detectable by UGS

Spina bifida	Open spinal cord
Anencephaly	Absence of the top of the head
Hydrocephalus	Excess fluid within the brain
Major congenital heart problems	Some defect in heart
Diaphragmatic hernia	A defect in the muscle which separates the chest and abdomen
Exomphalos/gastroschisis	Defects of the abdominal wall
Major kidney problems	Missing or abnormal kidneys
Major limb abnormalities	Missing or abnormal limbs
Cerebral palsy	Spasticity
Down syndrome	May be associated with heart and bowel problems

Fetal echocardiography is a test similar to an ultrasound. It may be advised in conditions where an Unborn child is at risk for a heart abnormality or other disorder or Couple already have a child with a heart condition, Mother has been exposed to medications that can cause heart defects (e.g. epilepsy treatment drugs), Medical conditions(including rubella, type 1 diabetes, lupus, or phenylketonuria etc).

In addition to above tests, NIPT(if required) can be performed in first trimester or second trimester.

Non invasive prenatal testing (NIPT)

This is done at 10-22 weeks of pregnancy, Blood sample of mother is sent to laboratory where it tests small amount of DNA of baby that is naturally found in blood of mother. It is performed for Down syndrome, trisomy 18, and hemophilia. This is a screening test. If result of the test is positive, amniocentesis (diagnostic test) is done to confirm the results.

Advantage-Detection rate for Down syndrome is better than other test

Disadvantage: it does not detect many chromosomal abnormalities.

Diagnostic tests

Chorionic villus sampling(CVS)

It is done between 10th -13th weeks of pregnancy. In this test, with the help of a needle sample is taken from chorionic villi (placenta tissue) of the growing fetus. Then the sample is sent to laboratory for the test e.g. karyotyping or enzyme analysis for Down syndrome. Approximate timing for result is 1-2 weeks for karyotyping and 1-2 days for FISH Test.

- Advantages – helps in early diagnosis and timely intervention.
- Disadvantages –Procedure related loss rate is < 1%.

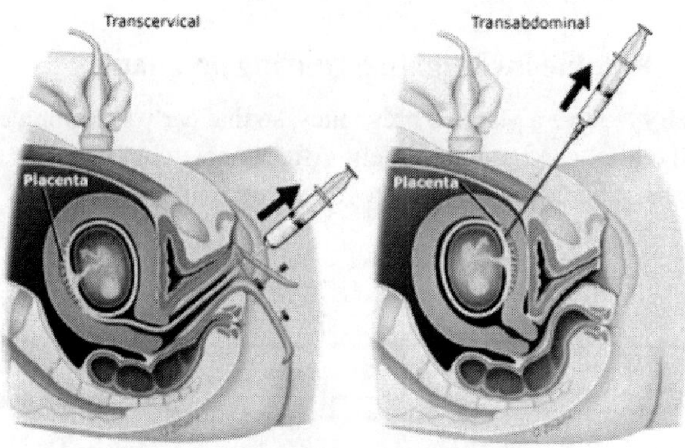

Chorionic villus sampling

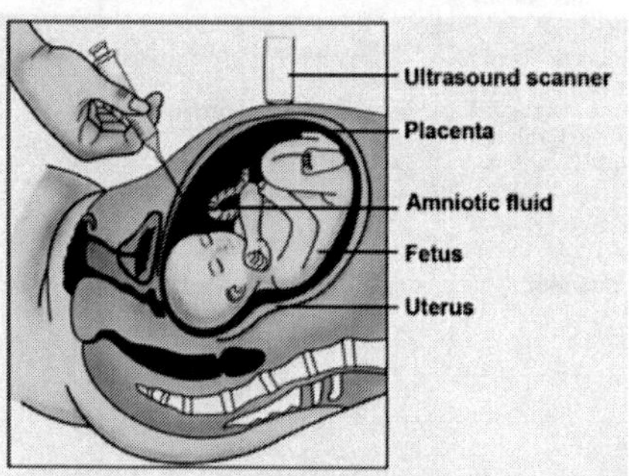

Amniocentesis

Amniocentesis

It is done between 15-20 weeks of pregnancy. In this test sample is taken from amniotic fluid present around the growing fetus. Ultrasound is used to help doctors to show location of baby and placenta so that needle could be inserted safely to the right place. Then the sample is sent to laboratory for the test, e.g. karyotyping for trisomy 18. Approximate timing for result is 2 weeks for karyotyping and 1-2 days for FISH Test.

Advantages– helps in early diagnosis and timely intervention.it is relatively safer.

Disadvantages–procedure-related loss rate is approximately 0.11%. Relatively late diagnosis.

Indications of diagnostic tests- Amniocentesis or CVS is typically offered for pregnancies at increased risk for chromosomal abnormalities.

Couple already having a baby with down syndrome.

Any genetic disorder history e.g. both the parents are carrier of thalasemia then CVS is a must for fetus.

Routine investigations during pregnancy

Always try to have a planned pregnancy, so that early screening could be done and folic acid can be done timely. After concieving there are specific routine tests must be followed by a pregnant women.

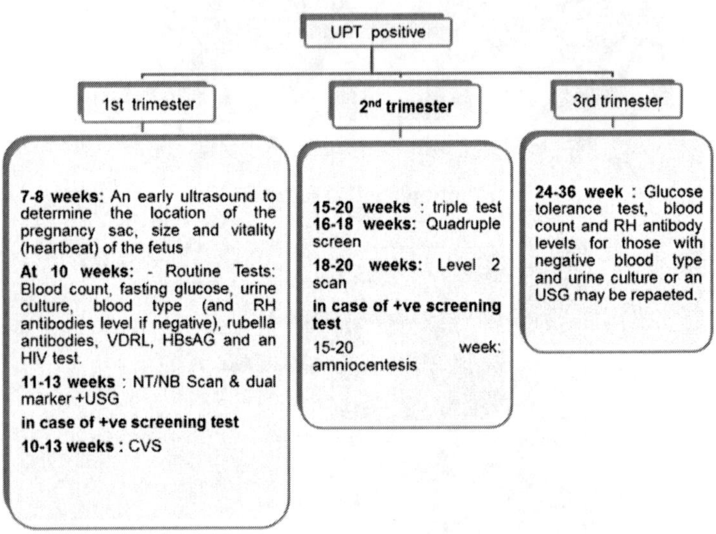

Preconceptional –Before planning preganncy every women should be screened for sexually transmitted infections (HIV/VDRL), Rubella and any other medical conditions (diabetes/thyroid). Beside this complete haemogram / blood group (Rh type)/ should be done. if a women it at risk for having a birth defect baby she must go for genetic screening e.g. thalassemia screening, karyotyping(both the partners).

Antenatal- After missed period, a urine or blood test can be performed to confirm pregnancy.

Test	*Approximate cost*		*Test is done for ??*
	In PGI(Rs/-)	*Outsisde(Rs/-)*	
Screening test			
Hemoglobin(Hb)	50 (appx.)	150 (appx.)	The hemoglobin test is used to check amount of hemoglobin in blood.
TSH	100(appx.)	280(appx.)	It is uded to detect thyroid disorders
Hb Electrophoresis	350(appx.)	1050(appx.)	This can detect HbS(sickle-cell disease),blood disorders such as beta thalassaemia and hemoglobin C
VDRL(Syphilis)	50(appx.)	170(appx.)	Assesses whether or not the patient has, a sexually transmitted infection (STI) e.g.Syphilis
Dual Screen	Not available	2400(appx.)	Dual marker(Blood test for HCG and PAPP-A)+ NT For Down's syndrome
Triple screen	Not available	AFP-900(appx.) HCG-775(appx.) ESTRIOL-750(appx.)	Blood test for AFP, hCG, and estriol to detect Down syndrome, Trisomy 18, Neural tube defects etc.
quad screen	Not available	INHIBIN A-2100(appx.)	Blood test (measures AFP, hCG, estriol, and inhibin-A)for Down syndrome, Trisomy 18, NTD etc.
Level 2 scan	100/-	1800(apprx.)	Detects certain birth defects in baby.
NIPT	Not available	25,000(appx.)	it tests small amount of DNA of baby that is naturally found in blood of mother for Down syndrome, trisomy 18, and hemophilia
Diagnostic tests			
CVS	Not available	Karyotyping-11,000(apprx.) FISH-13,000(appx.)	Sample is taken from chorionic villi of the growing fetus. and sent to laboratory for the test e.g. karyotyping or enzyme analysis for Down syndrome.
Amniocentesis	Not available	Karyotyping-12,000(apprx.) FISH-11,000(appx.)	Sample is taken from amniotic fluid present around the growing fetus e.g. karyotyping , FISH for trisomy 18.

Ethical issues of prenatal testing

The option left after prenatal testing is either to continue or terminate the pregnancy.

Patient must have complete information about the tests done.

Confidentiality should be respected.

Informed consent must be taken.

After confirmation of diagnosis for birth defect whether it is lethal (can cause death) or not ,in India after 20 weeks MTP is not allowed. E.g. in a recent news it was heard that the court declined a woman's plea to abort her 26 week old fetus detected with Down's syndrome. The court denied the plea by saying that the fetus poses no danger to the woman's life. The child with this syndrome is not as seriously handicapped as it to be terminated.

Detection of birth defectafter delivery (in child)

Certain birth defects are diagnosed only after the birth of baby. Early neonatal screening plays a important role in this. Sometimes, the birth defect is seen immediately at birth (club foot). In other cases birth defects might not be diagnosed until later in life (heart defect).

Whenever there is a health problem in a child, the doctor/nurse may look for birth defects by taking a medical and family history by asking questions. Doing a physical examination (anomaly detection) and sometimes recommending further tests (biochemical scrreening) may also be beneficial.

If the diagnosis is still uncertain, they might refer the child to a bigger hospital where a specialist in birth defects and genetics can deal with the patient. An exact diagnosis may not be made immediately because it takes time for further testing. Moreover there are many unknown causes which make diagnosis difficult.

For PKU, congenital hypothyroidism, and other inherited metabolic defects, neonatal screening is only option. It allows early dietary intervention for PKU and thyroid replacement therapy for hypothyroidism, both of which are critical to avoid mental retardation. Neonatal diagnosis of congenital hip dislocation provides the best chance for correcting this disorder through noninvasive techniques.

How to deal with birth defects after the confirmation of diagnosis

Not all birth defects are permanent or equally debilitating. Some are curable through early treatment, surgery, or therapies. However due to their disabling nature, some birth defects create a need for lifelong medical and supportive care for affected child. Certain conditions require very little additional expense to take proper care of the child.Others may require expensive medical equipment, extended hospitalization or repeated surgeries, or regular medication.This puts a lot of burden on the family.These also create various other social issues, e.g., stigmatization.

The first thing that most of the parent wants to know whether baby in the womb is healthy or not. So when they are told that their baby has birth defect they get shattered.

What to do If birth defect is detected during pregnancy (in fetus)

It is often difficult to take a decision in such situations. During thiss time couple should support each other and try to relax and feel normal.

Reliable and accurate information can help parents to take tough decisions well in time.(mtp <20 weeks). E.g. Women who come to know that fetus has thalassemia or Down syndrome may go for termination of pregnancy, if it is detected well in time.

If gestation age is more than 20 weeks you should continue routine antenatal checkup.

You must go for institutional delivery (in a hospital) so that newborn can get timely intervenion. e.g. Consider the case of heart problems, where a major artery may be connected incorrectly or a pumping chamber may be missing. Prenatal detection and immediate treatment at birth can prevent the sudden oxygen deprivation and shock at the time of birth. If the doctor is already aware of the finding and he can well manage the things in time.

What to do if birth defect is detected after delivery (in child)

As already discussed early neonatal screening can provide an opportunity to get an early treatment. E.g. pacemaker for a heart problem, surgery for anal atresia etc.

Many birth defects have no specific treatments. But the developmental delays that occur in first 3 years of life can be dealt with a multidisciplinary approach. Often the defects diagnosed in the baby at some later stage of life can cause irreversible life-long mental, physical, auditory or visual disability. e.g. a baby with congenital hearing loss can have delayed speech and language development if diagnosed later in life. Early detection through prenatal testing can help early management.

Early intervention services can include feeding support, assistive technology (tools, devices, and aids that make everyday tasks easier for people with disabilities), occupational therapy, physical therapy, speech therapy, nutrition services, and social work services

Parents sometimes over-protect their children out of a desire to keep them safe and healthy. However, over-protection can make a child feel that he is incapable of making good decisions. This can have unintended negative consequences as children become adults and need to care for themselves. Parents need to understand that, as much as possible, children with birth defects should be made to feel "normal"—like any other kid.

Steps for Management of birth defects

Careful clinical evaluation of pregnancy.

Review of family, prenatal history, and perinatal history.

Laboratory studies: Chromosome, DNA, biochemical assays

Imaging studies: USG,Echo, X-rays

Medical management and genetic counseling

Autopsy and specific pathological analyses if still birth/early neonatal death so that next pregnancy could be managed properly.

Visit to social worker and support groups for emotional support.

Role of parents

Parents must acknowledge their emotions of grief, anger or shock and talk about them with spouse/partner and other family members. A very heart touching example of a NGO "Sadhna Society" Chandigarh can be quoted here . Dr. Bhawna Tyal director of the society got inspiration to start this society from her own daughter with Down's syndrome. At present she is taking care of so many special children in her society .

Get support from healthcare professionals about their queries and find out the support group.

Let themself enjoy the welcome of their baby with birth defect in the same way any parent would do with a normal health baby.

Steps to be followed by parents of child with birth defect

Parents are often worried about the next baby. These fears are natural. But instead of worrying parents should go for investigation of the cause of defect so that in next pregnancy this factor could be taken care of .

Parents should visit a genetic counselor and educate themselves with the knowledge gained after discussion with doctor.

Parents should seek for early intervention, e.g., aids to make everyday tasks easier for children with birth defects, occupational therapy, physical therapy, speech therapy, etc.

Role of family

Family undergoes psychological and emotional burdens when they have a child who has a birth defect. There are many factors that can impact family finances such as travelling, medical costs and other health-care related costs as well as specialized child care management.

Siblings and other children in the family often feel neglected. These feelings may be justified but result in behavioral issues and depression.

Families should understand the difficulties parents and child are facing and provide emotional support to them.

Family members should support parents in every possible way, psychological or financial, to the possible extent .

Families should encourage parents of such babies for early consultation. They should provide support in follow-up visis if needed.

They should love the child with birth defect just like a normal baby. It is good if they interact with the baby as much as possible. The family should assist the parents in other household works as parents have to visit hospitals with their child every time

Family members can take care of siblings when the parents go to the hospital.

Prevention of birth defects

Prevention is better than cure

Birth defects have a serious physical, psychological and financial impact for the family. Cause of more than 60% of birth defects is unknown. Yet certain measures can be taken in to reduce the risk of their occurrence.

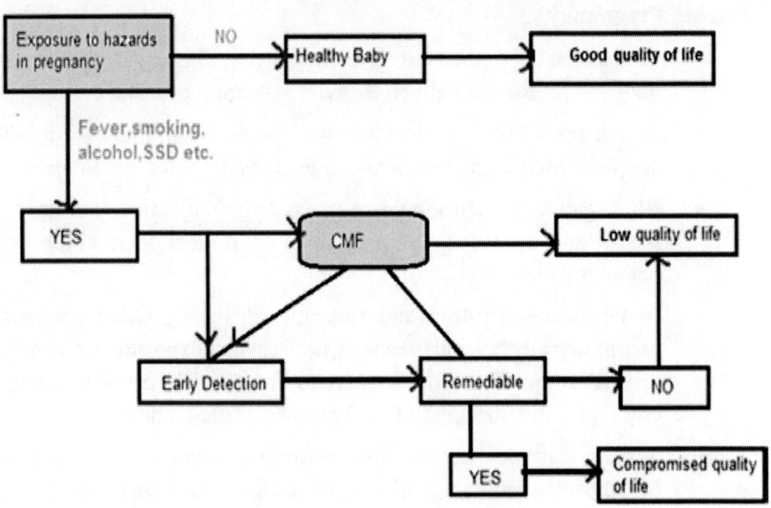

Before pregnancy

Marriage between very close blood relations like uncle- niece, aunt-nephew, among cousins should be avoided.

Avoid pregnancies before the age of 18 years and after the age of 35 years.

Rubella infections are cause of birth defect. Vaccination programs in several, mostly developed, countries prevent virtually all cases of congenital rubella. Giving measles-mumps-rubella (MMR) vaccine to girls prevents congenital rubella syndrome in baby born to women after marriage.

Optimization of medical disease before planning pregnancy e.g. epilepsy, diabetes. Avoid unnecessary intake of medicines, specially anticonvulsants, anticoagulants, thalidomide and misoprostol (When planning to conceive or during early pregnancy).

Consult a doctor before planning the pregnancy; if

(a) There is incidence of birth defects in your family.

(b) You have had difficulty in conceiving or have had a series of miscarriages, still births, twins, delivery by operation (Caesarean), obstructed labour/prolonged labour (more than 12 hours) and/or severe bleeding in previous pregnancy.

(c) You have Rh-negative blood type or You have diabetes/other chronic disease.

During Pregnancy

- Woman having frequent pregnancies, having a history of miscarriage/abortion/premature deliveries, must get expert prenatal care
- Proper intake of folic acid and well-balanced and nourishing diet supplemented with green leafy vegetables, proteins and vitamins.
- Rh Negative women should be given Anti D injection at around 28 weeks and 36 weeks of pregnancy to protect their child from hemolytic diseases.
- Avoid unnecessary drugs and medications, smoking, chewing tobacco, consuming alcohol and narcotics, unnecessary exposure to chemicals and radiations (X-rays), exposure to illnesses like measles, mumps, etc. especially during the first 3 months of pregnancy.
- Take precautions against lead poisoning (Lead is found in lead-based paints, including paint on the walls of old houses and toys)
- Prenatal diagnosis for familial disorders by e.g. Ultrasonography and maternal serum screening can be used to detect serious fetal anomalies, including neural tube defects and chromosomal disorders.

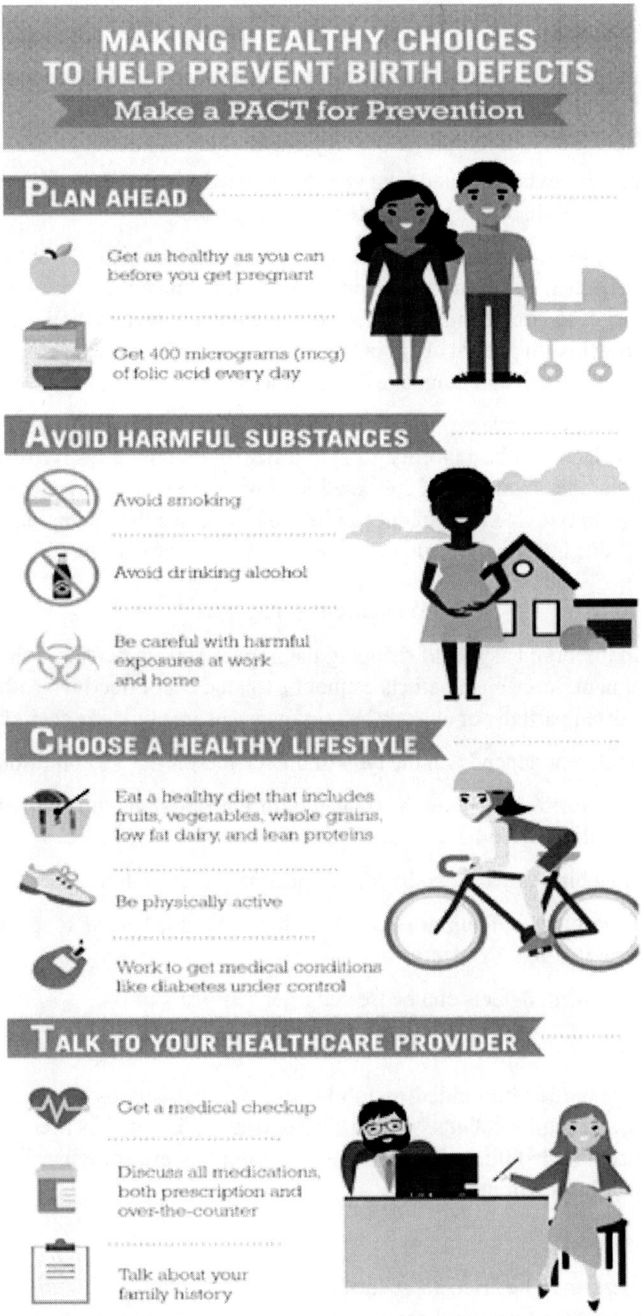
MAKING HEALTHY CHOICES TO HELP PREVENT BIRTH DEFECTS
Make a PACT for Prevention
PLAN AHEAD
Get as healthy as you can before you get pregnant
Get 400 micrograms (mcg) of folic acid every day
AVOID HARMFUL SUBSTANCES
Avoid smoking
Avoid drinking alcohol
Be careful with harmful exposures at work and home
CHOOSE A HEALTHY LIFESTYLE
Eat a healthy diet that includes fruits, vegetables, whole grains, low fat dairy, and lean proteins
Be physically active
Work to get medical conditions like diabetes under control
TALK TO YOUR HEALTHCARE PROVIDER
Get a medical checkup
Discuss all medications, both prescription and over-the-counter
Talk about your family history

After birth

Early neonatal screening can be implemented to avoid the complications of birth defects.This increases an affected child's possibilities of a better quality of life.

Infants can be screened for a variety of genetic, hematological, metabolic, and hormonal disorders to provide early diagnosis.

Early detection and treatment of birth defects can help prevent physical and intellectual disabilities. E.g. congenital hearing impairment can result from a number of environmental or genetic causes. Without early testing, a diagnosis of hearing loss might not occur until a child is two or three years old, resulting in delayed speech and language development.

Another example is phenylketonuria (PKU), which is an inherited disorder characterized by the inability to synthesize the amino acid tyrosine from phenylalanine. Treatment of this condition involves a diet low in phenylalanine and high in tyrosine. Treatment results are best if this diet is implemented at birth. If this is done the child can lead a relatively normal life.

Treatment strategies

An important aspect of reducing the impact of birth defects is the access to treatment.Some birth defects cannot be treated cost-effectively, others can be corrected partially or entirely by therapies that are clinically cost-effective.

Treatment depends on the type of defect and the baby's condition.

Some birth defects can be treated before birth (spina, bifida) but that is rarely available in India.

Some birth defects can be treated or repaired at the time of birth.(CHD)

Some birth defects are so small that they don't need to be treated. (periauricular tags, syndactyly)

Some birth defects can be treated after few years of life.

Home Care

Parents may be guided to follow specific instructions for monitoring, feeding and bathing infants with the birth defects. Although they need specialist guidance for rehabilitation, but to follow the guidelines to practise the child is a hometask for parents too.

Medicines

These may be used to reduce complications that arise due to certain defects.In some cases medication may also be prescribed to mother to correct an abnormality before the birth of baby. Cystic fibrosis would involve a multidisciplinary team (physician, physiotherapist, nutritionist, and social worker) to provide conventional therapy (antibiotics, pancreatic enzyme replacement by ingestion of capsules with meals, and nutritional support) and treatment for associated complications. Another example is of use of biotin in high doses for treatment of biotinidase deficiency.

Surgery

Surgery is also an option to treat many birth defects, e.g., cleft clip or cleft palate. Prenatal heart and renal tract defects are often treated surgically while the child is still unborn.Although these are not used on a wide scale in India. Operation of affected organ is also done after birth of the baby. This reduces harmful symptoms in children who have some physical birth defect (Plastic surgery for either cosmetic or health benefit).

Rehabilitation of children with birth defect

Many infants with severe birth defects experience lifelong disability requiring long-term treatment or rehabilitation. They may have serious lifelong consequences for both the patient and the family. Those afflicted require psychological, emotional, and social support on a continuing basis; this support should include referral to and assistance from social services such as education and social welfare. e.g., a child born with Down's syndrome has low IQ level. A child may need physical, occupational, and speech therapy for his or her development.

In many cases, appropriate education and rehabilitation for children and adults substantially increases their ability to function independently and contribute to family and community responsibilities.It also helps to overcome the isolation and stigmatization experienced by people with disabilities and encourages those with disabilities to live lives that are as normal as possible and are integrated into society.

Child may need different rehabilitation services depending upon the type of birth defect.

- Assistive technology (devices a child might need)
- Audiology or hearing services
- Speech and language services
- Counseling and training for a family
- Medical services
- Nursing services
- Nutrition services
- Occupational therapy
- Physical therapy
- Psychological services

Early screening& intervention focuses on helping eligible babies and toddlers learn the basic and brand-new skills that typically develop during the first three years of life

physical (reaching, rolling, crawling, and walking)
cognitive (thinking, learning, solving problems)
communication (talking, listening, understanding)
social/emotional (playing, feeling secure and happy)
Self-help (eating, dressing).

A successful story of a NGO in India helping special children

The occurrence of a shocking incident sometimes makes you stronger and inspires you for Noble task. As it is true of "Sadhna Society" for mentally handicapped where overwhelmed with the deep feelings for their own Children, few parents of children with intellectual disability got self-motivated to serve similar children in society and joined their hands to conceive Sadhna Society for the mentally handicapped. For the purpose to educate and train the special children Sadhana society started their Institute 'Sadhana vocational training institute' for the mentally handicapped in Chandigarh. The institute opened up new avenues for intellectually disabled under the expert guidance of educators, physiotherapist, speech therapist, yoga and dance teachers and the parents working voluntarily hard. Children are put to various schemes and programmes with the scientific approach apart from the basic academic.

Our students do us proud in Olympics every year by winning in different sports at zonal and national levels. They have brought us proud by winning awards in music and dance competitions Tejaswani Sharma the Music Prodigy is the star of our Institute. Not only intellectually disabled but also suffering from cerebral palsy and visual problems is star or miracle of god blessed with the rare gift of singing. Restricted to the age of 8, unable to walk, talk or even blink her eyes she struggled for life since her birth, but it is music that revived Tejaswani when she was 11. Her mother during the car drive suddenly noticed her humming the tune been played on the car stereo that was a momentus occasion for the family. To encourage her talent she was enrolled in a Music Academy where she learnt number of bhajans, ghazals and classical and folk song. Thereon it was her continuous journey towards her goal to be a

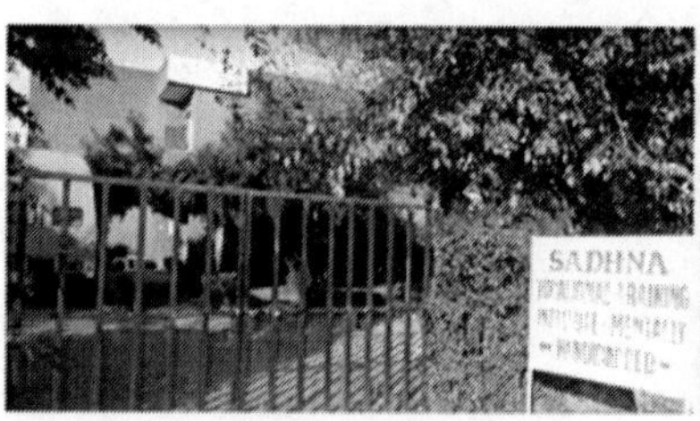

Sadhna society

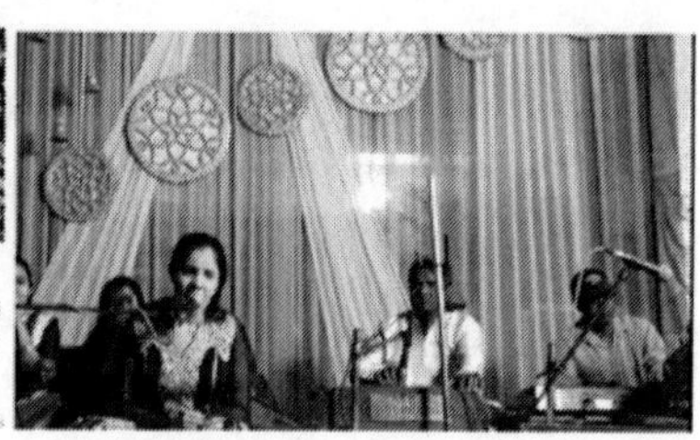

Tejaswini sharma singing performance

Dr. Bhawna Tyal, Director, Sadhna society NGO,Chnadigarh

professional singer, when she grows up. And today, her dreams have come true she has become a world famous singer apart from winning a number of music competition she got many awards.

Treatment options available for specific birth defects

Talipes or clubfoot

Early intervention is critical to correcting the condition and obtaining a foot that is supple, painless, plantigrade, and of normal shape and function.

Deformity can be resolved through manipulation and passive stretching,

By 12 weeks of age, the soft tissues of the infant foot are far less pliable, so only surgery can correct the condition.

More severe cases require treatments like plaster casts, splints, special shoes, and sometimes surgery followed by exercises

Baby should be encouraged to promote normal growth and development, including sitting up and crawling, while the foot is immobilized.

Cleft lip and/or cleft

Prenatal detection of the condition, available in some urban areas, can help parents to prepare for feeding and other special care of their child.

Support and education are key components of ongoing care.

Surgical repair of the lip can be done at 3 months and palatal repair at 6 months of age.

Comprehensive treatment can include speech and language therapy, preventive and restorative dental care, orthodontics, secondary surgery, otolaryngology for hearing problems, and psychological counseling.

Congenital heart disease (CHD)

Depending on severity, these are typically treated with surgery, drugs, or a mechanical aid like a pacemaker.

For example, medicines can control an irregular heartbeat, coarctation of the aorta, or tetralogy of Fallot.

Heart catheterization, where the doctor threads a thin, flexible tube called a catheter through a blood vessel in the groin, may also be used to repair a defect. Others may be helped by surgery e.g. closing holes in the heart with stitches or a patch, repair or replace heart valves, widen arteries or openings to heart valves, repair of complex defects.

Developmental dysplasia of the hip

Simple, noninvasive postural treatments can prevent a severe and crippling condition.

This requires a series of complicated surgeries and rehabilitations. Treatment appears to be equally effective at 6 weeks and can be undertaken successfully in children up to 2 years age.

Early treatment maintains the thighs in a flexed and partly abducted position so that the head of each femur remains deep within the acetabulum, encouraging it to encompass the femoral head more completely. To maintain this position, the thighs are splinted for weeks to months (up to a year).

Spina Bifida

Severe cases require surgery within 48 hours of birth, followed by special exercises.

The child may still need to use leg braces and crutches.

Missing limbs

Parents are referred to an orthopedic specialist who helps fit the child with a prosthesis as early as possible.

Intense physical therapy follows to help him or her learn to use it.

Down Syndrome

As such there is no treatment for this syndrome, as it cannot be "cured," but medical therapies may be necessary for accompanying visual or hearing impairments.

In addition, early intervention therapies like speech therapy and physical therapy help advance development

Thalassemia

Child requires regular blood transfusions combined with iron chelating therapy. This regime allows many people with the disorder to survive into their twenties and thirties.

A more expensive and higher-risk option is stem cell transplant from bone marrow or cord blood. This can cure the disorder but is not affordable in low-income populations.

Without diagnosis and treatment, patients with ß-thalassemia major usually die early in childhood.

Glucose-6-phosphate dehydrogenase deficiency

Interventions focus on reducing the occurrence and severity of hemolytic crises. These episodes can be precipitated by triggers for hemolysis such as infections such as hepatitis or pneumonia; exposure to certain chemicals and oxidative medications, including some antimalarial drugs; and consumption of fava beans.

In hemolytic crisis a blood transfusionmay be required.

Cystic fibrosis

An early diagnosis is the key for prevention of CF since many high-risk couples have a second affected child before the diagnosis has been established for the first child. Ideally, treatment of CF would involve a multidisciplinary team (physician, physiotherapist, nutritionist, and social worker) to provide conventional therapy (antibiotics, pancreatic enzyme replacement by ingestion of capsules with meals, and nutritional support).

Phenylketonuria (PKU)

Increased phenylalanine levels would be toxic to the fetus and cause severe mental retardation, birth defects, heart disease, and low birth weight. The mainstay of treatment is a phenylalanine-restricted diet. By limiting daily consumption to only 250–500 milligrams of phenylalanine per day, a positive nitrogen balance and safe plasma levels of phenylalanine can be maintained. Reduced phenylalanine levels improves IQ and neuropsychological outcome.

Hemophilia A and B

A series of exercises that facilitate absorption of the hematoma to improve joint range and strengthen muscles, which reduces the frequency of bleedingcan be taught to the patient.

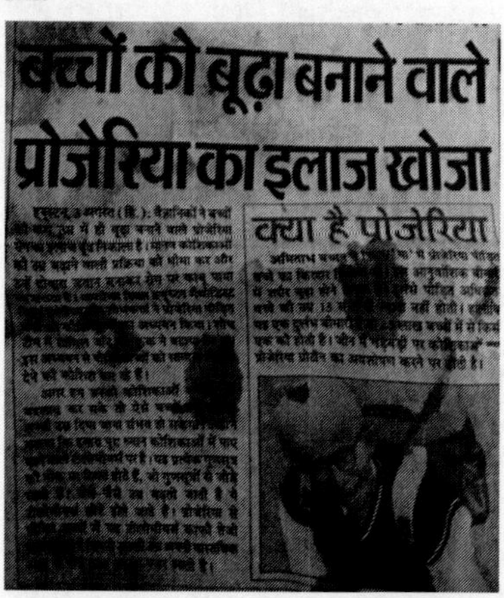

बच्चों को बूढ़ा बनाने वाले प्रोजेरिया का इलाज खोजा

क्या है प्रोजेरिया

Home care programs can be organized so that patients can administer their own Factor VIII infusions with the onset of symptoms.

गीतांजलि के सर्जन ने की 700 ग्राम वजनी नवजात की हार्ट सर्जरी

उदयपुर। गीतांजली हॉस्पिटल के कार्डियक थोरेसिक एवं वेसक्यूलर सर्जन डॉ संजय गांधी ने जयपुर के एक निजी हॉस्पिटल में 24 सप्ताह में जन्मे 700 ग्राम के नवजात की जटिल हृदय सर्जरी सफलतापूर्वक सम्पन्न कर नवजात को नया जीवन प्रदान किया। यह राज्य में ऐसा दूसरा सफल ऑपरेशन है जो जयपुर एनआईसीयू में किया गया है इससे पूर्व गीतांजली हॉस्पिटल में ऐसा ऑपरेशन हुआ था। जयपुर निवासी नेहा माथुर ने जयपुर के कोकून हॉस्पिटल में 700 ग्राम वजनी नवजात को जन्म दिया। नवजात के सांस लेने की परेशानी के चलते उसे एनआईसीयू में वेंटीलेटर पर लिया गया था। ईको-कार्डियोग्राफी में पता चला कि हृदय की दो मुख्य धमनियां आपस में जुड़ी हैं जिस कारण उसे वेंटीलेटर से हटाना संभव नहीं हो पा रहा। नवजात की नाजुक हालत को ध्यान में रखते हुए गीतांजली हॉस्पिटल के प्रशासन ने

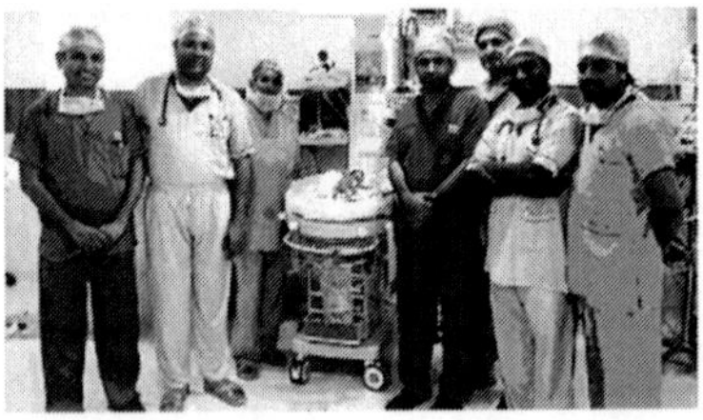

अपनी कार्डिक टीम को जयपुर भेजने का निर्णय लिया जिसके तहत डॉ संजय गांधी, डॉ अंकुर गांधी एवं समस्त ओटी स्टाफ कोकून हॉस्पिटल पहुंचे और रात करीब एक बजे एनआईसीयू में ही ऑपरेशन कर हृदय की जुड़ी हुई धमनियों को अलग किया। नवजात अब स्वस्थ है।

City doctors successfully perform genital reconstructive surgery

By Vikas Vaidya

BIRTH of a child in a family usually brings a delightful shower of happy moments. It was no different for a family from Nagpur when a girl child was born. As time passed by, the world of their little girl was filled with beautiful dresses and dolls and trinkets. But then one day, the reality hit the family like a bolt from the blue. There little girl, now 12, was, in fact, a boy!

It all started 12 years ago when Gopi (name changed) was born in a well-to-do family. She was developing normally and was a healthy child. She got good education and was also extraordinary in sports. The only concern of parents had been a swelling in her genital region and some atypical appearance. They discussed this with their doctor but were always reassured.

At the age of 12 years, Gopi started growing tall and muscular. Her voice was becoming a bit masculine and so was her behaviour. Her physical development is very different from girls her age. All this left Gopi's parents obviously panicky. They consulted Dr Hari Mangtani, Pediatric Endocrinologist of the city. He referred the case to Dr Dinesh Sarda, well-known Pediatric surgeon and Pediatric Urologist. After a complete work up what came to light shocked the parents to the core. It turned out that Gopi is, in fact, a male child internally with 46XY chromosomes.

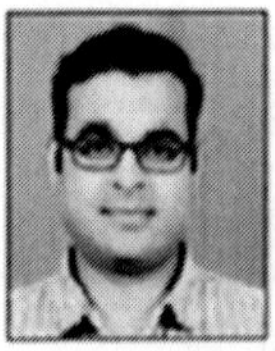

Dr Hari Mangtani

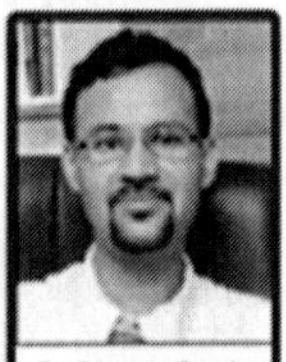

Dr Dinesh Sarda

The swelling in the genital region, that the parents had discussed with the doctor then, was in fact one of the testes.

Once the diagnosis was confirmed, it was thoroughly discussed with the parents and it was decided to give Gopi her real identity as a boy. Pediatric Pschycologist Dr Manju Giri came into the secene and had a tough task making the child understand what had happened and how to embrace the change. Meanwhile, the most challenging part for the doctors now was to make the genitalia appear as that of a male. This reconstructive surgical challenge was taken up by Dr Dinesh Sarda at his Ketki Nursing Home, Dhantoli. Presently Gopi is undergoing psychosocial and behavioral training to face the world afresh as a boy. The family members are happy that even if it took so many years, the psychological ordeal that Gopi would have had to face lifelong potraying what he is not, is now over.

(Contd on page 3)

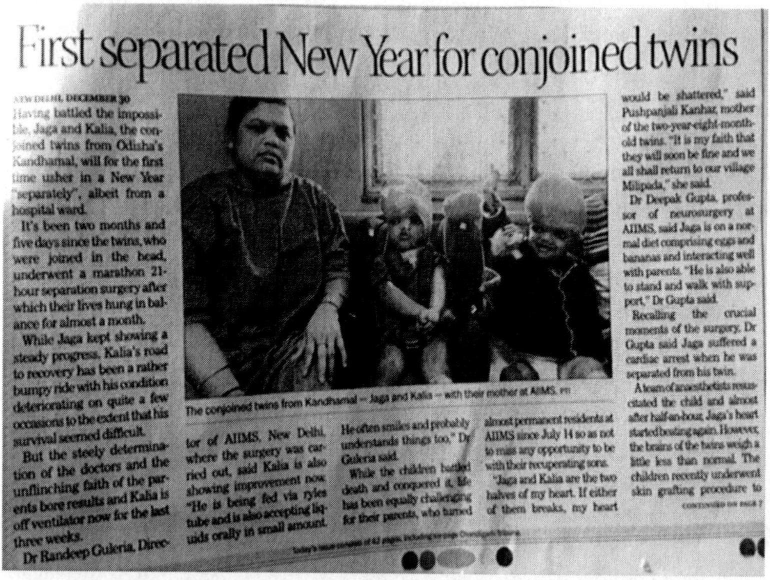

First separated New Year for conjoined twins

NEW DELHI, DECEMBER 30

Having battled the impossible, Jaga and Kalia, the conjoined twins from Odisha's Kandhamal, will for the first time usher in a New Year "separately", albeit from a hospital ward.

It's been two months and five days since the twins, who were joined in the head, underwent a marathon 21-hour separation surgery after which their lives hung in balance for almost a month.

While Jaga kept showing a steady progress, Kalia's road to recovery has been a rather bumpy ride with his condition deteriorating on quite a few occasions to the extent that his survival seemed difficult.

But the steely determination of the doctors and the unflinching faith of the parents bore results and Kalia is off ventilator now for the last three weeks.

Dr Randeep Guleria, Director of AIIMS, New Delhi, where the surgery was carried out, said Kalia is also showing improvement now. "He is being fed via ryles tube and is also accepting liquids orally in small amount. He often smiles and probably understands things too," Dr Guleria said.

While the children battled death and conquered it, life has been equally challenging for their parents, who turned almost permanent residents at AIIMS since July 14 so as not to miss any opportunity to be with their recuperating sons.

"Jaga and Kalia are the two halves of my heart. If either of them breaks, my heart would be shattered," said Pushpanjali Kanhar, mother of the two-year-eight-month-old twins. "It is my faith that they will soon be fine and we all shall return to our village Milipada," she said.

Dr Deepak Gupta, professor of neurosurgery at AIIMS, said Jaga is on a normal diet comprising eggs and bananas and interacting well with parents. "He is also able to stand and walk with support," Dr Gupta said.

Recalling the crucial moments of the surgery, Dr Gupta said Jaga suffered a cardiac arrest when he was separated from his twin.

A team of anaesthetists resuscitated the child and almost after half-an-hour, Jaga's heart started beating again. However, the brains of the twins weigh a little less than normal. The children recently underwent skin grafting procedure to

CONTINUED ON PAGE 7

The conjoined twins from Kandhamal — Jaga and Kalia — with their mother at AIIMS. PTI

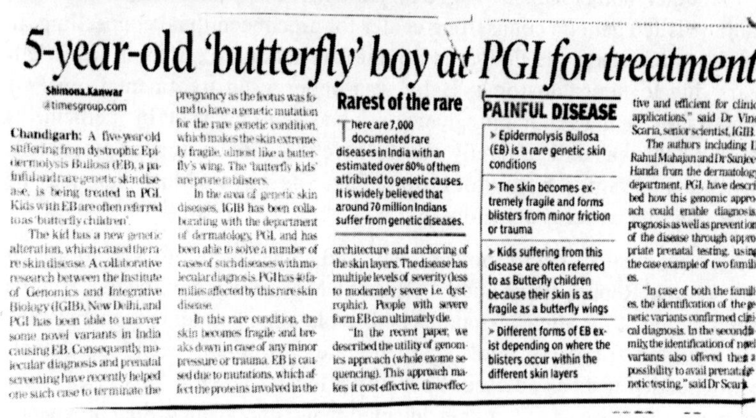

5-year-old 'butterfly' boy at PGI for treatment

Shimona.Kanwar
@timesgroup.com

Chandigarh: A five-year-old suffering from dystrophic Epidermolysis Bullosa (EB), a painful and rare genetic skin disease, is being treated in PGI. Kids with EB are often referred to as 'butterfly children'.

The kid has a new genetic alteration, which caused the rare skin disease. A collaborative research between the Institute of Genomics and Integrative Biology (IGIB), New Delhi, and PGI has been able to uncover some novel variants in India causing EB. Consequently, molecular diagnosis and prenatal screening have recently helped one such case to terminate the pregnancy as the foetus was found to have a genetic mutation for the rare genetic condition, which makes the skin extremely fragile, almost like a butterfly's wing. The 'butterfly kids' are prone to blisters.

In the area of genetic skin diseases, IGIB has been collaborating with the department of dermatology, PGI, and has been able to solve a number of cases of such diseases with molecular diagnosis. PGI has 40 families affected by this rare skin disease.

In this rare condition, the skin becomes fragile and breaks down in case of any minor pressure or trauma. EB is caused due to mutations, which affect the proteins involved in the architecture and anchoring of the skin layers. The disease has multiple levels of severity (less to moderately severe i.e. dystrophic). People with severe form EB can ultimately die.

"In the recent paper, we described the utility of genomics approach (whole exome sequencing). This approach makes it cost-effective, time-effective and efficient for clinical applications," said Dr Vinod Scaria, senior scientist, IGIB.

The authors including Dr Rahul Mahajan and Dr Sanjeev Handa from the dermatology department, PGI, have described how this genomic approach could enable diagnosis, prognosis as well as prevention of the disease through appropriate prenatal testing, using the case example of two families.

"In case of both the families, the identification of the genetic variants confirmed clinical diagnosis. In the second family, the identification of novel variants also offered them a possibility to avail prenatal genetic testing," said Dr Scaria.

Rarest of the rare

There are 7,000 documented rare diseases in India with an estimated over 80% of them attributed to genetic causes. It is widely believed that around 70 million Indians suffer from genetic diseases.

PAINFUL DISEASE

- Epidermolysis Bullosa (EB) is a rare genetic skin conditions
- The skin becomes extremely fragile and forms blisters from minor friction or trauma
- Kids suffering from this disease are often referred to as Butterfly children because their skin is as fragile as a butterfly wings
- Different forms of EB exist depending on where the blisters occur within the different skin layers

Recent advances in treatment (available surgeries)

Some Case studies

Case study 1

Mother name A wife of B resident of Chandigarh visited genetic counselling center. She was referred from OBG, OPD. Parents already have a baby with Down Syndrome.her age is 30 years.

She has been booked at PGI for her antenatal care. She is gravida 3. In her first pregnancy in 2012 she had delivered a baby through emergency

Caesarean due to eclampsia. A female baby was born. Baby did not cry at the time of birth. Baby was diagnosed to have down syndrome at a later stage. Mother was told that her baby had low IQ. Baby expired at two years due to frequent seizures.

In 2015, by her second pregnancy she delivered a male baby through normal vaginal delivery. That baby is normal and is of 3 years now and living a healthy life.

For her current pregnancy she reported at PGI at 14 week. She had not taken periconceptional folic acid. Her family history was normal. There was no history of consanguinity of marriage. Her personal history indicated she had increased thyroxin level. She was on medication for this. However her other investigations of blood were also normal (Hb, HIV, HCV).

She was was advised for Amniosentesis and level 2 scan at 16 week. Fortunately test reports came out to be normal. she continued her pregnancy and delivered a healthy female baby.

Case study 2

Another mother named M aged 27 years wife of N resident of Roop Nagar, Punjab visited genetic counselling center for preconceptional counselling. In her first pregnancy she delivered a male baby. Baby expired at 4 and half years due to neuroblastoma. Baby was undergoing treatment from PGI Chandigarh. In her second pregnancy she had gone for MTP by medicine as her first baby was ill. Her family was not able to afford her second pregnancy. There was no family history of birth defect. She was told that there may be some risk in next pregnancy too.

At her visit to centre both mother and father were advised to go for karyotyping. Reports came out to be normal. Mother was advised to start folic acid and take it for atleast 3 months before planning her next pregnancy. She was advised for early booking in her next pregnancy and go for all recommended tests as advised. Specailly a level 2 USG at 18 week in next pregnancy. If any sort of tumor is detected in next pregnancy, then pregnancy can be terminated with MTP. Also after delivery they should go for ultrasonography of baby after every six months until baby achieves an age of one year. For now parents do not need to undergo any further test.

Case study 3

MotherS age 33 years wife of T village Roop Nagar visited genetic counselling OPD. In her first pregnancy, she had an abortion, at eight month of pregnancy. In her second pregnancy she delivered a male baby through normal vaginal delivery. This baby is of eight years and living a healthy normal life. In her third pregnancy she delivered a male baby by normal vaginal delivery but baby died after four days due to Glutaric aciduria type-1. She told that baby had stopped taking milk after two days of birth. Baby had seizures. Baby had difficulty in breathing and baby used to remain irritable. In her current pregnancy her POG is 19 week. There is no history of consanguinity of marriage. She has increased thyroid level. She had taken folic acid, iron and calcium during her current pregnancy. There was no history of preconception folic acid intake.Her ultrasonography report is normal. She has been referred for genetic counselling in view of her previous baby that got expired due to blue glutaric aciduria type-1.

No DNA testing was done in expired child. No karyotyping was done in parents too . But now as it is 19th week pregnancy, she is late for the test because report will take few weeks to come and if there is any problem in the report, it will be very late for doing MTP. As MTP is to be done till 20th week of preganncy. If she would have reported earlier at approximately sixth week of pregnancy required tests would have been conducted in time.

Although she was advised for some required tests but,she could only continue her current pregnancy. She delivered a male baby at PGI. Baby had normal morphological feaures at the time of birth. After after a few days baby stopped feeding. Baby was investigated for DNA testing. Again this baby too reported to have Glutaric aciduria type-1. Her early booking at PGI could have helped her for early diagnosis and timely intervention for MTP.

Case study 4

A female aged 33 years (Name P w/o Q,Punjab) visited genetic counseling room no 2036 ,PGI in March 2017. She was referred through General Gynaecology OPD to genetic counseling room i/v/o previous baby having congenital disorder. As per her obstetric history she was G3 P201. She is a known case of secondary infertility and oligomenorrhea. She is taking treatment for infertility. Her previous baby has epidermolysis bullosa. First baby (female wt- 2.6 kg) got delivered through cesarean section at a private nursing home in Ropar. The baby had skin lesion on face and foot. Baby was referred to skin department of PGIMER; Chandigarh on the day of delivery. Epidermolysis bullosa was diagnosed in the baby, by the doctors. Doctors advised her not to go for any test till baby is 45 days old.KMNO4 compressions were advised. However baby died after 1week. Mother of the baby had itching all over the body during pregnancy. Now the patient is planning for her next pregnancy and has come to PGI for infertility treatment. After her checkup she has been referred to dermatology department as there is some skin lesion in perineum. She has been advised for some routine investigations, i.e., blood group/TSH/FSH/LH/GTT/Montoux. She has been advised to start folic acid and tab fluconozole along with vaginal pessary.

As no autopsy report of the previous baby or any blood sample is available parents have been advised to go for karyotyping by genetic counseling in Room 2036. After the karyotyping it will be seen whether there is some affected gene present in the parents by DNA testing , the same will be tested in next baby also.But parents were not willing as they said they cant afford the test. so they were advised to continue folic acid atleast 3 months before pregancy as well as to continue even after conception. She has been advised for early booking in next pregancy.

Understanding the mechanism- How and why genetic disorders occur?

Each organ of human body is made up of cells. Each normal cell contains 46 chromosomes(23 pairs).

Normal cell - 22 pair of chromosomes + XX (female)

22 pairs of chromosomes + X Y (male)

Gamete cells (ovum and sperm) only contain 23 chromosomes (rod like structures present in the nucleus of cell , made up of DNA). Each chromosome contains thousands of genes.

When the genes and chromosomes are 'normal ' a healthy child is likely to be born. If there is some defect in these chromosomes, congenital disorder or genetic disorder may occur.

During intercourse husband's sperm (22 chromosomes + X or 22 chromosomes + Y) and wife's ovum (22 chromosomes + X or 22 chromosomes + X) meet.

Normal mating

Each cell has 46 chromosomes

Gametes(ovum/sperm)

Children are born

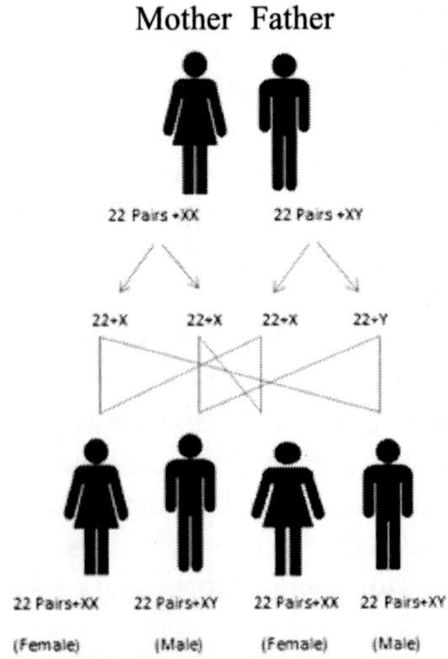

These two gametes merge into one zygote cell. The new zygote contains 23 chromosomes from father and 23 chromosomes from mother. Thus 46 chromosomes are attained in each cell.

Being male or female depends on whether we have XX or XY sex chromosomes as 23rd pair.

In newborn incidence of chromosomal anomalies is 5.6 per 1000 live births. They are of 2 types.

Numerical abnormalities – in Such cases whole chromosomes are either missing from normal sequence of 46 chromosome or is extra. For example Trisomy (three copies of a chromosome) instead of monosomy (single copy of a chromosome). Down's syndrome is probably the most well-known example. Besides trisomy 21, the major chromosomal aneuploidies seen in live-born babies are: trisomy 18, trisomy 13.

Structural abnormalities- when part of an individual chromosome is missing, is extra, switched to another chromosome, or turned upside down. Examples of structural chromosomal abnormalities include *cri du chat* or "cat cry" syndrome. Children with this syndrome have an abnormally developed larynx that makes their cry sound like the mewing of a cat in distress. They also have a small head, misshapen ears, and a rounded face, as well as other systemic defects. These children usually die in infancy. *Cri du chat* is caused by a deletion of a segment of DNA in chromosome no. 5.

Some Basic terms used in the context of genetics

Genotype : (Genetic constitution) -Tt

Phenotype: (outward expression)- tall

Homozygous: (when genes of a pair are alike)- TT or tt

Heterozygous: (when genes of a pair are different)- Bb or Tt

Dominant gene: In this the phenotype effect comes in both homo (TT) and heterozygous (Tt), i.e., both combinations will make a tall child

Recessive gene: In this effect comes only in homozygous (tt)- Short height. In Tt the effect of T will dominate over t = Tall Child

Autosomal: For abnormalities in non-sex chromosomes. Tt (Height character is transmitted through autosome)

Sex linked: X0Y/XX0- If the disease trait is present in X sex chromosome it will be known as X sex linked and if it is present in Y chromosome it will be known as Y sex linked.

Case: Presence of disease trait in one of the chromosome will make the male a case for that disease. (X0 Y), since disease causing Xo will dominate over normal Y) e.g. hemophilia

Carrier: As in a female there are two XX sex chromosomes. If there is Presence of a trait of disease in one X chromosome. Female will be carrier for that disease. Symptoms for that disease will not be present in the female (X0X). Since normal X will dominate over X= X0).

A clear example of the relationship between genotype and phenotype exists in cases where there are dominant and recessive alleles for a particular trait. This can be understood by a simple example.

A capital "T" is used to represent a dominant allele at a particular locus coding for "tallness" the lower case "t" is used to represent the recessive allele coding for "small height". Using this notation, a diploid plant will possess one of three genotypes: TT, Tt, or tt (the variation tT is identical to Tt). Although there are three different genotypes, but human will be either tall or short (two phenotypes). Human with a "TT" or "Tt" genotype are observed to be tall (phenotypically tall). Only those that carry the "tt" genotype will be observed to be short (phenotypically short). Figure -1

Another example may be of famous Bollywood star Amitabh and actress Jaya. (1st generation kids will be tall). Figure - 2

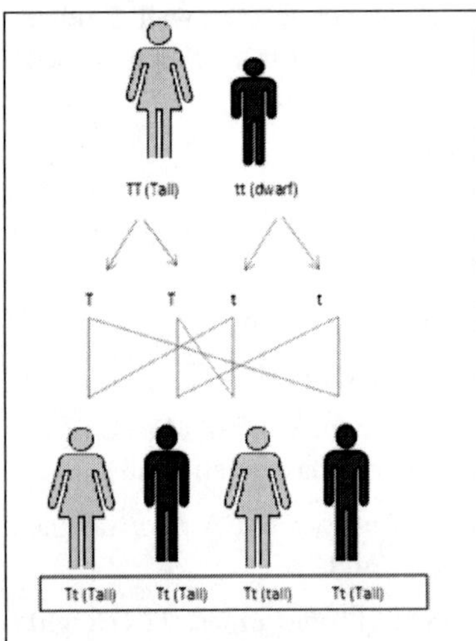

Figure 1

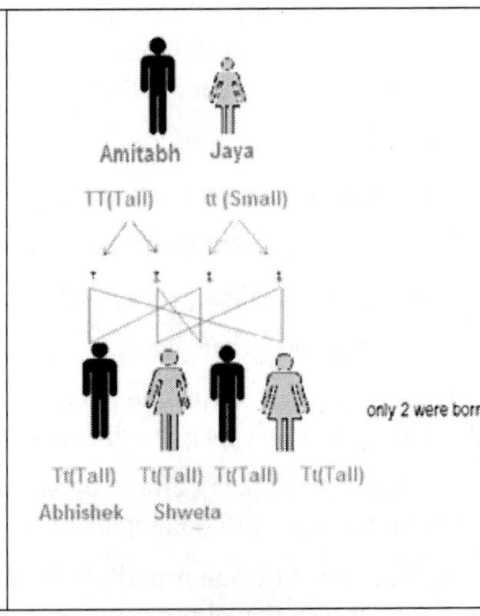

Figure 2

It can also be understood by another simple examplefor black colour of eyes. As it is known genes are always present in pairs. If mother and father both have black colour eyes (BB) all the babies will have black colour eyes. If mother and father have blue colour eyes (bb) all the babies have blue (bb) colour eyes.

To represent black colour of eyes we take B alphabet .so genotype will be BB. As B is dominant it will produce black colour eyes in BB and Bb pair. If it would have been recessive it would manifest only in bb.

In the first case we take black colour eye female (BB) dominant and blue colour eye male (bb) recessive. When we make a cross between them. We get the following results in the first generation kids. Bb is heterozygous and B is dominant and is present in all the four outcomes. So all babies with black colour eyes are produced. (Figure 3)

In the second case we consider female having black colour eye (Bb) and male with blue colour eyes (bb). Now in this case the following outcomes will be produced (Figure 4).We can see there are two Bb and two bb. Bb is heterozygous and B is dominant so they will have black colour eyes. Whereas bb is recessive and they will have blue colour eyes.

In the third case we consider female (Bb) black eyes and male also (Bb) black eyes. In this case one BB (black eyes) two Bb (black eyes) and one bb (blue eyes) are produced. There are chances of 3 babies with black eyes and one baby with blue eyes. (Figure 5)

Patterns of inheritance (see end of the chapter for illustrations)

Related to Autosomes

Autosomal dominant inheritance-When a single gene is present and expresses itself without regard to the other gene at that locus. It is said to be dominant.More than 700 such diseases are reported,e.g.,retinoblastoma, neurofibromatosis, Marfan syndrome achondroplasia, Huntington's chorea etc.

Each generation shows affected member (no generation is skipped).

Unaffected individuals do not transmit the trait to their offspring.

each of their offspring having a 50% chance of being affected.

Both sexes have equal chances of being affected.

This can be understood by the following diagram for a common autosomal dominant disease, .e.g. achondroplasia. Father is affected by the disease (one affected gene and another unaffected) whereas mother is not. There are equal chances of delivery of 50% male and 50% females.. In one male child affected gene may go and in another unaffected gene may go. Now in the male child that gets affected gene, disease will occur whereas the male child that gets unaffected gene, disease will not occur. It is to be noted here that in both male child the gene that comes from mother is normal.Now the female that gets affected gene from father becomes carrier for disease. It means symptoms will not express in the female child. However, symptoms may express in the next generations.

Autosomal recessive inheritance-When individual with one gene for the trait (carrier) does not express the clinical features. This is found more in cansanguineous marriages.

Only an individual who gets two genes for the trait has clinical manifestation.

On an average 25% of the offsprings of two carrier parents are affected.

Both sexes have an equal chance of being affected.

X linked recessive inheritance- The genes involved are located on X chromosome when the female carries a sex-linked recessive trait, she is a carrier. She does not exhibit clinical symptoms. This is because this gene is recessive to the normal alleles located on her second X chromosome.

However since male has only one X chromosomes. Therefore, only a single gene for a particular sex linked traits. All males who carry the defective genes will be affected.

With rarer exceptions only males are affected.

While the disease may appear to skip one or more generation, affected males are related through carrier females.

One half the sons of a carrier female will be affected e.g.Hemophilia acquired the name the royal disease due to the high number of descendants of Queen Victoria afflicted by it. This is assumed that a mutation occured in the sperm of the Queen's father, Edward Augustus, the Duke of Kent.

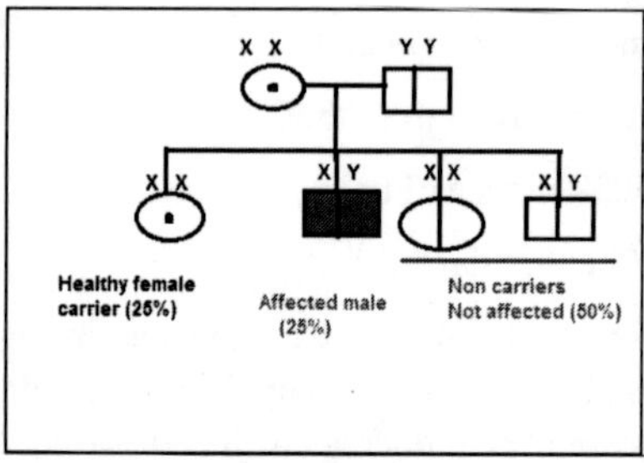

X linked recessive

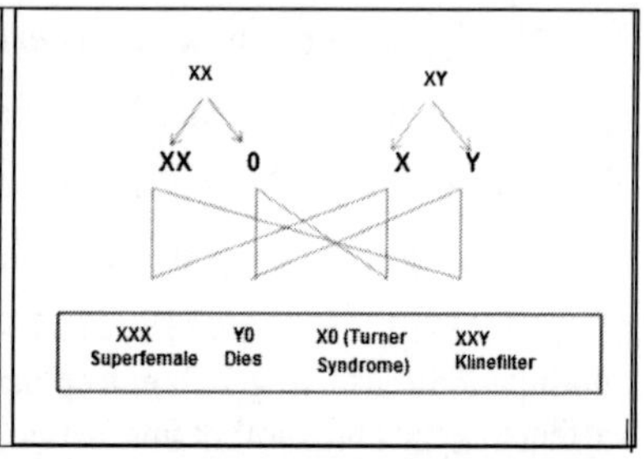

Problems related to sex chromosomes

If an affected male marries a healthy female carrier then there is 25% chance – affected female, 25% chance -affected male , 25% chance-unaffected healthy male and 25% chance – carrier healthy female. If he marries a normal healthy female 50%- carrier healthy female and 50% chance-normal healthy male.

(B) Related to sex chromosome

Klinefelter's syndrome- Person with this syndrome are abnormal male (XXY/XXXY). They have nonfunctional testis. Spermatozoa are absent in their ejaculations, growth of hairs on face, pubes, axillae is scanty. They can have gynaecomastia & mental retardation. Incidence 1/1000 male.

XYY Syndrome- Person is aggressive, antisocial, often criminal male. Main features are exceptional height (more than 6 feet), and personality/ behavior disorder.

Turner Syndrome- This is the most common chromosome disorder in humans . its incidence is 1 in 7500 live born girls. They have 45 chromosomes (Single X) instead of XX. They have short stature, infertility, primary amenorrhea; other features include, coarctation of aorta, pulmonary stenosis, and renal malformation. Persons suffering from this syndrome are apparent females with underdeveloped sex glands.

Super females (XXX/XXXX) They have underdeveloped external genitalia, uterus and vagina, and can be tall.

Table- List of chromosomal disorders

Autosomal dominant	Autosomal recessive
Achondoplasia,Huntington Chorea Neurofibromatosis, Polyposis Coli Brachydactyly, Marfan Syndrome Retinoblastoma	Fibrocystic Disease Of Pancreas Phenylketonuria, Albinism, Thalassemia, Color Blindness Microphthalmos, Infantile Amaurotic Idiocy Laurence-moon-Biedl-syndrome
X linked dominant Rickets-vitamin D resistant Hypophosphatemia, Blood group	Sex linked recessive Hemophilia, Agamma globulinemia Muscular dystrophy, Colour blindness-red green G6PD Deficiency

Medical Council of India sponsored CME on "A capacity building seminar for strengthening communication skills of doctors for counseling of parents regarding birth defects"

The seminar was organized with the objective of spreading awareness on birth defects. Birth defects are common, critical and costly conditions. They have a high impact in almost all spheres of our life like physical performance, competence and capability in case of major limb anomalies, central nervous system and cardiac anomalies. In some cases it makes a person dependent on others for whole life e.g. absence of limbs. Genetic counseling about various prenatal testing techniques helps a patient to know about possible risk and indication of the test. These tests give a clear and more accurate diagnosis at an earlier stage of pregnancy and parents get more time to seek proper advice.

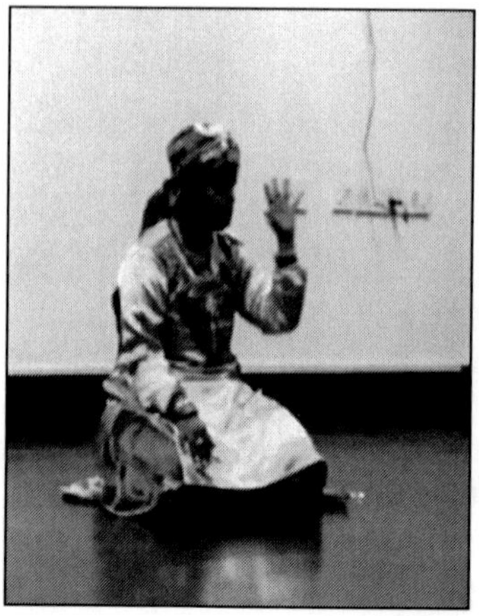

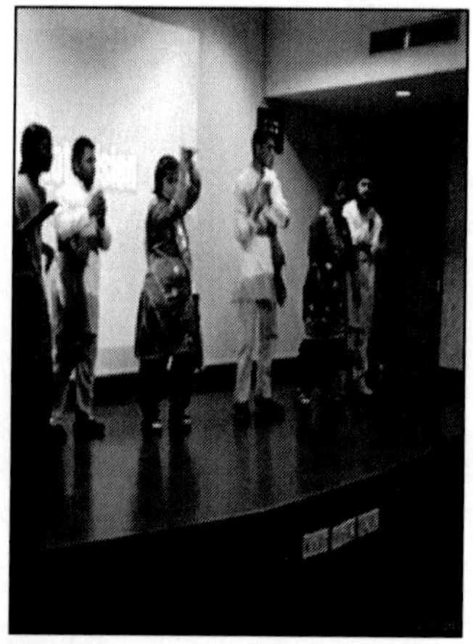

H.T. CHANDIGARH.

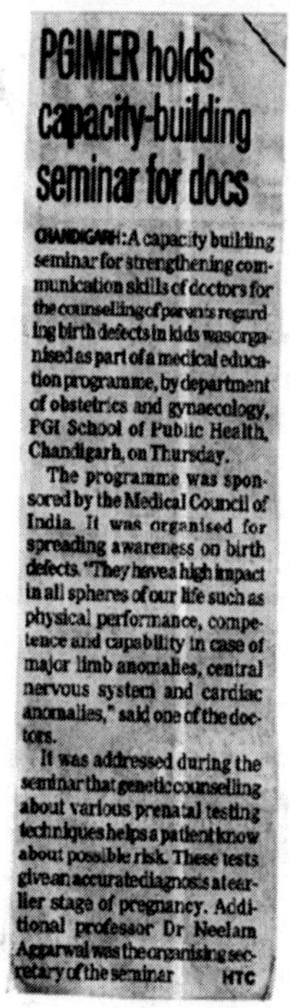

PGIMER holds capacity-building seminar for docs

CHANDIGARH: A capacity building seminar for strengthening communication skills of doctors for the counselling of parents regarding birth defects in kids was organised as part of a medical education programme, by department of obstetrics and gynaecology, PGI School of Public Health, Chandigarh, on Thursday.

The programme was sponsored by the Medical Council of India. It was organised for spreading awareness on birth defects. "They have a high impact in all spheres of our life such as physical performance, competence and capability in case of major limb anomalies, central nervous system and cardiac anomalies," said one of the doctors.

It was addressed during the seminar that genetic counselling about various prenatal testing techniques helps a patient know about possible risk. These tests give an accurate diagnosis at earlier stage of pregnancy. Additional professor Dr Neelam Aggarwal was the organising secretary of the seminar HTC

9-2-18

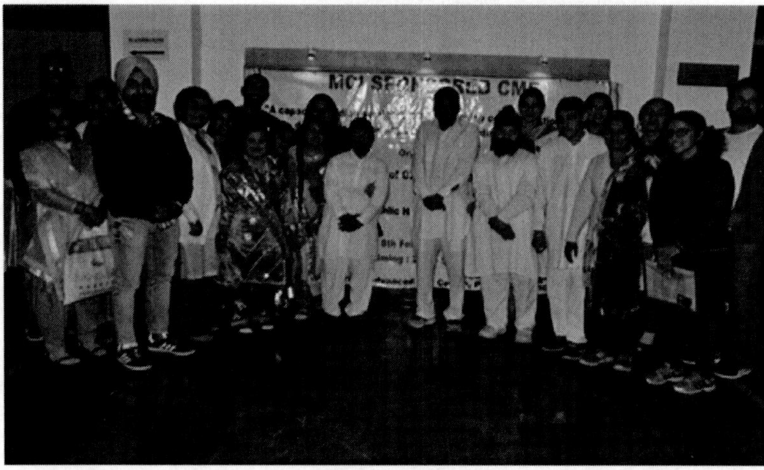

Dance performances by special children

Against this backdrop CMEentitled "A capacity building seminar for strengthening communication skills of doctors for counseling of parents regarding birth defects" was organized was organized to bring together various stakeholders on 8th February, 2018" at Auditorium-Advanced Eye Centre, 2-5 pm.

Dr. Neelam Aggarwal (Additional Professor, OBG Department, PGIMER) was the Organising Secretary to this Seminar. Dr. Amarjeet Singh (Professor, Department of Community Medicine) and Dr. Alka (Research Scholar, Centre for Public Health) were Convener and Co-convener to the seminar respectively.

Experts from various fields' i.e. Gynaecology, Pediatrics, community medicine, Nursing Institutes, Panjab University, Public health department participated in the seminar. Mrs. Bhwana Tyal, Director, Sadhna Society vocational training institute for mentally handicapped shared her experiences with Special Children. This was followed by performances by special children. Lecture of expert speakers was followed by interactive discussion with the audience. This initiative will help work towards removing barriers and making existing health care systems more inclusive and accessible to people having babies with birth defect.

This seminar is expected to ensure ears to needs of birth defect babies. Opinions of target group i.e. parents of birth defect babies will help identify gaps and priorities to reduce health inequalities and plan improvement for access and inclusion. This seminar will act as an advocacy mechanism for the needs of patients through discussion among experts.

Genetic counseling- where available

1. PGIMER, Chandigarh- Genetic clinic and prenatal counseling centre
2. AIIMS, New Delhi- Genetic Unit, Department of pediatrics
3. SGRH,Delhi- centre for medical genetics
4. SGPGIMS Lucknow- Department of genetics
5. Kasturba Hospital Manipal
6. Osmania university, Hyderabad
7. Nizam, Hyderabad
8. Centre for human genetics, Banglore
9. KEM Hospital,Mumbai
10. Koumundi Godbole, Pune

References

Acog.org. (2018). Screening Tests for Birth Defects - ACOG. [online] Available at: https://www.acog.org/Patients/FAQs/Screening-Tests-for-Birth-Defects [Accessed 23 Apr. 2018].

Addressing the public health challenge of birth defects in India. Available from: https://www.researchgate.net/publication/270105641_Addressing_the_public_health_challenge_of_birth_defects_in_India [accessed Apr 20 2017].

Bhat BV, BabuL.Congenital malformations at birth--a prospective study from south India.Indian J Pediatr. 1998;65(6):873-81.

Boyle, C. A., & Cordero, J. F. (2005). Birth Defects and Disabilities: A Public Health Issue for the 21st Century. American Journal of Public Health, 95(11), 1884–1886. http://doi.org/10.2105/AJPH.2005.067181

Centers for Disease Control and Prevention. (2018). Facts | Birth Defects | NCBDDD | CDC. [online] Available at: https://www.cdc.gov/ncbddd/birthdefects/facts.html [Accessed 3 Apr. 2017].

Centers for Disease Control and Prevention. Learn the signs. Act early. Available at: www.cdc.gov/actearly. Accessed March 4, 2017.

Centers for Disease Control and Prevention. Update on Overall Prevalence of Major Birth Defects–Atlanta, Georgia, 1978-2005. MMWR Morb Mortal Wkly Rep. 2008;57(1):1-5.

Centers for Disease Control and Prevention. (2018). Infographic: Make a PACT for Prevention | Birth Defects | NCBDDD | CDC. [online] Available at: https://www.cdc.gov/ncbddd/birthdefects/infographics/pact/index.html [Accessed 23 Apr. 2018].

Dshs.texas.gov. (2018). Birth Defects Glossary. [online] Available at: https://www.dshs.texas.gov/birthdefects/glossary.shtm [Accessed 15 March. 2017].

Genetic Alliance; The New York-Mid-Atlantic Consortium for Genetic and Newborn Screening Services. Understanding Genetics: A New York, Mid-Atlantic Guide for Patients and Health Professionals. Washington (DC): Genetic Alliance; 2009

Jul 8. APPENDIX K, BIRTH DEFECTS. Available from: https://www.ncbi.nlm.nih.gov/books/NBK115547/

Khurmi MS, Gupta M, Chaudhari G. Addressing the public health challenge of birth defects in India. Indian J Child Health. 2014;1(3):95-8.

March of Dimes (2006). Global Report on birth defects,the hidden toll of dying and disabled chidren, New Delhi: March of Dimes Birth Defects Foundation White Plains, New York. Available at https://www.marchofdimes.org/materials/global-report-on-birth-defects-the-hidden-toll-of-dying-and-disabled-children-full-report.pdf. [Accessed 15 March. 2017].

Mark A. Canfield, James L. Anderson, D. Kim Waller, Susan E. Palmer, Celia I. Kaye. MMWR Recomm Rep. 2002 Sep 13; 51(RR-13): 16–19.

Merriam-webster.com. (2018). Definition of BIRTH DEFECT. [online] Available at: https://www.merriam-webster.com/dictionary/birth%20defect [Accessed 12 june. 2017].

National Family Health Survey. Summary of findings, 2005-06; 35. Available from http://www.rchiips.org/nfhs/NFHS-3%20Data/VOL-1/Summary%20of%20Findings%20(6868K).pdf

Neogi S.B., Negandhi P.H., Ganguli A., Chopra S., Sandhu N., Gupta R.K. ,Zodpey S., Singh A., Singh A., Gupta R.Consumption of indigenous medicines by pregnant women in North India for selecting sex of the foetus: what can it lead to? BMC Pregnancy Childbirth. 2015;15:208

Operational Guidelines on Rashtriya Bal Swasthya Karyakram (RSBK). Ministry of Health and Family Welfare, Government of India; 2013. Available from: http://www.nrhm.gov.in/nrhm-components/rmnch-a/child-health-immunization/rashtriya-bal-swasthya-karyakram-rbsk/2013-12-19-08-30-24.html. [Last accessed on 2014 Sep 12].

Park K. Textbook of Preventive and Social Medicine.preventive medicine in Obstetrics,pediatrics and geriatrics.22rd ed. Jabalpur. BanarasidasBhanot Publishers, 2013; 13:531-534.

Parents. (2018). 9 Birth Defects and Their Symptoms and Treatments. [online] Available at: https://www.parents.com/baby/health/birth-defects/9-birth-defects-and-their-symptoms-and-treatments/ [Accessed 23 Apr. 2018].

Sharma R. Birth defects in India: Hidden truth, need for urgent attention. Indian J Hum Genet. 2013 Apr-Jun; 19(2): 125–129.

WHO (2014) Neonatal–perinatal database and birth defects surveillance,Report of the regional review meeting,, New Delhi. Available at http://apps.searo.who.int/PDS_DOCS/B5227.pdf [Accessed 12 june. 2017].

World Health Organization. (2018). Congenital anomalies. [online] Available at: http://www.who.int/mediacentre/factsheets/fs370/en/ [Accessed 23 Apr. 2017].

Chapter 5: Following pictures illustrate some **Examples of Congenital Malformations& their mode of transmission**

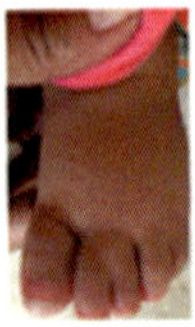	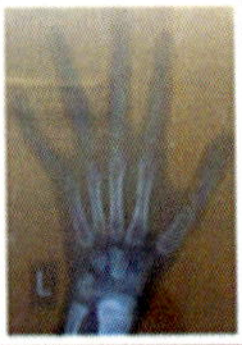	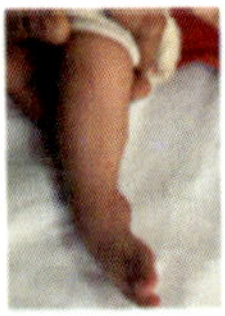	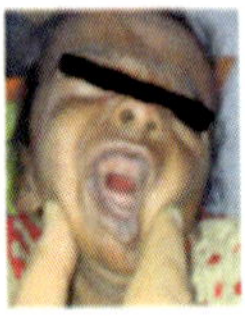	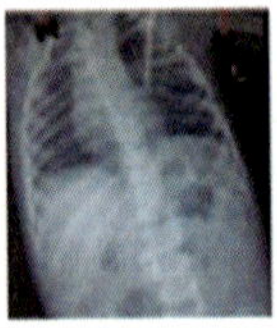
Syndactyly	Absent metacarpal bone	Right foot CTEV	Cleft palate	Spinal diastasis

Pix 1 : Examples of some birth defects.

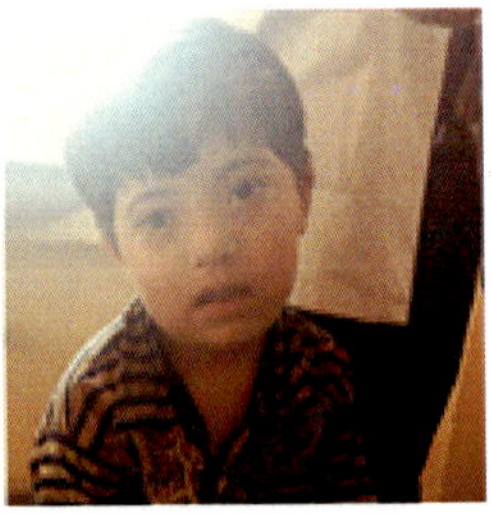

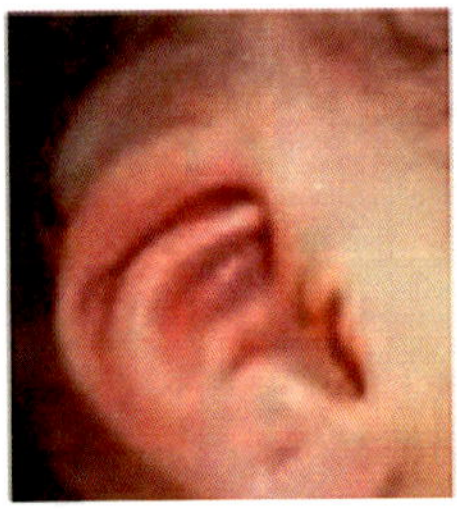

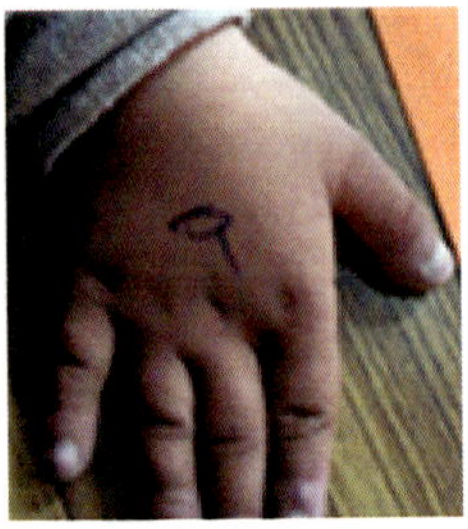

Pix 2: - Features of Down Syndrome- face / tops of ears may slightly fold over.

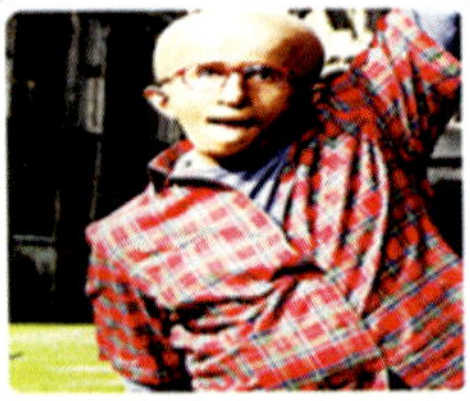

Amitabh Bachchan playing the role of a child who is suffering from Progeria, a genetic disorder which leads to quick acceleration of ageing process in children.

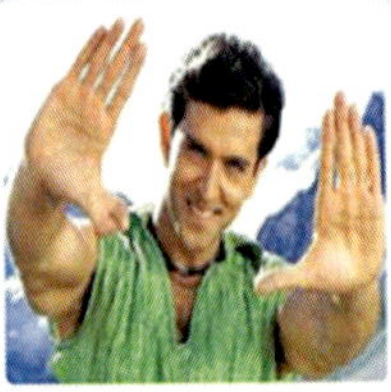

Hrithik Roshan has two thumbs on his right hand - and it concerns a rather complex combination of abnormalities: 'polydactyly' (= extra digits) + 'syndactyly'

(= fused digits).

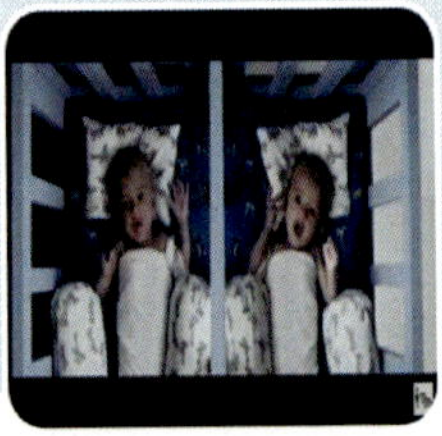

Varun dhawan as conjoined twins after surgery in Movie judwaa 2

Pix 3: Examples of some birth defects from Bollywood films.

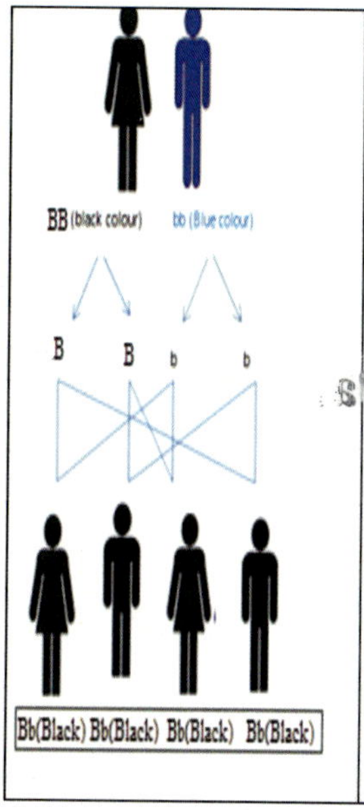

Figure 3

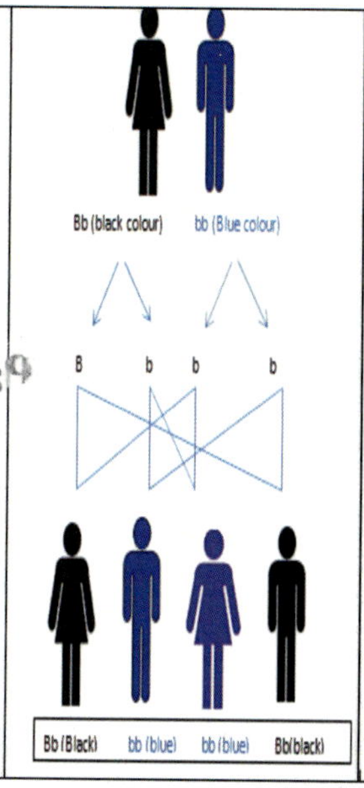

Figure 4

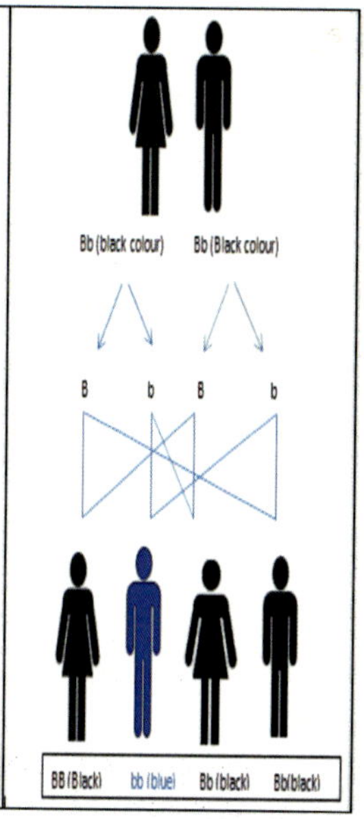

Figure 5

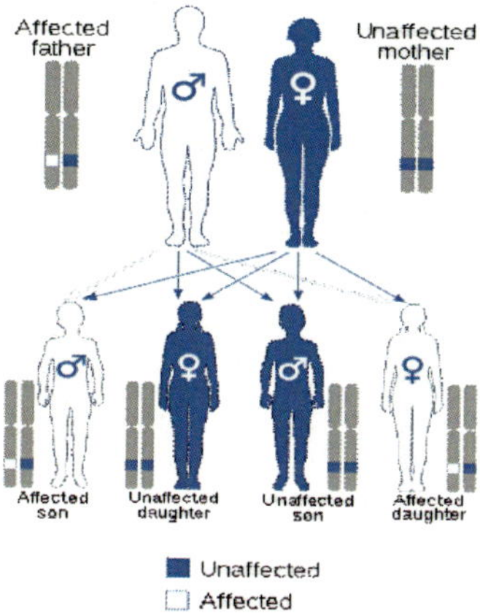

Autosomal Dominant

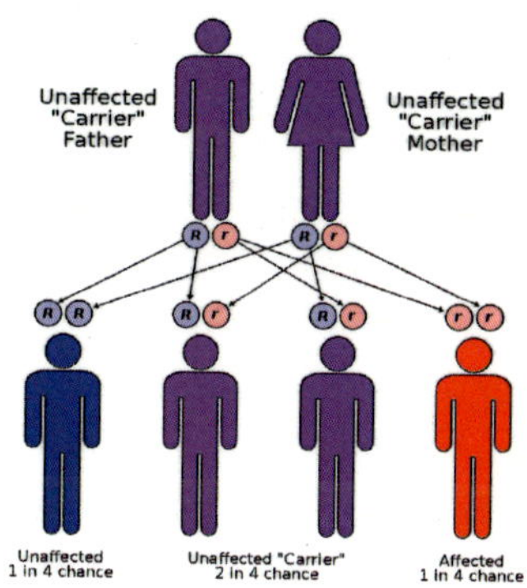

Autosomal Recessive

Chapter - 6

Care of Breast Cancer Patients after Surgery – A Guide for Women with Special Emphasis on Prevention of Shoulder Dysfunction and Arm Lymphedema

— Dr. Sukhpal Kaur, Dr. Gurpreet Singh,
Dr. Amarjeet Singh, Dr. Parul Sharma

Introduction

Breast cancer is the most commonly diagnosed cancerin women. Though it can be a fatal disease, still, breast cancer is considered as one of the "good" [illegible] woman" kind of malignancy as compared to other cancers of the body like blood cancer, lung cancer, liver cancer and cancer of gastro-intestinal tract. This is so because the prospects of cure of breast cancer are relatively much better after treatment. Usually, for cancers, success of therapy is evaluated in terms of 5 year survival. Patients with early breast cancer after proper treatment have about 90% chance of being alive after 10 years.

More than 1.2 million women are diagnosed with breast cancer annually worldwide. Global statistics show that the annual incidence of breast cancer is increasing. Breast cancer represents 10% of all the cancers diagnosed annually and constitutes 22% of all new cancers in women.The incidence of breast cancer is on the rise in India. It is rapidly becoming the number one cancer in females pushing the cervical cancer to the second position.

Statistics reveal:

- *Every 3 minutes a woman is diagnosed with breast cancer.*
- *Every 13 minutes a woman dies from breast cancer.*
- *Breast cancer accounts for 20% of the total cancer related diseases in India and is largely prevalent among urban women.*
- *Presently, nearly 100,000 new cases occur in Indian women every year.*
- *Over the course of a lifetime, 1 in 22 women will be diagnosed with breast cancer in India.*

Treatment of breast cancer: The treatment depends mainly on the stage of the cancer, the size of the tumor, the results of lab tests (the hormone receptor tests, HER2/neu test etc.), age, menopause, personal preferences and the general health of the patient. When cancer affects any body part like the breast, it may also spread in the advance stages to other parts of body like lymph nodes, bones, lungs, liver and brain. This spread is called **metastasis.**

Theaim of treatment for breast cancer is to:

- Remove the breast cancer.
- Destroy any cancer cells that might be left in the breast.
- Destroy any cancer cells that may have spread to the armpit.
- Destroy any cancer cells that may have spread in the body but cannot be detected.
- To try and prevent the disease from coming back.

Breast cancer treatment that is suitable for one woman may not be suitable for another. Most women need both local and systemic treatment.

(A) Local therapy: Here, breast surgery and radiation therapy are focused on the breast itself to remove or destroy the cancer cells confined to the breast.

1. Breast Surgery: Surgery is the most common treatment for breast cancer. Surgery can be done for removing cancer affected part. It can be of different types:

(a) Breast conserving surgery: It is also called lumpectomy, wide local excision, or partial mastectomy.This is an operation to remove only the breast tissue affected by the cancer but not the whole breast. This is done when disease is diagnosed at an early stage and is confined to a small area of breast. This has a cosmetic advantage.

(b) Totalmastectomy: This is also called simple mastectomy. This is an operation to remove the entire breast (or as much of the breast tissue as possible). This is done when cancer has affected a large area of the breast because the diagnosis was delayed. In some cases, because of cosmetic reasons a skin-sparing mastectomy may be an option. For this approach, the surgeon removes as little skin as possible (only internal tissue is removed).

(c) Radical/Modified mastectomy: This is a surgical procedure to remove the whole breast that contains cancer. Many of the lymph nodes under the arm, the lining over the chest wall, and the chest wall muscles under the breast are removed. This is done when cancer has spread to nearby lymph nodes and tissues (due to delay in diagnosis).

2. Radiation Therapy: It uses high-energy rays to kill cancer cells. It affects cells only in the part of the body that is treated. After surgery, going for radiotherapy reduces the chances of any cancer cells that are left behind which would trouble patients later. Radiotherapy is a must whenever breast conserving surgery is done. Selected patients may receive radiotherapy after mastectomy.

(B) Systemic therapy: Surgery and radiotherapy are effective for treating tumours confined to the breast but not for the cancer cells that have spread. In some cases, drug (systemic) therapy is needed. Drugs work systemically by entering the blood stream. That is, they kill cancer cells throughout the body rather than just in the breast or nearby tissues. The drug enters the bloodstream and destroys or controls cancer throughout the body. Different types systemic therapies include:

1. Chemotherapy: Here medicines are used to treat cancer. Many times this treatment is just called 'chemo'. Chemotherapy employs drugs called cytotoxic agents. They are given mostly by intravenous injection but sometimes orally.

2. Hormone therapy: The growth of some breast cancers is promoted by estrogen, one of the female hormones in the body. Most hormonal therapies work by decreasing the amount of estrogen in the body. Hormone therapies include:

(a) Anti-estrogens: These work by stopping cancer cells from getting estrogen. The most commonly used drug is Tamoxifen. It is taken as a tablet once a day, usually for 5 years. Anti-estrogens can be used by women of all ages.

(b) Ovarian treatment: Also called ovarian ablation, work by stopping the ovaries from producing estrogen. Ovarian treatments include:

- Radiotherapy to the ovaries.
- Surgery to remove the ovaries.
- Injection of drugs.

(c) Aromatase inhibitors: They work by stopping or inhibiting estrogen from being produced. Aromatase inhibitors are used as an alternative to anti-estrogens or after the use of anti-estrogens. Examples of aromatase inhibitors (drugs) in use are Anastrazole, Letrozole and Exemestane. These are used only in post menopausal women.

3. Biological therapy of breast cancer: Monoclonal antibody therapy is a cancer treatment that uses antibodies made in the laboratory. These antibodies can identify and attach to the receptors on cancer cells that help cancer cells grow. This way these kill the cancer cells, block their growth or keep them from spreading.

Various co-morbidities associated with breast cancer treatment: After treatmentmost women recover. However, there are many side effects of each and every treatment. The risks of any surgery include infection, bleeding, risks associated with general anaesthesia (for example, heart and lung problems) and reaction to medications. Risks specifically related to breast surgery in which the lymph nodes in the armpit (axillary lymph nodes) are removed include swelling of the arm called lymphedema and difficulties in the arm and shoulder movement called shoulder dysfunction. These can be prevented and managed. For this, certain specific exercises should be performed regularly. This book, however does not deal with other common problems reported during treatment of breast cancer.

Breast cancer affects many parts of your life. You have to cope with the emotional strain of the diagnosis and the discomfort of treatment, along with the stresses of everyday life. The treatment related events can have a significant impact on quality of life, overall well-being, including mental and physical health, ability to perform daily roles, sexual function, pain and fatigue. Breast cancer can affect how you feel inside and out. You may have short- and long-term side effects from the breast cancer itself as well as from the treatment. After treatment ends, health and non-health related issues (such as financial concerns) can impact your quality of life. Although you cannot get rid of all of these factors, there are ways to manage them and improve your quality of life.

Present book attempts to provide a guide to breast cancer patients. Women must not give up or think of being diagnosed with breast cancer as a death sentence. Although the news of being a breast cancer patient is not at all welcoming, it may act as a wakeup call. Your attitude towards life may change. You become more concerned and focused about the important things in your life. You may learn so much about yourself in a completely different light. Being a survivor also puts you in a unique position to help others affected by breast cancer.

Exercises after breast surgery

Mastectomy is a major surgical procedure. Recovery from this traumatic event can take lot of time and may be painful. After breast surgery, many people experience restriction in their ability to move their arm, chest area, shoulder and back on the affected side. When one of their breasts has been removed, many patients may not feel their body as balanced. The back and neck might become tense as the body tries to adjust to accommodate the change in the distribution of the weight. There may be a tingling sensation in the arm and fingers. The patient may also experience swelling in the arm and hand, if some of their lymph nodes have also been removed during surgery.

Role of exercise after breast surgery

A specific set of exercises may help to provide relief from the above mentioned problems which a patient may experience after breast surgery. **These exercises** are an important step in recovery of the patient. They can be used as a stepping stone to fit a new way of life and routine. The information given in this chapter regarding the exercises can help the patients in facilitating their recovery. Often, women have a variety of fears and misconceptions about exercising during their treatment or recovery. Failure to do the exercises may prolong the disuse of the arm. This can lead to the development of contractures. Regular exercises will also have a positive impact on the wellbeing of the patient.

Purpose of doing exercises after breast surgery: Performing regular exercises after breast surgery will:

- Increase the range of movement of arm and shoulder.
- Prevent any long-term problems after surgery, e.g. restriction in the arm and shoulder movement, stiffness in the arm and shoulderand problems with the posture.
- Reduce the risk of lymphedema (swelling caused by collection of lymph fluid).
- Improve the quality of life of the patients.
- Help to elevate mood, ease anxiety and improve your overall health.

General guidelines for doing the exercises

Following are certain points that you should keep in mind while doing the exercises.

- Always warm up before doing exercises.
- It may be helpful to do the exercises after a warm bath/shower when muscles are warm and relaxed.
- Wear comfortable, loose clothing while doing the exercises.
- Perform the exercises with your unaffected arm first and then with your affected arm.
- Do the exercises until you feel some stretch. Hold each stretch at the end of the motion and slowly count to 5. It is normal to feel some pulling as you stretch the skin and muscles that have been shortened because of the surgery.
- Do not bounce or make any jerky movements when doing any of the exercises.
- If you are doing exercises properly you should not feel pain as you do the exercises. Only gentle stretching should be there.

- If pain is there get a proper guidance from your doctor.
- Try to do each exercise correctly. If you have trouble with the exercises, talk to your doctor.
- Do the exercises twice a day until you get back to your normal flexibility and strength.
- Be sure to take deep breaths, in and out, as you do each exercise.
- Try to improve and achieve higher range of motion every day as you exercise.
- Do check your posture: it is important to have good posture while you are exercising. It is quite common to find postural changes after surgery. The best way to check postural changes is to do the exercises in front of a large full length mirror.
- Always do cool down exercises at the end of main session.

Concerns of the patients about exercises

It is normal for patient to feel apprehensive when she is told to do exercises after operation. Any person would feel that after operation exercises may harm the body as stitches might be raw. However, it is safe to do exercises. These would not harm the site of operation.

How hard are the exercises?

The exercises may seem uncomfortable at first. But the more you do them the easier they will become. While doing the exercises you may feel some pain. A stretching and pulling sensation is normal. It is important that you always complete the warm up at the beginning of exercise session and cool down at the end of each exercise session to help avoid injury and prevent stiffness. If, at any stage you become concerned about your range of movement or level of discomfort, report this to your doctor.

How long should a patient keep doing the exercises?

Muscles are prone to atrophy and stiffness if not used regularly. Arm stiffness or weakness can occur long after surgery and following radiotherapy. So, it is important to carry on with these exercises till your full range of movement and strength of muscles is achieved.

Types of exercises to be done by the patients

The various exercises which are to be carried out by the patients who have undergone breast surgery are grouped into two levels as under depending on their stage of recovery.

Level-I: Mobilization exercises

When to start: After 4 weeks of surgery, even if the removal of drains has not been done.

When to stop: Continue these exercises till you achieve your full range of motion.

Level-I exercises include:

1. Shoulder shrug
2. Shoulder flexion
3. Overhead reach
4. Open-close hand
5. Front wall slide
6. Side wall slide
7. Chest wall stretch
8. Back reach
9. Arm circles
10. Shoulder blade squeeze

Level-II: Strength training exercises

When to start: After 6 weeks of surgery, you should start doing strength training exercises along with the mobilization exercises.

When to stop: Continue these exercises till you achieve your full range of motion and strength.

Level-II exercises include:

1. Shoulder flexion with weights
2. Shoulder abduction with weights
3. Shoulder extension with weights
4. Chest wall strengthening with weights

All the exercises have been discussed in detail as follows:

Warm up Exercises

Before starting level-I exercises you should perform warm up exercises. Warm-up is one of the most important elements of an exercise program. It is particularly important to prevent injury. Warm-up is a low level activity, which should be completed prior to more strenuous exercise. The objective of the warm-up is to raise the muscle temperature and total body temperature to prepare the entire body for vigorous activity. The warm-up period prepares the cardiovascular system, respiratory system, nervous system and the musculoskeletal system for main set of exercises. Warm up helps by gradually increasing the demand on those systems so that they are able to accommodate the demands of more strenuous activity during exercise.

Risks of not performing warm up

- Exertion level increases
- Muscle cramps
- Muscle tear
- Muscle strain
- Faintness, dizziness

Two warm up exercises have been described. Do these exercises every time in the beginning of each exercise session. Same set of exercises can be done as cool down exercises.

1. **Walking**- Walking is a gentle, low-impact exercise which is accessible to everybody. It is very much safe and simple. It does not require any practice. Walking not only helps in a better metabolism by leading to a good digestion but also increases your appetite.

   Walk for five minutes slowly with your arms swinging freely by your sides.
2. **Deep breathing exercise**: This exercise is important for controlling pain, for relaxation and for relieving tightness in the chest and back. You can perform these exercises in the lying down or sitting position as per your comfort. Follow these steps:

   (a) While lying (Pix. 1a and 1b)

   - Lie down face up on a bed, head resting on a pillow and knees up (you can put a pillow underneath your knees).
   - Place your hand of the surgery side on your stomach and the other hand on your chest supporting the wound.
   - Breathe in deeply through the nose and feel your stomach rise (Pix 1a) with your hand.

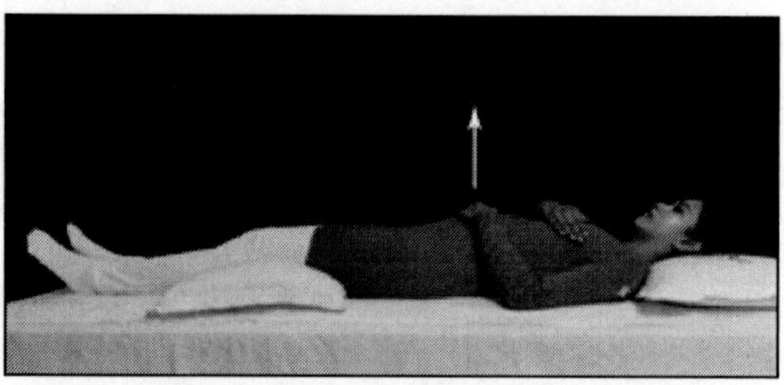

Pix. 1a: Belly rises as you inhale through nose.

- Breathe out through your mouth and feel your stomach fall (Pix. 1b)

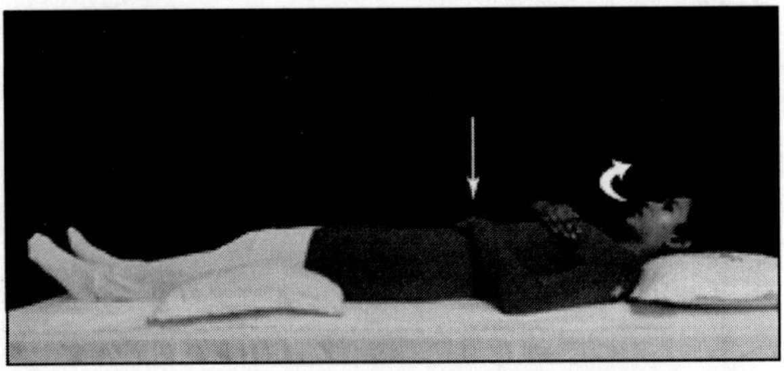

Pix. 1b: Belly falls as you exhale through mouth.

- Repeat for 10 times.

(b) While sitting down (Pix. 1c)

- Sit in a comfortable position on a stool, with your back straight and your feet flat on the floor.
- Place the hand of the surgery side on your stomach and opposite hand on your chest supporting the wound.
- Breathe in deeply through the nose and feel your stomach rise (Pix. 1c) with your hand.
- Breathe out through your mouth and feel your stomach fall with your hand.

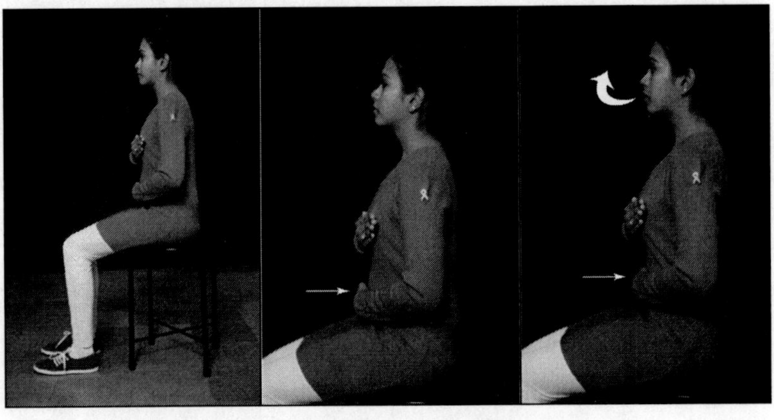

Pix. 1c: Deep breathing exercises while sitting.

- Continue to take deep breaths, concentrating on only moving your belly.
- Repeat for 10 times.

Tips for deep breathing exercises:

- ***If you are having trouble taking deep breathes, try breathing in through your nose and exhaling through your mouth normally.***
- ***To increase the whole duration you can slowly count to five in your mind as you breathe in and out and then increasing the number of counts to 6,7,8 till you reach your comfortable level.***

Level-I: Mobilization exercises

When to start: After 4 weeks of surgery even if the removal of drains have not been done.

This section consists of slow, controlled movements focusing on the upper body to help restore normal body and arm function after surgery. These 10 exercises aim to restore the movement in your shoulder joint. These should be done gently within your own comfort level.

All the exercises may be done first on the unaffected side and then on the affected

Before starting this section do warm up exercises, then do these 10 exercises and complete it with the cool down exercises. Even, if you are experiencing numbness over the chest, arm and armpit area, continue these exercises gently by supporting your wound and affected arm with your opposite hand. If you experience severe pain then do not persist with the exercises. At that time stop and do them gently later on during the day.

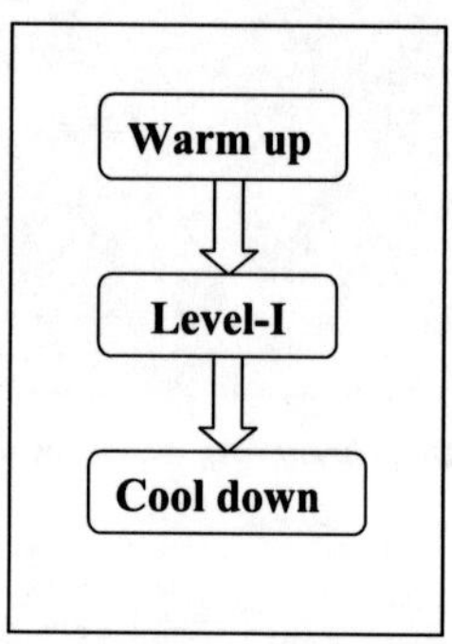

1. Shoulder shrug (Pix 2): This exercise increases shoulder elevation by moving the entire shoulder joint up to your ears. It also develops your upper trapezius, which is the broad, triangular muscle in your upper back and at the base of your neck.

- Stand with your feet about hip-width apart and back straight.
- Relax your arms by your sides so that the palms of your hands are facing the sides of your body as shown in Pix. 2.
- Lift your shoulders toward your ears as high as you are able to do.
- Hold this position for a slow count of 5.
- Lower your shoulders slowly down to the starting position.
- Repeat for 5 times to complete one set.
- Relax for short while and then repeat at least one more set.

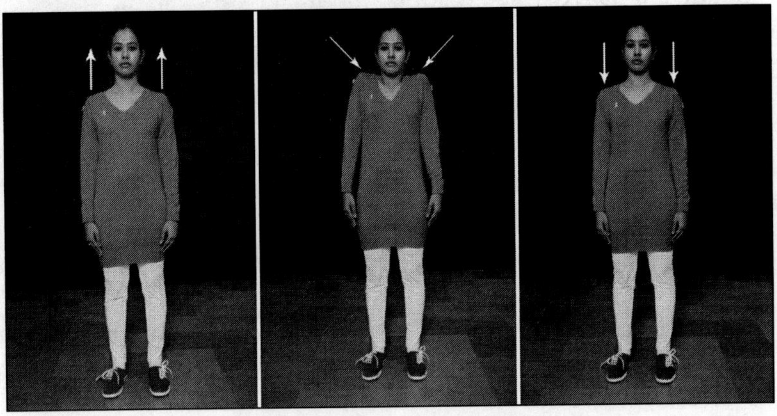

Pix. 2: Shoulder shrug exercise

Note:

- *Keep your arms relaxed at your side during the shrug.*
- *Do not lift your arms up in any way to assist your shoulders.*

2. Shoulder flexion (Pix. 3): It increases the mobility of the shoulder joint along with the strengthening of the shoulder flexor muscles.

- Stand comfortably with your feet about hip-width apart and back straight.
- Clasp your hands together in front as shown in Pix. 3.
- Straighten your arms and bring them steadily up in front of you- to about 90 degrees at shoulder height.

- Keep your elbows straight.
- Hold this position for a slow count of 5.
- Slowly return to the starting position.
- Repeat for 5 times to complete one set.
- Relax for short while and then repeat at least one more set.

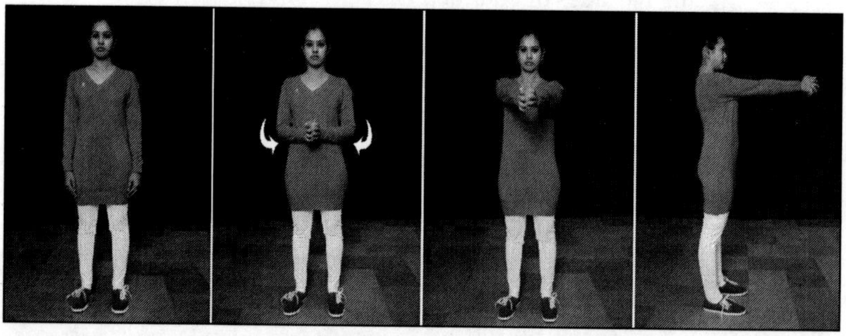

Pix. 3: Shoulder flexion (Front and side view)

3. Overhead Reach (Pix. 4): It stretches the muscles of your abdomen, back, shoulders and arms. It also stretches the underarm, which may feel tight after surgery.

- Stand comfortably with your feet about hip-width apart and back straight.
- Clasp your hands in front of you to about 90 degrees at your shoulder height (shoulder flexion position of previous exercise Pix.3).
- Keep your elbows straight.
- Slowly lift your arms up towards the ceiling upto the point of tightness.

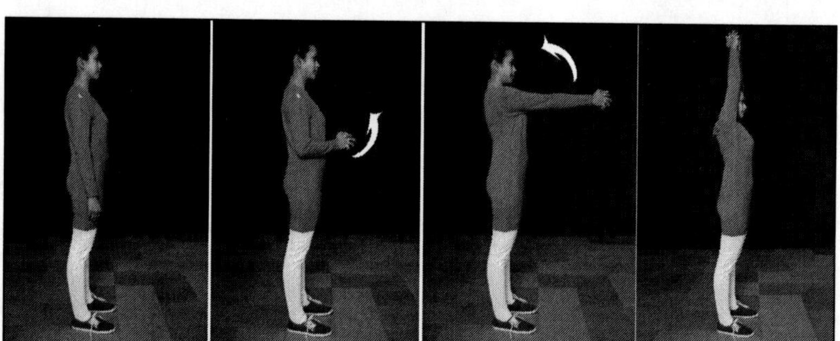

Pix. 4: Overhead reach (Side view)

- Hold this position for a slow count of 5.
- Slowly return to the starting position.
- Repeat for 5 times to complete one set.
- Relax for a short while and then perform one more set.

> Note:
> - *Support the affected arm with the unaffected arm while lifting up.*

4. Open-close hands: Opening and closing fist is known as the pumping motion. This primary pumping action is very useful for lymphatic and venous drainage. It pumps blood throughout the arm and helps in healing.

(a) At the level of waist (Pixs. 5a and 5b)

- Stand with your feet about hip-width apart and back straight.
- Keep your arms at your sides with elbows flexed and touching your body.
- Make a tight fist and slowly count to 5.
- Open up your fingers and hold this position for a slow count of 5.
- Repeat this pumping motion for 5 times to complete one set.
- Relax for a short while and then perform at least one more set.

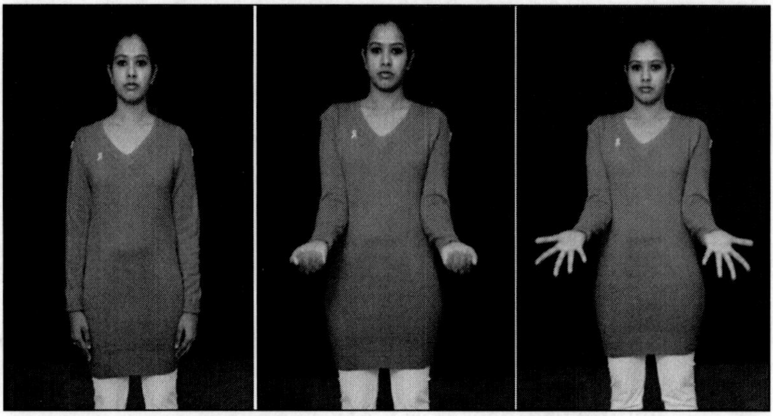

Pix. 5a: Fist closed at waist level ***Pix. 5b: Fist opened at waist level***

(b) Above your head (Pixs. 5c and 5d)

- Stand with your feet about hip width apart and back straight.
- Keep your elbows fully extended with arms placed overhead.
- Make a tight fist and slowly count upto 5.
- Open up your fingers and hold this position for a slow count of 5.
- Repeat this pumping motion for 5 times to complete one set.
- Relax for short while and then repeat at least one more set.

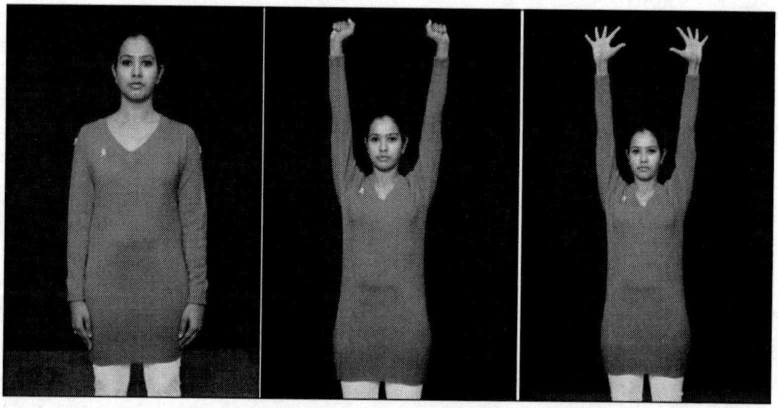

Pix. 5c: Fist closed overhead. ***Pix. 5d: Fist opened overhead.***

5. Front wall slide (Pix. 6): It stretches the muscles of the chest, shoulder, back as well as the underarm area. This improves your range of motion.

- Stand in a comfortable position facing the wall at a distance of 5-7 inches.
- Place the hands on the wall at shoulder level with elbows slightly bend.
- Keep your back straight.
- Slide your unaffected hand up on the wall then, try to reach this position with your affected hand.
- Gradually, slide your-hands up the wall as high as you can to the point of tightness.
- Move towards the wall as you go up.
- When your body comes in contact with the wall, hold the stretch for a slow count of 5.
- Slowly slide your hands down back to the starting position.

- Move away from the wall as you come down.
- Repeat for 5 times to complete one set.
- Relax for short while and then repeat at least one more set.

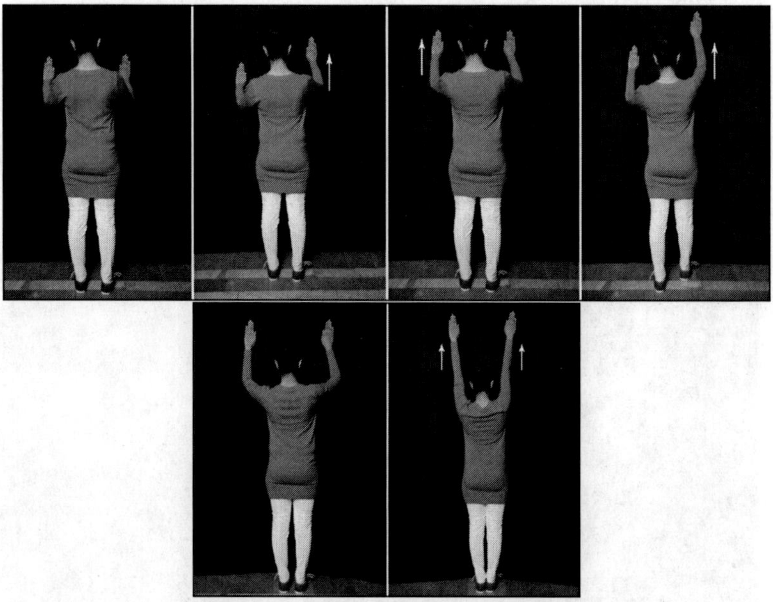

Pix. 6: Different positions of doing front wall slide exercise

6. Side Wall slide (Pix. 7): It stretches the muscles of the chest, shoulderand back as well as the underarm area. This improves your range of motion.

- Stand in a comfortable position at an arm's distance next to a wall.
- Keep your back straight.
- Place your one hand of unaffected side on the wall at shoulder height.
- Keep your elbow straight at an angle of about 90° with the wall.
- Slide your hand up the wall as high as you can upto the point of tightness.
- Move towards the wall as you go up.
- When your body comes in contact with the wall, hold the stretch for a slow count of 5.
- Slowly slide your hand back to the starting position, side by side move away from the wall.

- Repeat for 5 times to complete one set.
- Relax for short while and then repeat at least one more set.
- Alternate with the other hand.

Note:
- *You can do the exercise firstly with your unaffected hand and then with your affected hand.*

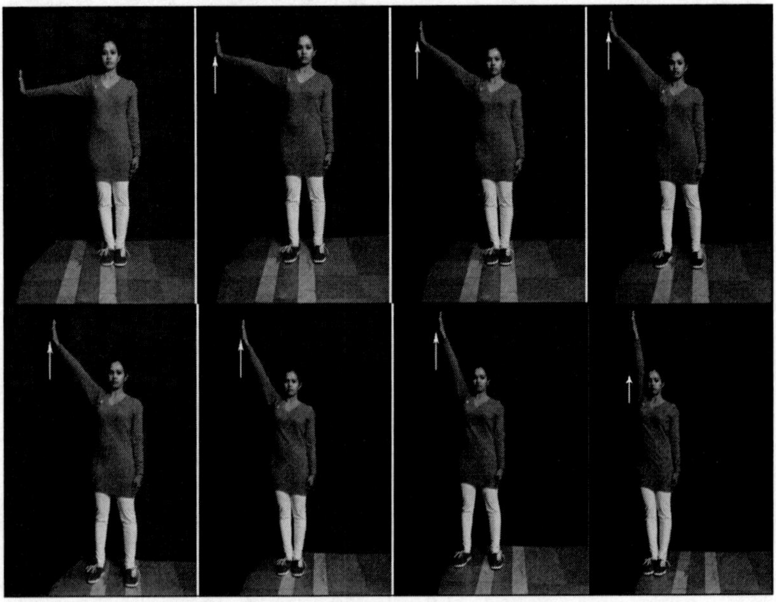

Pix. 7: Different positions of performing side wall slide exercise.

7. Chest wall stretch (Pix. 8): This exercise helps increase the mobility of the front of your chest and shoulder as it stretches the front muscles of chest.

- Stand in a comfortable position with your feet about hip width apart and back straight.
- Clasp your hands behind the neck with elbows pointing in front of the body.
- Gradually stretch your elbows backward.
- A stretch will be felt on the chest wall.
- Hold this position for a slow count of 5.
- Slowly return back to the starting position.

- Repeat for 5 times to complete one set.
- Relax for short while and then repeat at least one more set.

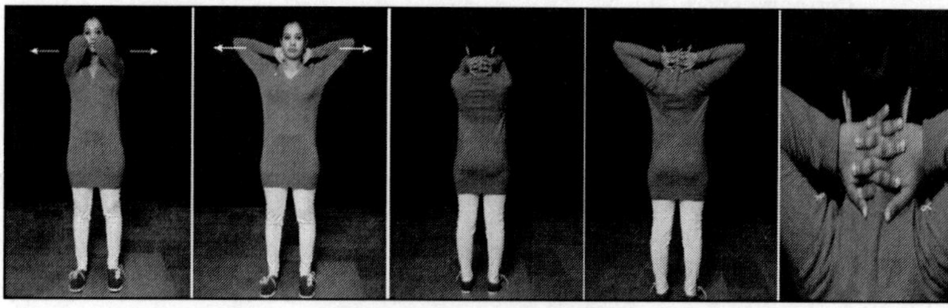

Pix. 8: Chest wall stretch front and back view

8. Back reach (Pix. 9): This exercise increases flexibility of arms and helps in gaining strength.

- Stand in a comfortable position with your feet about hip width apart and back straight.
- Place your hands behind your backand grasp your one hand with the other hand.
- Slowly slide your hands up towards the centre of the back as far as possible till you feel the stretch.
- Hold this position for a slow count of 5.
- Slowly slide down to the starting position.
- Repeat for 5 times to complete one set.
- Relax for short while and then repeat at least one more set.
- Alternate with the other hand.

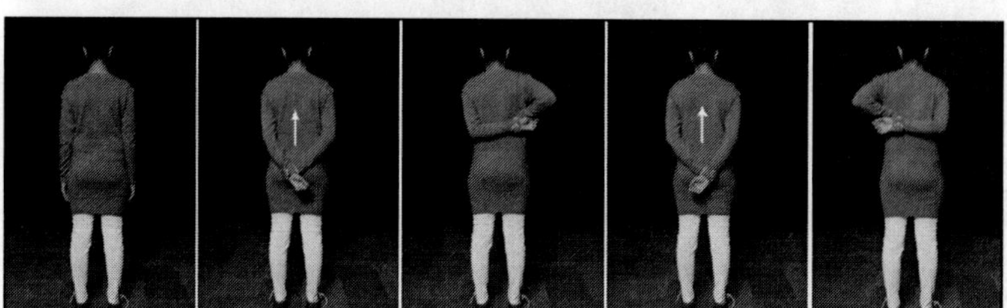

Pix. 9: Different positions of hand while performing back reach.

Note:

- *You can do the exercise firstly with your unaffected hand and then with your affected hand.*

9. Arm circles (Pix. 10): This exercise tones and tightens upper arm muscles and increases your range of motion.

- Stand in a comfortable position with your feet about hip width apart and back straight.
- Keep your arms at your sides.
- Raise your one arm out to the side at the shoulder height with your elbows straight.
- Make slow backward circles in the air with your arm.
- Return slowly to the starting position.
- Repeat for 5 times to complete one set.
- Relax for short while and then repeat at least one more set.
- Alternate with your other arm.

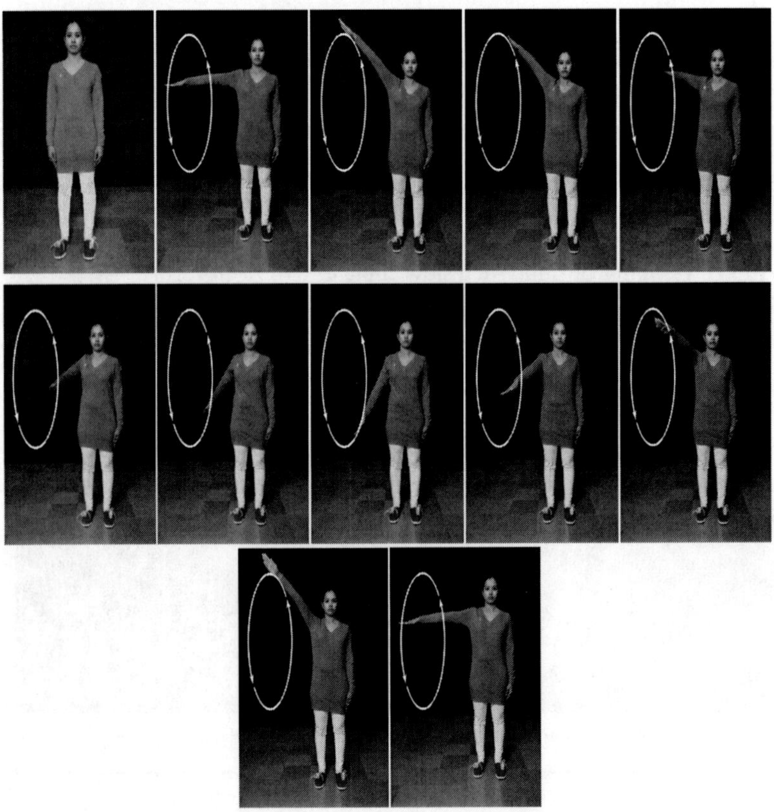

Pix. 10: Different positions of performing arm circles.

Note:

- *Be sure that the movement is occurring at the shoulder and not at the elbow.*
- *Increase the size of the circles until they are as large as you can comfortably make them.*
- *You can do the exercise firstly with your unaffected hand and then with your affected hand.*

10. Shoulder blade squeeze (Pix. 11): This exercise helps to increase shoulder blade movement. It engages the upper and middle back and improves shoulder mobility. It also opens up the chest, which is important for good posture.

- Stand in a comfortable position with your feet about hip width apart and back straight.
- Keep your arms at your sides with your elbows bent and palms facing down.
- Squeeze your shoulder blades together, bringing your elbows behind you. Palms come near your waist as you do so.
- Imagine you are trying to squeeze a pencil between your shoulder blades.
- Hold this position for a slow count of 5.
- Slowly return to the starting position.
- Repeat for 5 times to complete one set.
- Relax for short while and then perform at least one more set.

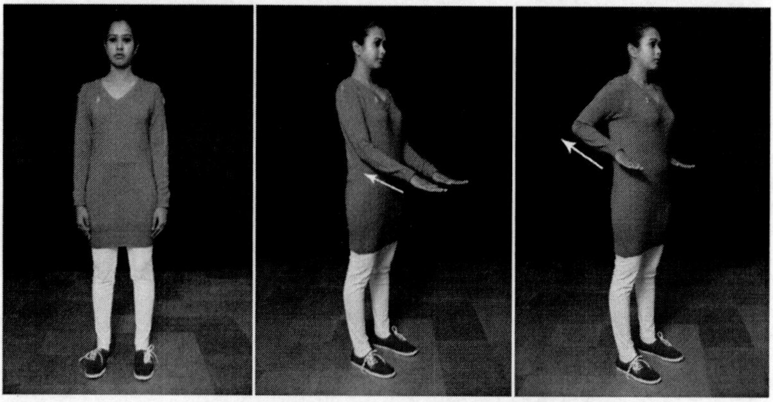

Pix. 11: Shoulder blade squeeze exercise.

Note:

- *Do not lift your shoulders up toward your ears as you squeeze your shoulder blades together.*

Level-II Strength training exercises (6 weeks after surgery and onwards)

When to start: After 6 weeks of surgery along with level-I you should start level-II exercises.

This section includes 4 well-designed strength-training exercises which can provide huge benefits. Strength training not only builds stronger muscles, but also builds stronger connective tissues and increases joint stability. This acts as reinforcement for the joints and helps prevent injury. Strength training improves balance and decreases your risk for injury. Strength training has been effective in increasing bone density and strengthening tendons and ligaments. Developing strong bones reduces the risk of developing osteoporosis and decreases the risk of bone fractures. Lifting weights can also improve your posture taking strain off your spine. Strength training improves your ability to lift objects of daily use. Despite the proven benefits of strength training, many women do not lift weights for the fear of developing large muscles and gaining weight which is a misconception.

Start with warm up, do Level-I, and then do these 4 strength training exercises of level-II completing the work up with cool down exercises.

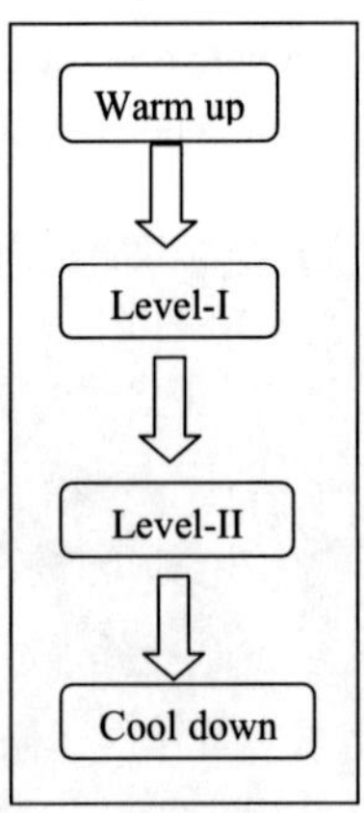

General instructions:

- Do these strength training exercises three days per week, with a day of rest in between.

- Perform every exercise at a slow, controlled and consistent rate of speed throughout the movement.
- Breathe through each exercise, inadvertently holding your breath while strength training can cause excessive stress to your heart.
- Do these exercise firstly with your unaffected arm and then try to do the same with your affected arm.
- For these strength training exercises you will require two dumbbells of 1 kg.
- If dumbbells are not available you can replace dumbbells with 1 Litre filled water bottles or you can use measuring weights of 1kg.

1. Shoulder flexion with weights (Pix. 12)

- Stand with your feet joined and back straight.
- Hold dumbbell of 1 kg. in your one hand.
- Raise this arm at shoulder level in front of you at about 90 degrees.
- Keep your elbow straight.
- Hold this position for a slow count of 5 and feel the stretch.
- Slowly return back to the starting position.
- Repeat for 5 times in one set.
- Rest for a while and perform one set with your other arm.
- Now again rest for a while and perform one set with both the arms together.

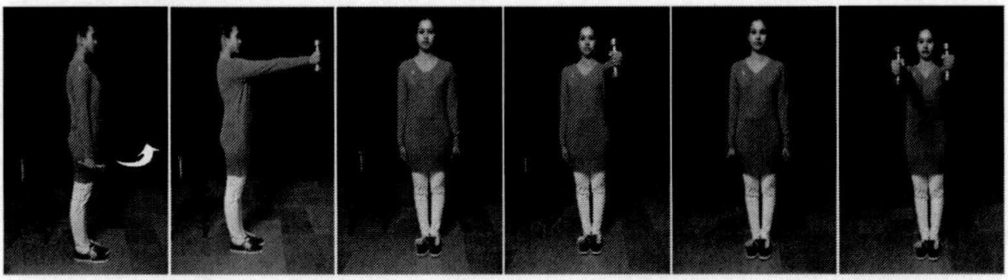

Pix. 12: Different positions of performing shoulder flexion with weights.

Note:

- *If you are not able to do the exercise with your affected arm for the first time holding weights, do it without weights for 5 times and then try to carry weights and do the same exercise.*
- *If dumb bells are not available with you, use 1 Lt. filled water bottle or 1kg of measuringweights.*

2. Shoulder abduction with weights (Pix. 13):

- Stand upright with your feet joined and back straight.
- Keep your arms to your sides and hold 1 kg. dumb bell in one hand.
- Raise this arm to your side at shoulder level.
- Keep your elbow straight.
- Hold this position for a slow count of 5.
- Slowly return back to the starting position.
- Repeat for 5 times in one set.
- Rest for a while and perform one set with your other arm.
- Now again rest for a while and perform one set with both the arms together.

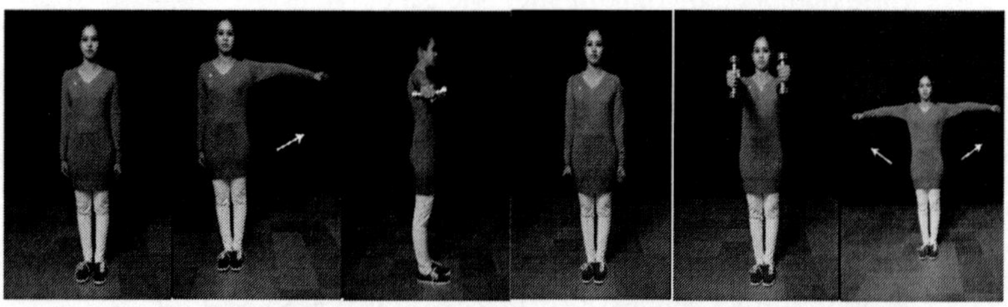

Pix. 13: Shoulder abduction exercise with 1 kg. dumbbell front and side view

Note:

- *If you are not able to do the exercise with your affected arm for the first time holding weights, do it without weights for 5 times and then try to carry weights and do the same exercise.*
- *If dumb bells are not available with you, use 1 Lt. filled water bottle or 1kg of measuring weight.*

3. Shoulder extension with weights (Pix. 14):

- Stand upright with your feet joined and back straight.
- Hold 1 kg. dumbbell in one hand.
- Take this arm back as far as possible till you feel the stretch.
- Keep your elbow straight.
- Hold this position for a slow count of 5.
- Slowly return back to the starting position.
- Repeat for 5 times in one set.
- Rest for a while and perform one set with your other arm.

- Now again rest for a while and perform one set with both the arms together.

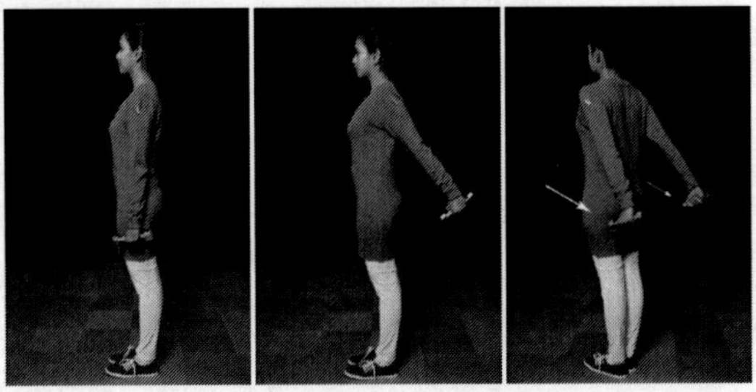

Pix. 14: Shoulder extension exercise with 1 kg. dumbbell

Note:

- *If you are not able to do the exercise with your affected arm for the first time holding weights, do it without weights for 5 times and then try to carry weights and do the same exercise.*
- *If dumb bells are not available with you, use 1 Lt. filled water bottle or 1kg of measuring weight.*

4. Chest wall strengthening with weights (Pix. 15):

- Stand upright with your feet joined and back straight.
- Hold 1 kg. dumb bell in one hand.
- Raise this arm at shoulder level at about 90° in front of you (shoulder flexion position Pix.14).
- Keep your elbow straight.
- Gradually take this arm away from your body to your side at shoulder level keeping elbow straight.
- You will feel the stretch at chest wall.
- Hold this position for a slow count of 5.
- Slowly return to the starting position.
- Repeat for 5 times in one set.
- Rest for a while and perform one set with your other arm.
- Now again rest for a while and perform one set with both the arms together.

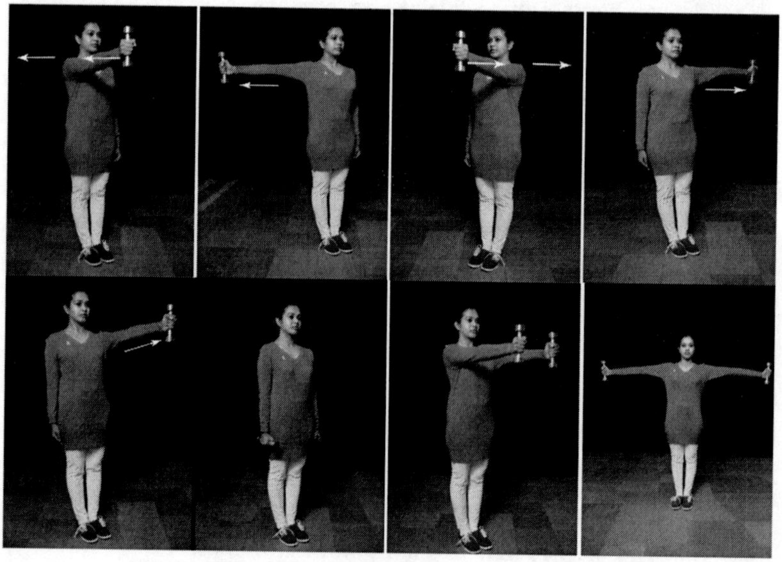

Pix. 15: Chest wall strengthening with the help of weights

Note:
- *If you are not able to do the exercise with your affected arm for the first time holding weights, do it without weights for 5 times and then try to carry weights and do the same exercise.*
- *If dumb bells are not available with you, use 1 Lt. filled water bottle or 1kg of measuring weight.*
- *Keep the elbow straight.*

Cool Down

After performing level-I and level-II exercises always perform cool down exercises. Cooling down is equally important. It helps your heart rate and breathing to return towards resting levels gradually. It helps to avoid fainting or dizziness, which can result from blood pooling in the large muscles of the legs when vigorous activity is stopped suddenly.

Risks of not performing cool down
- Exertion level increases
- Muscle cramps
- Muscle tear
- Muscle strain
- Faintness, dizziness

These exercises have been explained in detail in warm up section. Do these exercises at the end of every exercise session as cool down:

1. Walk for 5 minutes
2. Perform deep breathing exercise

Some important key points to remember regarding exercise

Do's:

- Exercise in pain free range.
- Exercise 2-3 times daily, if you can.
- Contact your doctor if you experience unexplained swelling or pain.
- Consult your doctor if your shoulder movements remain tight or if you experience swelling in your hand or arm even after exercising.
- Use your unaffected arm (on the side where surgery was not done) for injections, blood test and to check blood pressure.
- Use your unaffected arm to carry heavy items.
- Avoid tightly fitting jewellery and cuffs.
- Use your affected arm (on the side where surgery was done) as you normally would when you comb your hair, bathe, get dressed and eat.
- Try walking around with the natural swing of the arm after surgery, even though you feel tightness in the arm and around the wound.

Don'ts:

- Do not wear clothes like *duppatta* or *sari* while doing exercises as they can entangle or interfere in the movement.
- Do not over exercise.
- Do not hesitate to contact your doctor if you have a question.
- Do not let mastectomy arm hang down, especially when holding or carrying objects.
- Do not move arm quickly, or with jerking, pulling motions. Learn to move slowly and smoothly, especially when changing positions, lifting bags, opening doors, etc.
- Do not wear shoulder bags on the affected arm. The pressure of the strap on the shoulder can cause lymphedema. Avoid use of shoulder bags indefinitely.
- Do not continue an exercise upon unusual discomfort or persisting pain.

- Do not continue an exercise upon unusual fatigue. Rest for a moment, breathe, relax, and then continue slowly and carefully. If fatigue persists, stop exercising.
- Do not ever give up!

Prevention of arm lymphedema

In our body blood is circulated through arteries and veins. There is another channel of thin tubes for transport of lymph known as the lymphatic system consisting of lymph vessels and lymph nodes. Lymph is the fluid that carries immune cells (mostly lymphocytes) and proteins found in the blood throughout the body. Lymph nodes are located at focal points in this network of lymph vessels. Basically the lymphatic system carries our disease fighting immune cells to all parts of body. Lymph nodes capture disease causing bacteria. When we have infection lymph nodes get enlarged. This lymphatic system can be blocked due to various reasons. This leads to lymphedema. Arm lymphedema is an abnormal buildup of fluid (lymph) that causes swelling in the arms. This happens in breast cancer cases also. Lymphedema is a side effect of breast cancer surgery because the lymph nodes in the axilla are removed. The addition of radiotherapy to surgery increases the chances of developing lymphedema. Because of these, lymph is not removed from the arm. It starts accumulating and leads to swelling in the arm. Lymphedema in the arms and hands occurs in about 5% to 40% of women who have had a breast removal (mastectomy) with removal of all the axillary (underarm) lymph nodes.

Signs and symptoms of lymphedema: In the initial stage, it may be difficult to notice lymphedema. However, if the patients may experience following symptoms, it may be a hint that lymphedema has developed:

- Feeling of tightness in the shoulder, arm or hand.
- Movements in the joints such as shoulder, hand or wrist become restricted.
- Joints feel less flexible.
- Changes in the skin texture.
- Skin may feel tight, hard or may look red.
- Feeling of discomfort in that area.
- Difficulty fitting into clothing in one specific area of arm.
- Weakness in the arm.
- Tight-fitting bracelet, watch, or ring that was not tight before.

Following factors may increase chances of lymphedema after breast surgery

- During breast cancer treatment, if the patient received radiation therapy or had lymph nodes removed.

- Trauma to the muscles or skin of the arm that can lead to infection. These include scratches, insect bites, sunburn, kitchen burns, garden cuts, plant rashes, and skin dryness.
- Gaining a lot of weight after breast cancer treatment.
- Very hot weather and sitting in hot tubs while taking tub bath can cause lymphedema. Heat widens up blood vessels. It allows more fluid to collect in an area. This increases the risk of swelling.

Prevention and control of lymphedema: Although, it is not possible to predict who will develop lymphedema, certain steps can be taken to reduce the risk of its development. Some basic guidelines to lower the risk of lymphedema are as follows:

1. **Avoid infections:** Good hygiene and careful skin care may reduce the risk of lymphedema. So, practice the following measures:
   - Frequently wash your hands with soap and warm water, especially before preparing food, after using the bathroom and after touching soiled linens or clothes.
   - Protect your skin from scratches, sores, burns and other irritations that might lead to infection.
   - Use insect repellents to prevent insect bites.
   - Immediately report any signs of infection to your doctor.
   - Keep your arm always clean.
   - Wear protective gloves when doing household chores that use chemical cleansers or steel wool, while gardening or doing yard workand while washing dishes.
   - Wear a thimble/rubber finger when sewing to prevent cuts from needle and pin pricks to your fingers.
   - If you are stung by a bee or insect on the affected arm, clean and put ice on that area and raise the arm above your head. Keep it clean and consult your doctor if the sting shows any signs of infection.
   - Avoid extreme cold.
2. **Avoid burns and high heat:** Burns can cause extra fluid to build up and cause swelling when lymph nodes have been removed or damaged.
   - Protect your arm from sunburn.
   - Use oven mitts that cover your lower arm.
   - Avoid oil splash burns from frying; burns from microwave cooked foods or boiling liquids.

- Avoid high heat, such as from hot tubs and saunas.
- Do not use heating pad on the affected areas.
- It is better to avoid such tasks which involve working with high heat. Get these done by others (maids, relatives).

3. **Avoid constriction in the affected arm:** Squeezingof arm may increase pressure in nearby blood vessels. This may lead to increase fluid and swelling. Follow these simple steps to avoid it:
   - Wear loose jewellery, clothing and gloves.
   - Avoid anything that forms a snug band around your arm or wrist.
   - Do not use shoulder straps when carrying hand bags and purses.
   - Wear loose fitting bra with padded straps that do not dig into your shoulder.
   - After surgery, use light weight prosthesis (breast form). A heavy prosthesis may put too much pressure on the affected area.
   - Have your blood pressure taken on the unaffected arm. If both arms are affected, blood pressure can be taken on your thigh.
4. **Avoid muscle strain:**It is important to use your affected arm for daily activities. It will help you heal properly and regain strength. This includes doing things like combing your hair, bathing, dressing up, eating etc. Using your muscles help in avoiding strains and also helps to drain lymph fluid from your arm. Some tips to follow:
   - Use your affected arm as normally as you can. Once you are fully healed you can begin to go back to all activities you did before your surgery.
   - Exercise regularly.
   - Before doing any exercise, talk with your doctor. They can help you set goals and limits so that you can work at the level of activity that is right for you.
   - If your arm starts to ache, lie down and raise it above the level of your heart.
   - Avoid vigorous, repeated activities.
   - Avoid lifting or pulling loads.
   - Use your unaffected arm or both the arms to carry heavy packages, groceries, handbags, or children (use strolley or wheelers).

5. Avoid gaining weight*:* Extra fat requires more blood vessels. This means more fluid in the arm and chest area which places a greater burden on the lymph vessels that are left after surgery. Women who are obese are more likely to have severe lymphedema. Some tips to follow:

- Agood diet and regular exercise can help you maintain a healthy weight.
- Try to reduce the stress in your life.
- Get enough sleep too.

6. Maintain good nutrition: During and after treatment try to take healthy and balanced diet. For details on nutrition and diet please refer to Chapter-4 of this book.

7. Exercise regularly: To avoid problems like shoulder dysfunction, arm lymphedema and overweight do regular exercises. For details on exercises to be done after surgery please refer to Chapter-2 of this book.

8. When to contact doctor: You should immediately inform your doctor if you notice any of these symptoms:

- Redness, swelling, a skin rash, or blistering on the side of your body where you had surgery, or if you have a temperature greater than 100.4 degree F (38 degrees C).
- These warning signs of infection could be an early sign of lymphedema and should be treated immediately.

Some important Do's and Don'ts for preventing lymphedema

Do's:

- Moisturize your skin frequently and regularly.
- Keep your hand and arm extra-clean, but do not use harsh soaps.
- Wear protective gloves while gardening and doing other yard work outside.
- Take more frequent rest breaks when scrubbing, mopping, cleaning, or while doing other vigorous or repetitive activities, especially if your arm feels tired, heavyor achy.
- Wear oven mitts when handling hot foods.
- Use insect repellents which do not dry out the skin. Avoid brands that contain a significant amount of alcohol.
- Apply antibiotic ointment to any insect bites or torn cuticles (as long as you are not allergic to its contents).
- Protect your arm from sunburn with sunscreen. Use a product with a minimum SPF of 15, although SPF 30 is much better.
- Use a thimble when you sew.

- Rest your arm in an elevated position. But do not hold up your arm without support for a long time because your muscles will tire or strain.
- Control your blood sugars very carefully if you have diabetes, to minimize the danger of damage to the small blood vessels and infection.
- Wear compression bandages or a compression sleeve and glove on the affected arm when flying in airplanes (if you already have arm swelling).

Don'ts

- Do not take unusually hot baths or showers.
- Do not go from extreme hot to cold water temperatures when you bathe or wash dishes.
- Do not go into high-heat hot tubs, saunas or steam baths.
- Do not apply heating pads or hot compresses to the arm, neck, shoulder or back on the affected side.
- Also, be cautious of other heat-producing treatments provided by physical; occupational; or massage therapists; such as ultrasound, whirlpool, fluidotherapy or deep tissue massage. Heat and vigorous massage encourages the body to send extra fluid into the compromised area.
- Do not carry heavy objects with your affected arm, especially with the arm hanging downward.
- Do not wear heavy shoulder bags on the affected side.
- Do not wear clothing that has tight sleeves or that restrains movement.
- Do not wear watch or other jewellery on your affected hand or arm.
- Do not use heavy breast prosthesis after mastectomy. It may put excessive pressure on alternative routes of lymphatic drainage that are already doing double duty.
- Do not drink alcohol. Alcohol causes blood vessels to expand and leak extra fluid into the tissues.
- Do not smoke. Smoking narrows the small blood vessels, lessening the flow of fluids in the arm.
- Do not get manicures that cut or overstress the skin around the nails.
- Do not permit blood pressure testing on your affected arm. If you have breast cancer in both the breasts, get your blood pressure to be tested on your thigh. If this is not possible, ask the concerned person to measure your blood pressure by inflating the cuff only slightly

above your normal systolic pressure (the first, higher number of your blood pressure).

- Do not permit the skin of your affected arm to be pierced for any reason like injections, drawing blood or vaccinations. If you have had breast cancer in both breasts along with underarm lymph node dissections, blood should be drawn from another part of your body. If blood must be drawn from your arm, use your non-dominant arm (your left arm, if you are right-handed; your right arm, if you are left-handed). If your one side had no lymph node dissection, use the arm on that side, regardless of whether it is your dominant arm.

Nutrition for patients after breast surgery; Care of breast cancer patients undergoing chemotherapy/ radiotherapy

(see related chapter elsewhere)

Breast Self Examination

Post mastectomy breast self examination

If you have undergone mastectomy on one side, you may be at risk of having breast cancer in your other breast. So, you should continue your breast self examination of the other breast on a regular basis. Irrespective of mastectomy of single or of both sides, you should check the areas for any kind of abnormalities where your surgery was performed. This is also called post mastectomy self examination. It includes examination of the incision as well as other areas around it. While doing post mastectomy self examination, you should look for any persistent rash or irritation in the areas of your scar, redness, colour changes, any discharge, swelling and skin thickening at the site of surgery. The examination should be performed in a well lit room. After washing your hands properly with soap and water, you can use your three middle fingers together using light, medium and deep pressure to feel for any lump or thickening at the site.

The patients with reconstructive surgery should also examine the reconstructed breast for redness or colour changes, any discharge, swelling and skin thickening after washing their hands properly with soap and water. They should also continue their regular BSE of the normal breast.

What is Breast self examination?

Breast self-examination (BSE) is a procedure which is performed by a woman to physically and visually examine herself for any changes in the breasts and underarm areas of the body. It is a method which may be used to detect early breast cancer. In this the woman herself looks at and feels each of her breasts for possible lumps, distortions or swelling. BSE should be done in addition to Clinical Breast Examination (CBE) which is performed by a doctor.

What is the main goal of BSE?

The main goal of breast self examination is to get used to the way your breasts look and feel. Knowing your breasts will help you notice any abnormality immediately in a better way. If, you find any abnormality, you can take necessary steps to prevent and correct them.

What is the right time to do BSE?

Women can begin practicing BSE at about age of 20 years. They can continue this practice throughout their lives, even during pregnancy and after menopause.

For pre-menopausal women: If you still menstruate the best time to perform the breast self examination is about a week after your period ends. At this time, your breasts usually are not tender or swollen.

For post menopausal women: If you have attained menopause you can fix up a day for breast examination. It should be performed on the same day each month (e.g. 1st of every month or 1st Sunday of every month).

For pregnant and breast feeding women: Women who are pregnant or breast-feeding can continue to examine their breasts every month. Breast-feeding mothers can examine their breasts after feeding the baby so that the breasts have as little milk as possible. It will make the examination easier and more comfortable.

What should be focused on while examining breast?

You should look for the following changes in your breasts while performing BSE.

- Development of a lump or thickening of breast.
- Sticky or bloody discharge from your nipples.
- Swelling of the breast.
- An unusual increase in the size of one breast.
- Skin irritation or dimpling.
- Nipple abnormalities (such as pain, redness, scaliness, turning inward).

How to perform BSE?

There are certain steps of carrying out BSE. Follow these steps:

- Step 1-3 should be performed in the standing or sitting posture.
- Step 4 should be carried out in the lying down position.
- During all the steps there should be no clothes, above the waist.

Steps	

Step 1
➢ Stand in front of the mirror.
➢ Keep your shoulders straight
➢ Place your hands on your waist.
➢ Look at your breasts in the mirror for the following changes:
    ➢ Dimpling, puckering, or bulging of the skin.
    ➢ Nipple pushed inward.
    ➢ Redness, soreness, rash or swelling
	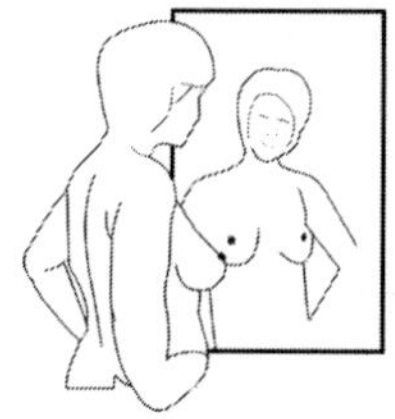
	Fig. 1: Hands on the waist

Step 2 ➢ Raise your arms. ➢ Clasp your hands above head. ➢ Look for the above said changes again.	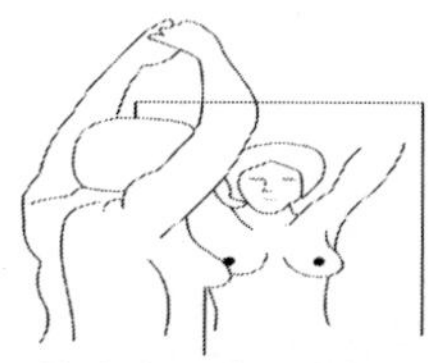 Fig. 2: Arms above the head
Step 3 While you are in front of the mirror, gently squeeze each nipple between your fingers and thumb and check for any nipple discharge (this could be a watery, milky or yellow fluid or blood).	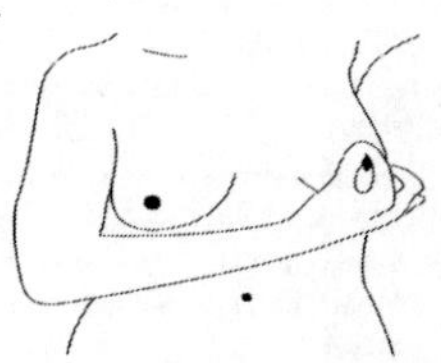 Fig. 3: Squeezing the nipple

Step 4
➢ Lie down
(In lying down position the breast tissue spreads evenly over the chest wall and is as thin as possible. It becomes much easier to feel all the breast tissue)
➢ Place a small pillow under your left shoulder.
➢ Keep your left arm behind your head (Fig 4).
➢ Use the finger pads of the 3 middle fingers of your right hand as shown in the figure to feel for lumps in the left breast (Fig 5).
➢ Use 3 different levels of pressure to feel all the breast tissue.
    ➢ **Light pressure** is needed to feel the tissue closest to the skin;
    ➢ **Medium pressure** to feel a little deeper and
    ➢ **Firm pressure** to feel the tissue closest to the chest and ribs.
➢ Follow a pattern to be sure that you cover the whole breast.
➢ Cover the entire breast. From top to bottom i.e. from your collarbone to the top of your abdomen and side to side i.e. from your armpit to your cleavage.
➢ For the circular movements (spiral pattern) begin at the nipple, moving in larger and larger circles until you reach the outer edge of the breast (Fig.6).
	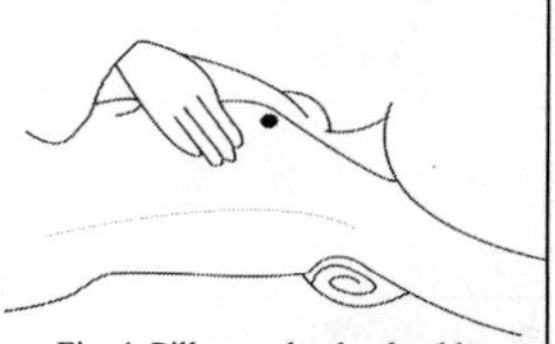
	Fig. 4: Pillow under the shoulder and left arm above the head
	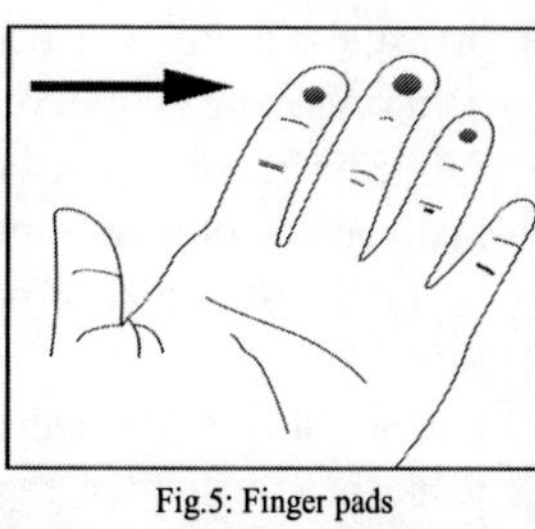
	Fig.5: Finger pads

- For the vertical movements (top to bottom and vice versa) start in the armpit and work down to the bottom of the bra line. Move one finger-width toward the middle and work up to the collarbone. Repeat until you have covered the entire breast (Fig 7).
- Repeat all these steps for the other breast.

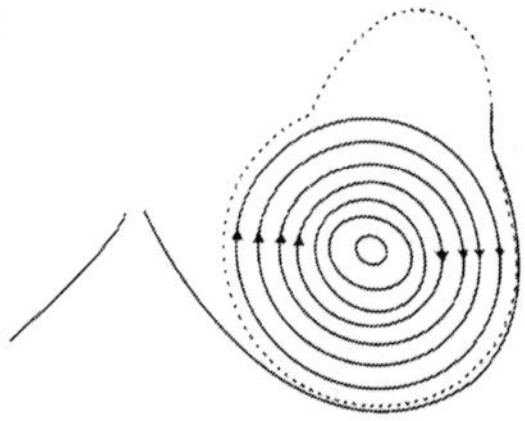

Fig. 6: circular movements

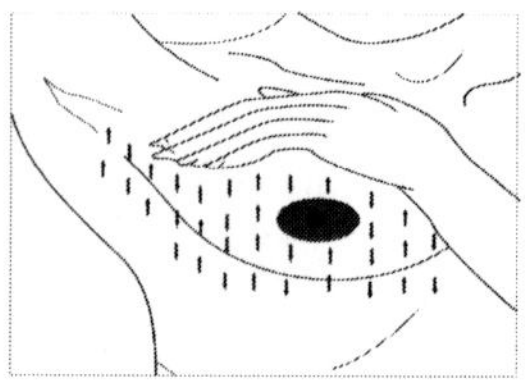

Fig. 7: Top to bottom and vice versa movements

Step 5: Many women find that the easiest way to feel their breasts is when their skin is wet and slippery, so they like to do this step in the shower. Actually soapy fingers slide easily across the breast and may increase your chances of detecting a change.

- While standing in the shower, place one arm over your head and lightly soap your breast on that side.
- Using the flat surface of your fingers, cover your entire breast, using the same hand movements as described in step 4.

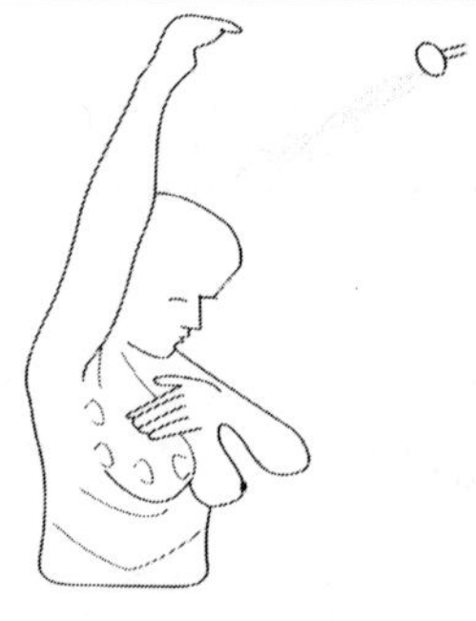

Fig. 8: BSE under the shower

Remember:

- While performing step 1 to 3, make sure there is good lighting.
- While performing step 4 and 5 i.e. examining your breast, complete with one breast first and then the second one. If you are starting with your right breast, put a pillow under your right shoulder, raise your right arm, place your right hand behind your head and use your left hand to feel your breast.
- While examining your breasts, do not take your hand off your breast so that you do not miss a spot.
- You may use lotion or powder to help your fingers glide easily over the skin.
- If you notice any change in any of your breast, do not panic, do not be tense, but consult the experts immediately.

Some experiences of breast cancer survivors

While writing this booklet we met many breast cancer patients who are living completely normal life after their treatment. They have won this battle of breast cancer by their will power, timely treatment and adopting certain strategies in their lives. We have put some of these real life stories of breast cancer survivors in this chapter to motivate and encourage patients.

Survivor: 1, Age: 41

I being the pampered queen of my hubby and loving mother of two daughters was enjoying my life. My job was my passion. Time was flying and I had no time to look around. But, my sixth sense was warning me time and again that something is going to be wrong somewhere, but what is that I could not realise. However, I was very conscious about my health, weight and especially about the breast cancer. One day while I was performing regular breast self examination in front of the mirror, I found a big dark patch on my back which was not there earlier. I showed it to the physician who said it may be due to tanning. Suddenly, one day in October 2010, I found a lump near my right arm pit. It gave me a huge shock. I started exploring internet and came to know that all the lumps are not malignant. Some lumps are benign. These types of lumps may appear during the periods and vanishes on their own. I waited till the start of my next menstrual cycle. But the lump still persisted.

My sixth sense started giving me alarming signals. I went to a nearby gynaecologist. She told me to go for mammography without any delay. Immediately, I went to the radiologist and within 2-3 hours it was confirmed that something was actually wrong. It was suggested that FNAC was the next step to know about the cancer stage. The whole world was shattered. I and my husband went for FNAC. I was very scared. On seeing tears in my eyes the doctor's words were "Madam, don't cry, you are not the only one and you are not the last one". During the procedure of FNAC he told me that malignancy is confirmed and instead of crying I should be prepared for its treatment and prognosis. On the funnier side, I told the doctor that it is not the disease which is scaring me, but it is the hospital, big machines, injections, operation procedure and stitches etc. which are troubling me. I, searched through the internet, talked to so many people and survivors. Ultimately, we narrowed down to PGI for its treatment.

Dr.Gurpreet Singh's name was recommended by a family friend who himself is an Oncologist at Delhi. Luckily Dr. G. Singh was available who, otherwise had a plan to attend a conference overseas. During my visit a very scary question was posed to me by the doctor- whether I want Lumpectomy or Mastectomy. I was at loss as I didn't know the answer. Then my doctor asked me to sit down calmly. Very politely, he explained me the pros and cons of both the procedures. Ultimately, it was decided that lumpectomy will be done. We decided to go first for surgery and then Chemotherapy. I was operated on 27th Dec, 2010. During my treatment I realised, that if you are aware about your disease and keep yourself updated then the things become very easy for you and for your doctors.

There was always a full support from my family and few very close friends. We all had decided that I will be allowed to meet and talk to only those people who see the positive side of life; to keep me positive. To avoid infection, I use to meet only few people. Everyone in PGI was very co-operative though at one time I had thought them to be as persons from different planet and those who didn't have any emotions. My two lymph nodes out of 23 were found to be infected in the biopsy test. FISH test was also done for HER2 protein which was found to be negative. I was diagnosed as a triple negative case. So, my chemo was decided accordingly.

After 03 weeks of the surgery, I went for Chemo port implantation. It was a havoc experience worse than the surgery. Anyhow, I was to be given eight cycles of chemo - four sets of each. In the meantime, my close friends kept on boosting my morale. First 3 days, after my first chemo were very troublesome. But, instead of popping in lots of relieving medicines, I opted for yoga and breathing exercises. I read, the '*Chicken Soup Series*' during my treatment which I found to be very encouraging. By the end of the first chemo, my hair fall started and it was a paining experience. To get over this, I decided to get my head shaved off. As the depression was gripping, friends and husband suggested that I should try to keep myself busy with the things I like the most. Since my work was my passion I decided to join back my office on the 3rd day after my first Chemo. Now, time started flying with my 9-5 job. My family and my friends took special care and made it sure that I should not think negatively. I was given complete home cooked food, abundance of fruits, coconut water, pomegranate and soya milk every day. I took wheatgrass juice throughout my treatment. My menstrual cycle ceased after Ist chemo. I started doing regular exercises, so that I should not put on much weight. After 8 cycles of Chemo, I was told that 25 cycles of radiotherapy and then booster doses will be given. The spirit of "*I can have cancer but cancer cannot have me*" was boosting me up. I usually, went for radiotherapy from my office and then return back to work. After one year of my surgery, no cancer cells were found in mammography. Today, I am following the proper schedule of follow ups. Since I was a triple negative case so Tamoxifen was not for me and I was given only Calcium and multivitamin. Except for few tit-bits, today I am living normal life. My periods started again after one year and are normal now. The pigmentation on my back is also gone. With full support of my husband, kids other members of my family and friends now only few traces of this bad dream are left. Positivity and indulgence in your passion plays the key role.

As a survivor I can suggest:

- Keep yourself update about your disease and treatment.
- Read motivational books like I read.
- Indulge in your passion.
- Trust your doctor.
- Do regular exercises.
- Have home cooked food and include lots of fruits and vegetables in your diet.
- Always be positive.

Survivor: 2, Age: 63

It has been five and half years, my body and mind faced a grave challenge of breast cancer. It was a very painful experience, but I gained a lot of experience from this; I learnt a lot. Now, by associating with 'Chandigarh Breast Cancer Trust' I am boosting the morale of women facing this challenge, encouraging them to maintain their strong will power on the basis of my experiences. I also thank God who provided me relief after tormenting me.

It was one morning of March, 2006 while taking bath; I experienced a kind of stiffness and a nodule on the lower part of my left breast. The difference became clear when I moved my hand over my right breast with a doubt. A myth was broken that treatment of menopausal symptoms is a guarantee of safety from cancer. I had to go with Gargi to Allahabad to participate in '*Hindi Sahitya Sammelan, Prayag*' on March, 26-27. Although my mind was full of doubts and I was sad still, I went there and spent three days among various authors and writers and had a good time. On 28th of March we had a plan to roam in *Benaras*, we even went but had to return because of Gargi's illness.

After returning back to Chandigarh the rounds of hospital started. I went to Sector-22 Polyclinic. They told me that the nodule was of course there but there was nothing to worry about. They advised for mammography. We got it done, but the report was not clear. Even needle test did not reveal anything. The surgeon at the Polyclinic was satisfied with the report and wrote a prescription of 15 days. I also thanked God. I shared my experience with my brothers and sisters-in-law. Even after 15 days of medication the nodule persisted. It could not be postponed anymore. I reached PGI, OPD alone on Wednesday morning at 8.30 am during summer vacations. I wanted to face the challenges of my condition on my own strength without doubting the love and understanding of my friends and siblings.

After my check-up first by a junior doctor and then by the senior Dr. Gurpreet Singh I was advised to go for biopsy on the same day. I got the needle and syringe from Sector-11 and deposited the requisite fee at the counter. I had to wait for the biopsy till 3 p.m. Dr. Preetish took 4 samples from the site of nodule and asked very politely, ‘Ma, did my injection cause a lot of pain?’ I laughed and said, ‘Needle prick will pain of course’. I submitted this sample along with the form in the lab of Research block-A and had lunch at 4 p.m. after returning home.

During the ensuing period of apprehension the checking of answer sheets helped me in involving myself in some activity. The report was expected only after 10 days. Before starting the treatment, I honoured my work commitments by checking 700 answer sheets continuously. I got the report on 19th of May, which confirmed the diagnosis of cancer. Then, I started having endless cooperation from my sisters, brothers, sisters-in-law and friends. One of my friends Mrs. Neeta Sehgal whose treatment was already being continued gave me many suggestions for enhancing encouragement. Sharing of the experiences by the sufferers gave me assurance that now cancer is treatable. From U.S. the husband of one of my cousin provided me the literature from ‘World Cancer Society’. My younger brother obtained full details on this disease from Dr. Gurpeet.

I was eager to start treatment early. The only worry was the ever extending strike of doctors on the issue of OBC reservation. Dr. Gurpreet assured that my treatment will start on 31st, of May whether strike continues or not. When I asked him, ‘If I would be O.K.’, he said, ‘We will only treat you, the will power to get well is to be displayed by you only’. Last scan was done on 30th of May and on 31st of May I got the first injection of chemotherapy. My long tresses and my figure which used to be appreciated by people were now the target of unknown enemies. I had always got pleasure and good results in all my struggles. I combated with my full self respect every challenging circumstance or untoward incidence in this ruthless world. So, I had developed a kind of faith that whatever happens is always for the good. I had penned following lines in one such phase of my life when I faced difficulties.

“I was thoroughly sidelined but, I had so much internal strength that every sideline become my supporter’

From 31st May to 13th of September I got 6 injections at the interval of 20 days each. Every injection process was of two and half hour ordeal. After first injection, I had to go to toilet every 15 minutes on first night. I started having nausea, vomiting, uneasiness and constipation from second evening onwards. After every injection I went to my brother’s place for 4-5 days and then return to my home. Anita took care of me like my daughter. My friends and neighbours never let me worry about how time passed.

All my hair disappeared from my head by the time I received my third injection. Throughout the day, I use to be busy arranging for my meals and for treatment of side effects of Chemotherapy. I massaged my injection arm with coconut oil 3-4 times; I use to do cold fermentation at night; I applied *Navratan* oil to my head and did mustard oil massage on legs and my back. I put cucumber slices on my eyes since these felt heavy. When my soles had a burning sensation I managed these with bottle gourd. I went for morning walks; in the evening I did acupressure. I did mild exercises and meditation. I also continued my academic work and reading as far as possible. Usually I went to sleep chanting '*Namaskar/Gayatri Mantra*' at night.

I had determined that I will win this battle with the help of my will power and through cooperation of friendly doctors. I came to know through cancer related literature that tomatoes, lemon, oranges has to be avoided and banana, potato, rice etc. are to be taken. My taste was altered. Sweet things tasted bitter and salt tasted tangy. I had nausea whenever I looked at chapattis. I survived on *Khichari, dalia*, bread, *suji* rusk, potato and fruits. In the evenings, I had soup of Bengal gram (*Kala Chana*). At night, I had *Isabgol* husk with luke warm milk. In the morning, I had *giloy* and wheat grass juice; then *gond katira* in milk; *awala murrabba* (Gooseberry), almonds etc.

All throughout the day, I ate something or the other. Apart from dietary supplements, I utilised whatever knowledge, I gained through reading cancer literature. Otherwise,mainstay was allopathic treatment. For example, I applied ginger juice on cancer affected area. I exposed the cancer point to early morning sun rays. After fourth injection, the nodule disappeared completely but still the whole process of treatment was to be continued. Six chemo injections; then operation (partial mastectomy); then 16 sittings of radiotherapy and yes I did not have to take temoxifen or any other medicines for five years.

Now, I am alright but by the last chemo my Hb went down to 8.9 gms and weight reduced to 48 kgs. Slowly, everything became ok. Hair became long and dense as before. Hb and weight all returned to normal.I Still include *gur*, *kala chana*, *moongfali*, *akhrot*, *badam*, *awala*, *paneer*, *ankurit moong*, green leafy vegetables and fruits in diet. Simultaneously, I also take vitamins, calcium and iron tablets. Even, after the treatment was over my digestion was fragile. But now, I have forgotten all this. This is also true, that whenever, anything happens to me I think about cancer only. The fear is not of the death, but what I am afraid of is running around for treatment. I wish no one gets any disease. But, when we have our bodies some or other disease will be there. Whenever, we have any problem we have to bear it, but, with the determination to get well.

Some suggestions:

- Regularly have an informal self check-up of your body.

- Instead of being afraid of disease, get yourself checked up whenever, you have a little doubt.
- Start treatment early, since cancer cells grow fast.
- On being diagnosed with cancer, rather than panicking try to remain happy, maintain your will power and take care of your diet.
- Main treatment of cancer is only in allopathy other modalities can only be assistive therapy not the main remedy.
- Cancer can reappear or cancer means death- such thoughts should not be the cause of your worry.
- Adopt the philosophy of living as for now and for today.
- Even if you don't have any problems, take complete care of your diet and health.
- Have a balanced diet.
- It is better to avoid non-seasonal fruits and vegetables.
- Spare sometime from your daily schedule for walks.
- Also do breathing exercises along with physical workouts.

I hope my experiences will enlighten other women, since this disease is affecting many women. I salute the doctors and my will power which helped me get rid of this disease!

Survivor: 3, Age: 30

It's a story of bon voyage – The story which changed my whole world. By profession, I am a nurse in army. The word cancer was not new to me and I knew its consequences very well. I had worked in oncology ward for quite a long time. But, now the person who is the victim of this disease was no one else, it was me.

I was practicing self breast examination since, I was 20 years of age. I learnt this technique during one of my nursing class and I have taught this to many of my patients too. One fine morning, while taking bath, I was examing my breasts. I was doing this as a part of my monthly routine. To my surprise, I found a small lump in my right breast which was not there earlier. On the very next day, I went to general surgeon. He told me that this may be due to my menstrual cycle and there is nothing to worry about. But, I was not satisfied and insisted him for FNAC which he agreed for.

I was in great stress throughout the week. After one week, I went to collect the report. Doctor called me personally to his chamber. On founding me all alone, he was bit hesitant. I, instantly got the clue and smiled at him saying, 'Why are you scared to tell me that I have cancer? He nodded and said, 'please take care and have faith in God.'

From that very moment, I was determined to take good care of myself and came out as winner from this battle of breast cancer. Though, the thought was shaking me inside out. Time and again I was thinking about my parents and my best friend. I am eldest in the family of two siblings. My younger brother is suffering from Bipolar Affective Disorder (BPAD). My parents bank upon me for whole support. I want to fulfill all their dreams. When, I shared this news with my mom she was shattered completely. But, I told her and all my family members to be my support. I assured them that together we will fight it. I got whole hearted support from my all family member and my husband who was posted in J & K at that time. He came down to Kolkata for my treatment. We planned to go to Tata Memorial Hospital, Mumbai for my treatment.

My treatment started, lab tests confirmed that I am triple negative. Date of my surgery was fixed. Breast surgery at such a young age just two years after my marriage, not even having kids as yet was giving tremors to me. Though, I was pretending to be brave but deep inside I was losing myself and one most feminine part of my body. Question of body image was big for me. But, I was determined to save my life. Breast surgery is one of the treatments which can give me life. I will still be a woman. This is how I struggled during the morning of my surgery. After surgery, I was scared to look at my operated sight. Later on, I found that they did not remove my whole breast and only a little lower section of my right breast was removed.

After two weeks of surgery, my chemotherapy was planned. I was given 6 cycles of chemo with 21 days of gap in between. After chemotherapy, 31 cycles of radiotherapy was given to me. All these treatments affected my life tremendously. But, every time I faced certain problem my determination increased to fight and conquer them. I quit my army job. But, I am a kind of person who cannot sit idle so I thought of starting a new course. I joined B.sc nursing (post basic) course.

I studied hard and kept myself always engrossed in books. I topped in my post basic nursing. Though, my life has changed drastically but I have coped very well with all my problems. Today, I am doing masters in nursing. I am counted as one of the best students in my class. I have won many competitions and awards. Although, life was not at all easy for me but, I choose to smile and fight. Today my cancer is completely gone but, I take utmost precautions wherever possible.

Being from an army background and nurse by profession has helped me sail through this journey with ease. I have changed my lifestyle according to my needs. Here are few simple strategies, I wish to share with you which I used in my life:

- I performed regular exercise as prescribed by doctor. Even, when I did not feel like doing.

- I kept my life as normal as ever. I was very much self reliant and tried to do all my personal work myself.
- Even during my treatment days I went for shopping, driving, attended family functions, gathering etc.
- I read and learnt everything regarding my disease and treatment. Knowledge and attitude matters a lot.
- I always sleep with my arm raised above my head supported with pillows.
- I keep myself warm during cold days by using electric blanket. This helped me in combating body pains also.
- I never wear any jewellery on my affected hand and arm.
- I have changed my wardrobe according to my new hair style and looks.
- I shaved all my head before starting chemotherapy. So, that hair fall does not affect me.
- I changed my clothes and bed linen every day.
- I used separate bathroom during my treatment.
- I used Colgate presensitive toothpaste along with sensitive tooth brush to avoid mouth problems.
- I used homemade mouth wash. You can prepare your own mouthwash by boiling guava leaves and salt in water. Strain this brown colored liquid in bottle and warm it every time before you use. This has a very refreshing taste.
- I always had healthy, nutritious and high protein diet. I never skipped any of the meal. Even nausea and vomit was also no excuse for me. I use to take food again even after vomiting.

Some food related recommendations:

- Always take fruits and vegetable after peeling their skin for e.g. fruits like mango, papaya, banana etc. Never take those fruits and vegetables whose skin you cannot peel for e.g. grapes, cabbage, capsicum etc.
- To make food taste good, I use to add lemon juice in it. I even prepared a special pickle with no spices which I use to take every time with meals. To make pickle – cut green mangoes and lemon into small pieces, add some green chilies, salt and mustard oil. Put this preparation in sunshine for 15-20 days and your home made less spicy pickle is ready. Use it with every meal to add taste.
- I use to add garlic cloves in my every dish.

You too can win this battle just like me by taking good care of yourself. Always be positive and never lose your mental strength.

Survivor: 4, Age: 42

Needless to say, the moment you receive the diagnosis is the worst moment of your life. But the sooner you accept it and move on to facing the long journey that the treatment entails, the better you are. Try to focus on the treatment you are to receive and tell yourself you are going to move beyond this phase of your life. These are few tips to get along:

Dealing with the diagnosis:

1. Try to gather as much information as you can for yourself. This will help you to understand what is being done, its importance and what you need to do, to be an active member of the team.
2. Beyond that, ask questions to understand what is being done, what to expect and how to handle it.
3. Communication is very important.
4. Make sure you can get across that you want to get better no matter what. Do not put on any pre- conditions on the doctors, so that they can go all out to treat you.
5. Think positively about the future and more towards achieving that because your small daily choices and your well being depend on that.

In short, your behavior, clear headed and focused attitude will help you and your doctor to reach the finish line.

Before you meet the doctor:

1. Make a list of your doubts and questions so that you can quickly ask the doctor and not forget something important.
2. Be ready to write down what the doctor is telling you. You may not remember it all the moment you step out.
3. Speak up about your concerns.
4. Speak up about any symptoms bothering you so that they can be handled well in time.

Every patient is different and reacts in a different way to the treatment. So unless you tell the doctor and ask you may not get your answers.

Getting on with the treatment:

Remove any elements of anger and focus on your treatment and remaining well. Do not feel guilty when you see other people sail through the treatment moving around, working, shopping, etc.

1. Eat easy to digest nutritious foods.
2. Listen to your body, when to rest, what to eat, when to eat.
3. Keep mentally alert as far as possible. Pick up skills if you can not go out by:
    - Reading books
    - Writing
    - Cooking (with care)
    - Watching T.V.
    - Working on the computer
4. Do exercises as prescribed by doctor.
5. Spend some time on meditation.

Beyond the treatment:

1. In case your treatment has made you prone to lymphedema (arm swelling), you can develop problems even years afterwards and your arm will never feel the same again. So, take immense care of the arm and hands particularly, since they are prone to injury.

- Avoid any cuts, burn and splinters.
- Wear gloves for washing, driving, cooking, etc.
- Avoid lifting grocery and other weights from affected side.
- Avoid sudden jerks and pulls.
- Massage without undue pressure.

2. In case you develop a tingling or numbness in the hand or arm, taking a multivitamin may resolve the problem.

3. When in the sun, cover the arm with a loose cotton sleeve or covering to keep it cool.

The role of the caregiver:

We cannot get through any major crises without family support and understanding. It is understanding that the patient needs, and not pity from people at home and outside.

The immediate caregiver can help in the following ways:

1. Help to ask the doctor the relevant questions and record answers.
2. Help to make a note of the symptoms so that they can be addressed.
3. Ask the doctor questions about the correct way to take medications.
4. Ask the doctor questions about a suitable diet at each stage of the treatment.

5. Do not force feed the patient.
6. Find and prepare the correct food choices:
   - Palatable
   - Easy to digest
   - Nutritious
7. At home, have a cool, quite and comfortable space for the patient to reduce irritability and anxiety.
8. Let the patient have any suitable distractions:
   - For some it may be meeting people (keeping infection control in mind)
   - Listening to music
   - Listening to religious discourses
   - Watching T.V.
9. It is most important to bide time suitably, comfortably and as productively as possible.